Sexual and Reproductive Health of Women

Pradip Chouhan • Avijit Roy •
Nanigopal Kapasia • Jayanta Das •
Margubur Rahaman
Editors

Sexual and Reproductive Health of Women

Dimensions and Perspectives

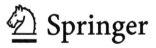

Editors
Pradip Chouhan
Department of Geography
University of Gour Banga
Malda, West Bengal, India

Avijit Roy
Department of Geography
Malda College
Malda, West Bengal, India

Nanigopal Kapasia
Department of Geography
Malda College
Malda, West Bengal, India

Jayanta Das
Department of Geography
Rampurhat College
Rampurhat, West Bengal, India

Margubur Rahaman
Department of Migration & Urban Studies
IIPS
Mumbai, Maharashtra, India

Govind Ballabh Pant Social Science
Institute (GBPSSI)
Prayagraj, India

ISBN 978-981-97-8417-2   ISBN 978-981-97-8418-9 (eBook)
https://doi.org/10.1007/978-981-97-8418-9

© The Editor(s) (if applicable) and The Author(s), under exclusive license to Springer Nature Singapore Pte Ltd. 2024

This work is subject to copyright. All rights are solely and exclusively licensed by the Publisher, whether the whole or part of the material is concerned, specifically the rights of translation, reprinting, reuse of illustrations, recitation, broadcasting, reproduction on microfilms or in any other physical way, and transmission or information storage and retrieval, electronic adaptation, computer software, or by similar or dissimilar methodology now known or hereafter developed.

The use of general descriptive names, registered names, trademarks, service marks, etc. in this publication does not imply, even in the absence of a specific statement, that such names are exempt from the relevant protective laws and regulations and therefore free for general use.

The publisher, the authors and the editors are safe to assume that the advice and information in this book are believed to be true and accurate at the date of publication. Neither the publisher nor the authors or the editors give a warranty, expressed or implied, with respect to the material contained herein or for any errors or omissions that may have been made. The publisher remains neutral with regard to jurisdictional claims in published maps and institutional affiliations.

This Springer imprint is published by the registered company Springer Nature Singapore Pte Ltd.
The registered company address is: 152 Beach Road, #21-01/04 Gateway East, Singapore 189721, Singapore

If disposing of this product, please recycle the paper.

Foreword

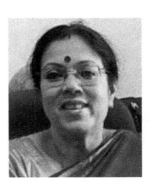

I am delighted to write the foreword for *Sexual and Reproductive Health of Women: Dimensions and Perspectives*, a comprehensive exploration of highly relevant and multifaceted topics. This book is the collaborative effort of esteemed scholars, namely Prof. Pradip Chouhan, Dr. Avijit Roy, Dr. Nanigopal Kapasia, Dr. Jayanta Das, and Mr. Margubur Rahaman. Their diverse expertise spans the humanities, the social sciences, and geography, enriching the book's content and perspective. Published by Springer, this edited volume, with its comprehensive overview of the complexities surrounding women's sexual and reproductive health, stands as a beacon of enlightenment and advocacy for an issue that is fundamental to societal, economic, and human development.

Women's health, particularly their reproductive health, has long been ensnared in a web of gender-based disparities, constrained healthcare decision-making, and socioeconomic vulnerabilities. The editors of and contributors to this volume have embarked on a quest not only to dissect these challenges but also to illuminate the paths toward equity, understanding, and improved health outcomes for women across diverse contexts. By adopting a holistic lens that encompasses societal, temporal, individual, spatial, and policy perspectives, this book offers a rich, nuanced exploration of sexual and reproductive health that is both timely and timeless.

The present volume is a collection of 24 research studies from across transdisciplinary communities. The significance of this work lies in its fearless confrontation of the disparities and difficulties that women face in accessing and exercising their reproductive rights. Through rigorous research, systematic approaches, and spatial modeling, the contributors provide insights into reproductive morbidity and the pressing need for policy attention in this domain. From the challenges encountered by homeless women and residents of slums to the unique circumstances of those in vulnerable communities and the unprecedented backdrop of the COVID-19 pandemic, no stone is left unturned in the quest to understand and advocate for better reproductive health outcomes for all women. As we stand at the crossroads of policymaking and health service delivery, *Sexual and Reproductive Health of Women: Dimensions and Perspectives* acts as not just a critical academic resource but also a clarion call for action. It is a testament to the power of collective knowledge and the urgent need for a concerted effort to address the reproductive health needs of women. This volume is an invaluable tool for academicians, researchers, health professionals, social scientists, and public health practitioners dedicated to making a difference in the lives of women around the world.

Centre for the Study of Regional Development,　　　　　　　　　　Anuradha Banerjee
School of Social Sciences
Jawaharlal Nehru University,
New Delhi, India

Preface

The journey to compile *Sexual and Reproductive Health of Women: Dimensions and Perspectives* began with a recognition of the profound complexities that define women's health issues, particularly sexual and reproductive health. As editors, we were driven by a shared commitment to illuminate the nuanced realities that women face across different societal contexts and the critical need for informed, empathetic policies that address these challenges head-on. This book represents a concerted effort to bring together diverse perspectives, research findings, and policy discussions to create a comprehensive resource that sheds light on the multifaceted nature of women's reproductive health.

Our motivation stems from an understanding that women's reproductive health is not merely a medical concern but also a reflection of broader societal, economic, and cultural dynamics. Gender-based disparities, limited access to healthcare, socioeconomic vulnerabilities, and the impacts of global crises like the COVID-19 pandemic significantly affect women's ability to exercise their reproductive rights and access the care they need. These challenges are further compounded for women living in marginalized communities, including those residing in slums and homeless populations and those facing intimate partner violence. In addressing these issues, *Sexual and Reproductive Health of Women: Dimensions and Perspectives* seeks to offer a holistic view of the factors influencing women's sexual and reproductive health. Through systematic research approaches, spatial modeling, and in-depth analyses, our contributors, comprising academicians, researchers, health professionals, and social scientists, have endeavored to provide insights that are both academically rigorous and practically relevant. Each chapter contributes a piece to the puzzle, exploring different dimensions of reproductive health, from rights and practices to maternal health, contraception, and sexually transmitted infections.

Our goal with this book is to inform and inspire. We aim to inform policymakers, health practitioners, and researchers about the pressing issues and potential interventions in women's reproductive health. Equally, we hope to inspire a new generation of health professionals and advocates to pursue innovative solutions and advocate for policies that improve health outcomes for women worldwide. This book is intended for a wide audience, including students, academics, professionals in the fields of public health and social work, and anyone else interested in the complexities of women's health. We believe that understanding and addressing the challenges in women's sexual and reproductive health requires a multidisciplinary approach and a commitment to equity and justice. The content of this book reflects on the diverse experiences of women globally and considers the role that you can play in shaping a healthier, more equitable future. Our collective efforts can and will make a difference in the lives of women everywhere.

Malda, West Bengal, India	Pradip Chouhan
Malda, West Bengal, India	Avijit Roy
Malda, West Bengal, India	Nanigopal Kapasia
Rampurhat, West Bengal, India	Jayanta Das
Mumbai, Maharashtra, India	Margubur Rahaman

Key Features

- The book offers comprehensive insights into women's sexual and reproductive health by integrating geographical, demographic, economic, and sociological perspectives.
- It highlights empowering narratives on women's reproductive rights, including abortion rights, family planning autonomy, and fertility behaviors.
- The book showcases methodological diversity by featuring cutting-edge social science research methods, including mixed-method spatial approaches and provides evidence-based recommendations to shape reproductive health policies and practices.

Acknowledgments

The creation of *Sexual and Reproductive Health of Women: Dimensions and Perspectives* has been a journey of collaboration, learning, and shared vision. As editors, we are profoundly grateful to a multitude of individuals and organizations whose support, expertise, and dedication have been instrumental in bringing this book to fruition. First and foremost, we extend our heartfelt thanks to all the contributors to this volume. Their rigorous research, insightful analyses, and commitment to advancing women's health have constituted the backbone of this work. Their willingness to explore complex and often-underrepresented issues has enriched the content of this book immeasurably. We are also deeply indebted to the peer reviewers, whose critical insights and constructive feedback have ensured the academic rigor and relevance of each chapter. Their expertise and meticulous attention to detail have significantly enhanced the quality of this publication. We extend our heartfelt appreciation to the University of Gour Banga, Malda College, Rampurhat College, and the International Institute for Population Sciences for their unwavering support of our contributors. These esteemed institutions have been crucial in providing essential resources and fostering an environment conducive to research. Beyond that, they have nurtured a culture of inquiry and advocacy, which has been fundamental to the depth and quality of the research presented in this book. We must also acknowledge the invaluable support of our publishing team. Jacqueline Eu, our editor in behavioral and health sciences at Springer Nature Singapore, and Kamesh Senthilkumar, our production editor for books, have been instrumental in elevating our manuscript. Their expertise in editing, design, and production has transformed our manuscript into a professional and accessible resource. Their patience and professionalism throughout the publication process have been exemplary. Special thanks are due to the families and communities of the women whose experiences and stories are reflected in this book. Their resilience and courage in the face of adversity are the true inspiration behind our work. We are committed to honoring their stories through our efforts to advocate for improved sexual and reproductive health outcomes for all women. Lastly, we express our appreciation to our own families, colleagues, and mentors for their support, encouragement, and belief in the importance of this project. Their understanding and sacrifices have not gone unnoticed and have been a source of strength and motivation throughout this endeavor. This book is a witness to the power of collective action and shared commitment to advancing women's health. Together, we hope to contribute to a future where every woman has the knowledge, resources, and support to make informed decisions about her sexual and reproductive health.

About the Book

Women's health is complex in nature due to the twin burden of reproductive health difficulties and general sickness. Women's reproductive health is essential for social, economic, and human development. But gender-based disparities in reproductive rights, tapered attitudes on healthcare decision-making, and poor livelihoods lead to risks in women's reproductive health. In this scenario, *Sexual and Reproductive Health of Women: Dimensions and Perspectives* is contextualized as a comprehensive guide to understanding the complexity of women's sexual and reproductive health, reproductive morbidity, and policy attention. The book highlights the multidimensional societal, temporal, individual, spatial, and policy perspectives of women's sexual and reproductive health, encompassing reproductive health rights and practices, maternal health, contraception, and sexually transmitted infections. Furthermore, it delves into the intricacies of reproductive health within underserved communities, examining the challenges faced by homeless people, those residing in slums, and individuals in vulnerable communities against the backdrop of the COVID-19 pandemic crisis. Adopting systematic research approaches and techniques in the social sciences and spatial modeling, this book offers a unique and insightful look into women's reproductive health and its implications for shaping health policies. *Sexual and Reproductive Health of Women: Dimensions and Perspectives* could be a vital resource for academics, researchers, graduate students, health professionals, social scientists, and public health scientists in the fields of women's reproductive health administration, health service research, community health, social work, and behavioral health.

Contents

Part I Women's Reproductive Health Matters

1 **Hypertension and Its Association with Anthropometry and Mental Health Among Adolescent Girls in Slum Areas** 3
Jay Saha, Abhishek Agarwalla, and Pradip Chouhan
  1.1 Introduction 4
  1.2 Data Sources and Methods 5
    1.2.1 Study Type and Design 5
    1.2.2 Sample Size and Sampling 6
    1.2.3 Methods of Sample Collection and Operational Definition 6
    1.2.4 Statistical Analyses 6
  1.3 Results 7
    1.3.1 Association Between Hypertension and Anthropometric Variables 7
    1.3.2 SBP and Anthropometric Variables 8
    1.3.3 DBP and Anthropometric Variables 9
    1.3.4 Correlation Matrix of Blood Pressure (SBP and DBP) with Different Anthropometric Measurement Variables ... 11
    1.3.5 Blood Pressure and Mental Well-Being 11
  1.4 Discussion 12
    1.4.1 Limitations 13
  1.5 Conclusion 14
  References 14

2 **Homeless Women's Multifaceted Vulnerabilities in India: A Research Roadmap Delineation** 17
Margubur Rahaman, Komal Sureshrao Gajbhiyeand, and Kailash Chandra Das
  2.1 Introduction 18
  2.2 Methodology 19
    2.2.1 Search Strategy 19

		2.2.2	Inclusion and Exclusion Criteria	20

	2.2.2	Inclusion and Exclusion Criteria	20

        2.2.2 Inclusion and Exclusion Criteria 20
        2.2.3 Data Extraction 20
    2.3 Results 20
        2.3.1 Prevailing Research Dimensions of Women's Homelessness 20
        2.3.2 Temporal Variability in Female Homelessness Research 21
        2.3.3 Livelihood Vulnerabilities Among Homeless Women 23
        2.3.4 Multifaceted Health Vulnerabilities Among Homeless Women 25
        2.3.5 Healthcare Behaviors and Barriers Among Homeless Women 26
        2.3.6 Discussion 27
                2.3.6.1 Limitations and Strengths of this Chapter 30
        2.3.7 Conclusion 31
    References 31

3 Menstrual Irregularities Among Women: A Literature Review 35
Mahashweta Chakrabarty, Subhojit Let, Sourav Chowdhury, and Vineet Kumar
    3.1 Introduction 36
    3.2 Procedures and Techniques 37
    3.3 Results 37
        3.3.1 Definitions and Prevalence 37
        3.3.2 Risk Factors 38
        3.3.3 Health Impacts 38
        3.3.4 Psychological and Quality of Life Impacts 38
    3.4 Conclusion 39
    References 39

4 Contextualising Anaemia Among Reproductive Women in West Bengal: Trends, Patterns, and Predictors 41
Subhojit Let, Seema Tiwari, and Aditya Singh
    4.1 Introduction 41
    4.2 Database and Methodology 42
        4.2.1 Database 42
        4.2.2 Dependent Variable 42
        4.2.3 Predictor Covariates 43
        4.2.4 Statistical Analysis 43
    4.3 Results 43
        4.3.1 Prevalence of Anaemia Among Respondents, According to Various Characteristics 43
        4.3.2 Illustration of Anaemia in West Bengal During 2015–2016 and 2019–2021 46
        4.3.3 Logistic Regression Results 48
    4.4 Discussion 53

	4.5	Conclusion	54
	References		54

5 Tracking the Changes in Socioeconomic Disparities in Menstrual Hygienic Product Use Among Young Women in Urban India: A Repeated Cross-Sectional Analysis ... 59
Mahashweta Chakrabarty and Aditya Singh
- 5.1 Introduction ... 60
- 5.2 Methods ... 61
  - 5.2.1 Data Source ... 61
  - 5.2.2 Variables ... 61
    - 5.2.2.1 Dependent Variable ... 61
    - 5.2.2.2 Independent Variables ... 62
  - 5.2.3 Statistical Analysis ... 62
- 5.3 Results ... 63
  - 5.3.1 Change in the Use of HPs by Wealth Quintiles ... 63
  - 5.3.2 Richest–Poorest Ratios in the Use of HPs Across Indian States from 2015–16 to 2019–21 ... 65
  - 5.3.3 Geographical Variation in Socioeconomic Disparity in HP Use Over Time ... 65
  - 5.3.4 Breaking Down the Socioeconomic Disparity in the Use of HPs Over Time ... 68
- 5.4 Discussion ... 70
- 5.5 Conclusion ... 71
- References ... 72

Part II Women's Reproductive Rights

6 Critics on Abortion Rights in India: Issues and Policy Perspectives ... 77
Parama Bannerji and Rohit Bannerji
- 6.1 Introduction ... 77
- 6.2 Material and Methodology ... 79
- 6.3 Results ... 79
  - 6.3.1 Historical Perspectives: Practice of and Attitudes Toward Abortion ... 79
  - 6.3.2 The Global Context of Abortion Rights and Associated Outcomes ... 80
  - 6.3.3 Abortion Practices in India ... 80
  - 6.3.4 Abortion Incidence in India ... 81
  - 6.3.5 Mortality and Morbidity in India from Unsafe Abortion ... 81
  - 6.3.6 Methods of Abortion in India ... 81
  - 6.3.7 The Issue of Gender-Selective Abortion in India ... 82

		6.3.8 Barriers to Abortion Service Delivery	83
		6.3.9 Abortion Policy Perspectives in India	83
		6.3.10 Challenges in Abortion and Abortion Care in India.	84
	6.4	Discussion	85
		6.4.1 Limitations	86
	6.5	Conclusion	86
	References		87

7 Linkages Between Women's Education and Family Planning 89
Jay Saha and Avijit Roy

	7.1	Introduction	89
	7.2	Data and Methods	91
		7.2.1 Study Design and Sample	91
		7.2.2 Outcome Variable	91
		7.2.3 Explanatory Variables	92
		7.2.4 Statistical Analyses	92
	7.3	Results	93
		7.3.1 Background Characteristics of the Respondents	93
		7.3.2 Prevalence of the Use of Family-Planning Methods Among Married Women in EAG States of India	94
		7.3.3 The Influencing Factors of the Use of Family-Planning Methods Among Married Women	95
	7.4	Discussion	96
		7.4.1 Strengths and Limitations	98
	7.5	Conclusions	98
	References		99

Part III Contraceptive Dynamics

8 Understanding the Dynamics of Modern Contraception Discontinuation Among Women in India 103
Nanigopal Kapasia and Swagata Ghosh

	8.1	Introduction	104
	8.2	Data and Methods	105
		8.2.1 Data	105
		8.2.2 Study Variables	105
		8.2.2.1 Explanatory Variables	106
		8.2.3 Statistical Analysis	106
	8.3	Result	106
		8.3.1 Distribution of Contraceptive Discontinuation	106
		8.3.2 Cause-Specific Discontinuation	107
		8.3.3 Geographical Variation in Causes for Contraceptive Discontinuation	107
		8.3.4 Prevalence Rate for Causes of Contraceptive Discontinuation Among Women Aged 15–49 Years in India	109
		8.3.5 Likelihood of Contraception Discontinuation	112

		8.3.6 Discussion	116
		8.3.7 Conclusion	117
	References		118
9	**Temporal, Spatial and Socioeconomic Dimensions of Hindu–Muslim Differences in Contraception Use in India**		121
	Mohai Menul Biswas		
	9.1	Introduction	122
		9.1.1 Rationale of This Study	123
	9.2	Data and Methods	124
		9.2.1 Outcome and Explanatory Variables	125
		9.2.1.1 Outcome Variable	125
		9.2.1.2 Explanatory Variables	125
		9.2.2 Methods	125
	9.3	Results	125
		9.3.1 Differentials in Trends of Contraceptive Use Between Hindus and Muslims	125
		9.3.2 Differences in Contraceptive Use Between Hindus and Muslims According to Background Characteristics	127
		9.3.3 State-Level Differences in Socioeconomic Correlates of Contraceptive Use	130
		9.3.4 Differences in Socioeconomic Correlates of Contraceptive Use Prevalence Between Hindus and Muslims	132
	9.4	Discussion	135
		9.4.1 Limitations of This Study	136
	9.5	Conclusion	136
	References		137
10	**Understanding the District-Wise Variation and Reasons of Low Fertility in West Bengal: A Cross-sectional Descriptive Study**		141
	Gita Naik, Astapati Hemram, Dinabandhu Patra, and Jagannath Behera		
	10.1	Introduction	142
	10.2	Data and Methods	143
		10.2.1 Study Setting	143
		10.2.2 Study Design and Study Population	144
		10.2.3 Dependent Variable	144
		10.2.4 Predictor Variables	144
		10.2.5 Statistical Analysis	144
	10.3	Results	145
		10.3.1 Change in Total Fertility Rate	145
		10.3.2 District-Wise Spatial Variation in Fertility	145
		10.3.3 District-Wise Contraceptive Use	146
		10.3.4 Contraceptive Use According to Background Characteristics	147
		10.3.5 Results from Multinominal Logistic Regression	151

10.4	Discussion	154
10.5	Conclusion	156
References		156

Part IV Sexually Transmitted Infections

11 Knowledge of Sexual and Reproductive Health Matters Among Girls in India: Does Parent–Adolescent Communication Play a Role? ... 161
Pintu Paul and Ria Saha

- 11.1 Background ... 162
- 11.2 Data and Methods ... 164
  - 11.2.1 Data Source ... 164
  - 11.2.2 Measures ... 164
  - 11.2.3 Analytical Strategies ... 165
- 11.3 Results and Discussion ... 165
  - 11.3.1 Knowledge of SRH Matters ... 165
  - 11.3.2 Knowledge of SRH Matters According to Socioeconomic Characteristics ... 168
  - 11.3.3 Parent–Adolescent Communication on SRH Issues ... 169
  - 11.3.4 Relationship Between Parent–Adolescent Communication and Girls' Knowledge of SRH Matters ... 171
- 11.4 Conclusion ... 173
- References ... 174

12 Do Menstrual Hygiene Practices Reduce Sexual Diseases? A Cross-sectional Study ... 179
Swagata Karjee and Prites Chandra Biswas

- 12.1 Introduction ... 180
- 12.2 Database and Methodology ... 181
  - 12.2.1 Sample ... 181
  - 12.2.2 Variables ... 181
  - 12.2.3 Statistical Analysis ... 181
- 12.3 Results ... 182
- 12.4 Discussion ... 185
  - 12.4.1 Limitations ... 186
- 12.5 Conclusion ... 186
- References ... 187

Part V Maternal Health: Key Issues

13 Maternal Healthcare Scenario in India: Evaluating Implications of the National Health Policy ... 191
Ankita Zaveri and Salim Mandal

- 13.1 Introduction ... 192

		13.2	Data Sources and Methods.	193
			13.2.1 Variables	194
		13.3	Results	194
		13.4	Discussion	200
		13.5	Conclusion	202
		References		203
14	Mental Health of Pregnant Women in Bangladesh During the COVID-19 Pandemic: A Cross-Sectional Study			207
	Sumaia Rahman, Ahammad Hossain, Al MuktadirMunam, Ayesha Akter Lima, Rejvi Ahmed Bhuiya, Jayanta Das, and Md. Kamruzzaman			
		14.1	Introduction	208
		14.2	Data Sources and Methods.	210
			14.2.1 Sample-Size Determination	210
			14.2.2 Measurement	211
			14.2.3 Data Collection	211
			14.2.4 Data Analysis	212
		14.3	Results	212
		14.4	Discussion	235
			14.4.1 Limitations	236
			14.4.2 Recommendations	237
		14.5	Conclusions	237
		References		238
15	Individual-and Community-Level Determinants of Maternal Healthcare Utilization in Afghanistan			243
	Aditya Singh, Sayed Ataullah Saeedzai, Ajit Kumar Jaiswal, Shivani Singh, and Rakesh Chandra			
		15.1	Introduction	244
		15.2	Data and Methods	245
			15.2.1 Ethical Statement	245
			15.2.2 Outcome Variables	246
			15.2.3 Exposure Variables	246
			15.2.3.1 Individual Level	246
			15.2.3.2 Community-Level Variables	247
			15.2.4 Statistical Analysis	247
		15.3	Results	249
			15.3.1 Profile of the Respondents	249
			15.3.2 Differentials in Maternal Healthcare Service Utilization	250
			15.3.3 Factors Associated with the Utilization of Maternal Healthcare Services	253
			15.3.3.1 Four or More Antenatal Care Visits ($\geq$ Four ANC Visits)	253
			15.3.3.2 Institutional Delivery	255
			15.3.3.3 Postnatal Care	258

	15.4	Discussion	261
	15.5	Conclusion	264
	References	265

16 Full Antenatal Care Service Utilization Among Tribal Mothers in India: A Multilevel Analysis 269
Aditya Singh, Mahashweta Chakrabarty, Sourav Chowdhury, Vineet Kumar, Rakesh Chandra, and Shivani Singh
- 16.1 Introduction ... 270
- 16.2 Data and Methods ... 272
  - 16.2.1 Data ... 272
  - 16.2.2 Sampling Design and Study Size ... 273
  - 16.2.3 Dependent Variables ... 273
  - 16.2.4 Independent Variables ... 274
  - 16.2.5 Statistical Analysis ... 274
- 16.3 Results ... 275
  - 16.3.1 Results of Multilevel Logistic Regression ... 280
- 16.4 Discussion ... 283
- 16.5 Conclusion ... 286
- References ... 287

17 Utilization of Maternal Healthcare Services Among Women in Urban Slums of Prayagraj City, India 291
Namrata Ahirwar, Vikesh Kumar, and Kunal Keshri
- 17.1 Introduction ... 292
- 17.2 Data Source and Methods ... 293
  - 17.2.1 First Step ... 295
  - 17.2.2 Second Step ... 295
  - 17.2.3 Selection of Study Area ... 296
    - 17.2.3.1 Prayagraj City (Erstwhile Allahabad) ... 296
- 17.3 Results ... 296
  - 17.3.1 Socioeconomic and Demographic Characteristics ... 296
  - 17.3.2 Utilization of Antenatal Care Services ... 299
  - 17.3.3 Utilization of Delivery and Postnatal Care Services ... 299
  - 17.3.4 Qualitative Findings ... 306
- 17.4 Discussion and Conclusion ... 312
- References ... 314

18 Inadequate Iron–Folic Acid Consumption Among Pregnant Mothers in India: A Spatial Analysis 317
Aditya Singh, Mahashweta Chakrabarty, Sourav Chowdhury, Shivani Singh, and Rakesh Chandra
- 18.1 Introduction ... 318
- 18.2 Data and Methods ... 319
  - 18.2.1 Data Source ... 319
  - 18.2.2 Outcome Variable ... 320

		18.2.3	Predictor Variables	321
		18.2.4	Statistical Analysis	321
	18.3	Results		322
	18.4	Discussion		327
	18.5	Conclusion		331
	References			332
19	**Maternal and Child Healthcare Utilization and Corresponding Expenditure in India**			**335**
	Rupa Dutta			
	19.1	Introduction		336
	19.2	Data and Methodology		338
	19.3	Results		339
		19.3.1	Coverage and Expenditure Related to Child Immunization	339
		19.3.2	Coverage and Expenditure Related to Pre- and Postnatal Care	340
		19.3.3	Coverage and Expenditure Related to Institutional Delivery Care	342
		19.3.4	Average Healthcare Expenditure by Medical Institutions	346
	19.4	Discussion		348
		19.4.1	Limitations	352
	19.5	Conclusion		353
	References			354

Part VI Societal Perspective of Women's Sexual and Reproductive Health

20	**Addressing Menstrual Stigma in South Asia: A Holistic Approach Toward Gender Equality and Public Health**		**359**
	Raka Sarkar, Puja Das, and Mahua Chatterjee		
	20.1	Introduction	359
	20.2	Understanding Menstruation Stigma	361
	20.3	Ritual Impurity and Social Exclusion	364
	20.4	Taboos and Restrictions	365
	20.5	Impact on Gender Dynamics	365
	20.6	Access to Menstrual Hygiene Products	366
	20.7	Challenges and Strategies	368
	20.8	Conclusion	369
	References		370
21	**Gender-Parity-Specific Fertility Decline in India: A Spatiotemporal Study**		**373**
	Kakoli Das and Saswata Ghosh		
	21.1	Introduction	374
	21.2	Materials and Methods	375

		21.2.1	Data and Variables	375
		21.2.2	Analytical Model	377
	21.3	Results		377
		21.3.1	Change in Completed Fertility and Desired Family Size from NFHS-1 to NFHS-5	377
		21.3.2	Gender-Parity Composition and Family-Size Choices	378
		21.3.3	Fertility Desires and Household Economic Conditions	378
		21.3.4	Influence of Women's Education on Changing Fertility Preferences Across Different Survey Rounds	379
		21.3.5	Influence of Spouse's Occupational Characteristics on Family-Planning Choices Between Survey Rounds	381
		21.3.6	Religious Affiliation and the Waning Desire for Another Child	382
		21.3.7	Current Working Status of Mothers and the Shifts in Their Desire for Future Children Between Survey Rounds	382
		21.3.8	Media Exposure and Changing Fertility Choices Among Mothers	383
		21.3.9	Region-Specific Decline in the Desire for an Additional Child	384
		21.3.10	Multivariate Analysis	385
	21.4	Discussion		388
	21.5	Conclusion		390
	References			391
22	**Intimate Partner Violence and Risk of Unintended Pregnancy: Findings from Rural India**			**395**
	Anshika Singh and Aditya Singh			
	22.1	Introduction		396
	22.2	Data and Methods		397
		22.2.1	Source of Data	397
		22.2.2	Dependent Variable	398
		22.2.3	Independent Variables	399
		22.2.4	Control Variables	399
		22.2.5	Statistical Analysis	399
	22.3	Results		400
		22.3.1	Respondent's Background Characteristics	400
		22.3.2	Physical IPV Among Currently Pregnant Women	402
		22.3.3	Sexual IPV Among Currently Pregnant Women	403

		22.3.4	Unintended Pregnancy Among Currently Pregnant Women..	404
		22.3.5	Association Between Intimate Partner Violence (IPV) and Unintended Pregnancy (UP).................	404
	22.4	Discussion..		408
	22.5	Conclusion...		410
	References..			411
23	**Male Involvement in Maternal Healthcare (MHC) Services: A Religious Differential Approach**............................			**413**

Bikash Barman and Koyel Majumder

	23.1	Introduction...		414
	23.2	Data Source and Methods.......................................		416
		23.2.1	Data..	416
		23.2.2	Methods...	416
		23.2.3	Variable...	416
		23.2.4	About the Study Area.......................................	418
	23.3	Results..		420
		23.3.1	Sociodemographic Characteristics of Men in Maldah...	420
		23.3.2	Knowledge About MHC Services......................	420
		23.3.3	Knowledge About Danger Signs During Pregnancy...	420
		23.3.4	Reasons for Not Visiting a Health Facility for ANC Visits..	422
		23.3.5	Pregnancy Care Given to a Wife by Her Husband.....	423
		23.3.6	Preparation for Delivery During Pregnancy.........	423
		23.3.7	Determinants of Male Involvement in the Utilization of MHC Services...............................	424
			23.3.7.1 Determinants of Male Involvement in the Utilization of ANC Services..............	424
			23.3.7.2 Determinants of Male Involvement in the Utilization of Delivery Care Services......	426
			23.3.7.3 Determinants of Male Involvement in the Utilization of Postnatal Care Services	429
	23.4	Discussion..		432
	23.5	Conclusion...		433
	References..			434
24	**A Survey on Awareness of Ongoing Family-Planning Programs and Policies Among Teacher Educators in Odisha, India**..........			**437**

Tanushri Mohanta, Chaitali Sarangi, Moumita Pradhan, and Agradeep Mohanta

| | 24.1 | Introduction... | | 438 |
| | 24.2 | Methodology.. | | 441 |

		24.2.1	Population	441
		24.2.2	Sample	441
		24.2.3	Tools	441
	24.3	Results of Analyses		442
		24.3.1	Major Findings	444
	24.4	Discussion		445
		24.4.1	Chapter Limitations and Strengths and Recommendations for Future Research	448
	24.5	Conclusion		449
	References			450
Index				451

Editors and Contributors

About the Editors

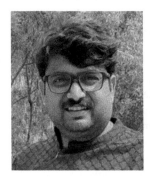

Pradip Chouhan is a professor at the Department of Geography, University of Gour Banga, Malda, West Bengal, India. Earlier, he was an assistant professor at the Department of Geography, Jadavpur University, Kolkata. His areas of research interest include fertility behavior, public health, maternal health, and child health. Actively engaged in teaching and research in population geography for nearly two decades. Prof. Chouhan has published more than 50 research papers in Scopus- and Web of Science–indexed journals, edited three books and authored one book. He is an academic editor of *PLOS One* and the *Scientific Reports Journal* and a reviewer of Scopus- and Web of Science–indexed journals. He has completed four research projects funded by the ICSSR (02), DST (01) and UGC (01). He has successfully supervised seven PhD and eight MPhil scholars.

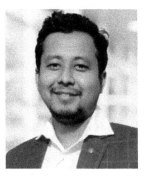

Avijit Roy is a state-aided college teacher in the Department of Geography at Malda College in Malda, West Bengal, India. He teaches courses related to population geography, gender studies, regional planning, urban geography, social, and cultural geography. Dr. Roy completed his PhD in geography at the University of Gour Banga. He conducts research in a range of settings across the globe. His current research interests lie in women's sexual and reproductive health, maternal morbidity and mortality, newborn health, geriatrics, healthcare services, child marriage, violence against women, and spatial analysis. His work in the global health arena has focused on key debates and emerging tools in the campaigns to improve women's healthcare and reduce maternal morbidity in low-resource settings.

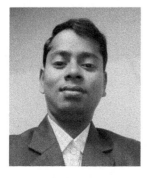

Nanigopal Kapasia is an assistant professor in the Department of Geography at Malda College, Malda, West Bengal, India. He has completed his PhD degrees at the Department of Geography and Applied Geography, University of North Bengal, India. His research field of interest is social and cultural geography especially on public health, maternity care services, and the emerging challenges related to women's health. Dr. Kapasia has published more than 20 research articles in reputed national and international journals.

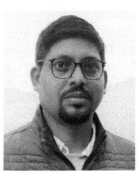

Jayanta Das is an assistant professor at the Department of Geography in Rampurhat College, University of Burdwan, West Bengal, India. He has completed his postgraduate and PhD degrees at the Department of Geography and Applied Geography, University of North Bengal, India. His research interests include agricultural modeling and sustainable management studies, groundwater, flood, drought analysis, climate change, watershed management, hydrological modeling, water quality, geospatial data analysis, data mining, and GIS applications, with more than 15 academic years of experience. Dr. Jayanta Das has published more than 50 scholarly articles in peer-reviewed journals, focusing mainly on climate change, agricultural suitability analysis, natural and human-caused hazard analysis, risk management, and spatial data analysis. He has been reviewing many journals such as *Advances in Space Research*, *Natural Hazard*, the *Arabian Journal of Geosciences*, the *Archives of Agronomy and Soil Science*, *Climatic Change*, *Environment, Development and Sustainability*, *Geo Journal*, *Sustainability*, *SN Applied Sciences*, *Geocarto International*, *Environmental Science*, and *Pollution Research*. Dr. Das has also published three edited books with Springer Nature. He has served as an editor for the *Journal of Water* and as a guest editor for *Environmental Science and Pollution Research* (*ESPR*), published by Springer. His academic endeavors are further highlighted by his leadership in organizing international seminars and receiving prestigious awards for his research contributions.

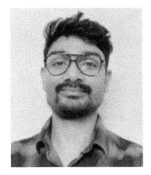

Margubur Rahaman is a senior researcher fellow at the Department of Migration & Urban Studies, International Institute for Population Sciences (IIPS), Mumbai, India and currently serves as a research associate at the Govind Ballabh Pant Social Science Institute, India. He is also an editorial board member of BMC Public Health (Springer Nature) and an academic editor of PLOS ONE. He has completed his masters in population studies and MPhil degrees at the Department of Migration & Urban Studies, International Institute for Population Sciences (IIPS), Govandi Station Road, Deonar, Mumbai, India. With advanced degrees in Population Studies (MPhil, Master's) and Geography, his doctoral research focused on reproductive health issues among pavement-dwelling women. His expertise spans sexual and reproductive health, child and elderly health, health inequality, gender-based violence, traditional and alternative medicine, and labor migration. Proficient in both quantitative and qualitative research methods, his work often integrates socio-economic, demographic, and climatic dimensions to address health and social issues.

Contributors

Abhishek Agarwalla University of Gour Banga, Malda, India

Namrata Ahirwar G B Pant Social Science Institute, Prayagraj, India

Parama Bannerji Nababarrackpur Prafulla Chandra Mahavidyala, Kolkata, India

Rohit Bannerji ESI-PGIMSR Medical College and Hospital, Joka, India

Bikash Barman Malda Women's College, Malda, India

Jagannath Behera Fakir Mohan University, Balasore, India

Rejvi Ahmed Bhuiya University of Rajshahi, Rajshahi, Bangladesh

Mohai Menul Biswas International Institute for Population Sciences, Mumbai, India

Prites Chandra Biswas Acharya BrojendraNath Seal College, Cooch Behar, India

Mahashweta Chakrabarty Department of Geography, Banaras Hindu University, Varanasi, Uttar Pradesh, India

Rakesh Chandra Tata Institute of Social Sciences, Mumbai, India

Mahua Chatterjee Lady Brabourne College, Kolkata, India

Pradip Chouhan Department of Geography, University of Gour Banga, Malda, India

Sourav Chowdhury Department of Geography, Raiganj University, Raiganj, West Bengal, India

Jayanta Das Rampurhat College, Rampurhat, West Bengal, India

Kailash Chandra Das International Institute for Population Sciences, Mumbai, India

Kakoli Das Institute of Development Studies, Kolkata, India
Vidyasagar University, West Medinipur, West Bengal, India

Puja Das University of Gour Banga, Malda, India

Rupa Dutta Ministry of Commerce and Industry, New Delhi, India

Komal Sureshrao Gajbhiye International Institute for Population Sciences, Mumbai, India

Saswata Ghosh Institute of Development Studies, Kolkata, India

Swagata Ghosh University of Gour Banga, Malda, India

Astapati Hemram Cooch Behar Panchanan Barma University, Cooch Behar, India

Ahammad Hossain Varendra University, Rajshahi, Bangladesh

Ajit Kumar Jaiswal International Institute for Population Sciences, Mumbai, India

Md. Kamruzzaman University of Rajshahi, Rajshahi, Bangladesh

Nanigopal Kapasia Department of Geography, Malda College, Malda, India

Swagata Karjee Cooch Behar Panchanan Barma University, Cooch Behar, India

Kunal Keshri International Institute for Population Sciences, Mumbai, India

Vikesh Kumar International Institute for Population Sciences, Mumbai, India

Vineet Kumar Department of Geography, Banaras Hindu University, Varanasi, Uttar Pradesh, India

Subhojit Let Department of Geography, Banaras Hindu University, Varanasi, Uttar Pradesh, India

Ayesha Akter Lima Varendra University, Rajshahi, Bangladesh

Koyel Majumder University of Gour Banga, Malda, India

Salim Mandal Darjeeling Govt. College, Darjeeling, India

Agradeep Mohanta The Maharaja Sayajirao University of Baroda, Vadodara, India

Tanushri Mohanta Institute of Advanced Studies in Education, Cuttack, India

Al Muktadir Munam Varendra University, Rajshahi, Bangladesh

Gita Naik Fakir Mohan University, Balasore, India

Dinabandhu Patra Fakir Mohan University, Balasore, India

Pintu Paul Ashoka University, Sonipat, India

Moumita Pradhan Institute of Advanced Studies in Education, Cuttack, India

Margubur Rahaman Department of Migration & Urban Studies, IIPS, Mumbai, India

Govind Ballabh Pant Social Science Institute (GBPSSI), Prayagraj, India

Sumaia Rahman Varendra University, Rajshahi, Bangladesh

Avijit Roy Department of Geography, Malda College, Malda, India

Sayed Ataullah Saeedzai Ministry of Public Health, Kabul, Afghanistan

Jay Saha University of Gour Banga, Malda, India

Ria Saha Business Development & Research Intelligence, Somerset Council, UK

Chaitali Sarangi Institute of Advanced Studies in Education, Cuttack, India

Raka Sarkar Jawaharlal Nehru University, New Delhi, India

Aditya Singh Banaras Hindu University, Varanasi, India

Population Council, New York, NY, USA

Anshika Singh Banaras Hindu University, Varanasi, India

Shivani Singh Independent Researcher, Lucknow, India

Seema Tiwari Mahila Maha Vidyalaya, Varanasi, India

Ankita Zaveri University of Gour Banga, Malda, India

Abbreviations

AB-HWCs	Ayushman Bharat–Health and Wellness Centres
ADHD	Attention deficit hyperactivity disorder
AIC	Akaike Information Criterion
AIDS	Acquired immunodeficiency syndrome
AMB	Anemia Mukt Bharat
ANC	Antenatal care
AOR	Adjusted odds ratio
ARHCs	Affordable rental housing complexes
ASHA	Accredited social health activists
BiLISA	Bivariate local indicators for spatial association
BLR	Binary logistic regression
BMI	Body mass index
BP	Blood pressure
BPHS	Basic package of health services
CC	Concentration curve
CI	Concentration index
CI	Confidence interval
CMPNDs	Communicable, maternal, perinatal, and nutritional conditions
CMR	Child mortality rate
CPR	Contraceptive prevalence rate
CSO	Central Statistics Organization
CVD	Cardiovascular diseases
DALYs	Disability-adjusted life years
DASS	Depression, Anxiety, and Stress Scale
DBP	Diastolic blood pressure
DHS	Demographic and Health Survey
DM	Diabetes mellitus
EAGs	Empowered action groups
EBM	English Bazar Municipality
EPHS	Essential package of hospital services
FGD	Focus group discussion

FP-LMIS	Family Planning Logistics Management Information System
GHQ	General Health Questionnaire
GoI	Government of India
HG	Hyperemesis gravidarum
HIV	Human immunodeficiency virus
HP	Hygienic products
HTN	Hypertension
ICC	Intraclass correlation
IFA	Iron and folic acid
IGUC	Indian government's Union Cabinet
IIPS	International Institute for Population Sciences
IMR	Infant mortality rate
IoE	Institute of Eminence
IPV	Intimate partner violence
IRB	Institutional Review Board
IUD	Intrauterine devices
JSSK	Janani Shishu Suraksha Karyakram
JSY	Janani Suraksha Yojana
KSY	Kishori Shakti Yojana
LH	Luteinizing hormone
LMICs	Low and middle-income countries
MCH	Maternal and child health
MCoC	Maternal continuum of care
MDGs	Millennium Development Goals
ME	Marginal effect
MHC	Maternal healthcare
MHM	Menstrual hygiene management
MHS	Menstrual hygiene scheme
MMR	Maternal mortality rates
MoHFW	Ministry of Family and Health Welfare
MSPSS	Multidimensional Scale of Perceived Social Support
NFHS	National Family Health Survey
NGOs	Nongovernmental organizations
NNMR	Neonatal mortality rate
NSS	National Sample Survey
OBC	Other backward class
OLS	Ordinary least squares
OOPEs	Out-of-pocket expenses
PCA	Principal component analysis
PCOS	Polycystic ovary syndrome
PMMVY	Pradhan Mantri Matru Vandana Yojana
PMSMA	Pradhan Mantri Surakshit Matritva Abhiyan
PNC	Postnatal care
PPs	Percentage points
PRHDs	Pregnancy-induced hypertensive disorders

PRISMA	Preferred Reporting Items for Systematic Reviews and Meta-Analyses
PSUs	Primary sampling units
QoL	Quality of life
RA	Rheumatoid arthritis
RCH	Reproductive and child health
REC	Research ethical committee
RKSK	Rashtriya Kishor Swasthya Karyakram
RMNCH+A	Reproductive, maternal, newborn, child, and adolescent health
RRR	Relative risk ratio
RTIs	Reproductive tract infections
SBA	Skilled birth attendance
SBP	Systolic blood pressure
SC	Scheduled Caste
SD	Standard deviation
SDGs	Sustainable Development Goals
SEM	Spatial error model
SES	Socioeconomic status
SEs	Standard errors
SLM	Spatial lag model
SRH	Sexual and reproductive health
SRS	Sample Registration Survey
ST	Scheduled Tribe
STDs	Sexually transmitted diseases
STIs	Sexually transmitted infections
TFR	Total fertility rate
TT	Tetanus toxoid
UDAYA	Understanding the lives of adolescents and young adults
UGC	University Grants Commission
UNICEF	United Nations International Children's Emergency Fund
UP	Unintended pregnancy
UTs	Union Territories
VIF	Variance inflation factor
VPC	Variance partition coefficient
WHO	World Health Organization
WRA	Women of reproductive age

Part I
Women's Reproductive Health Matters

Chapter 1
Hypertension and Its Association with Anthropometry and Mental Health Among Adolescent Girls in Slum Areas

Jay Saha ⓘ, Abhishek Agarwalla ⓘ, and Pradip Chouhan ⓘ

Abstract According to up-and-coming preliminary evidence, primary hypertension or near-to-high blood pressure (BP) is clearly detectable in adolescent girls and generally occurs as an underdiagnosed problem. Both prehypertension and depression are due to low mental health and are common disorders. This study aimed to determine the relationship of BP with anthropometry and mental health among adolescent girls aged 12–18 in the English Bazar Municipality (EBM) of Maldah District. This study sample was taken using the random sampling method. This study was conducted among 380 adolescent girls aged 12–18 from randomly selected slums of the EBM of Maldah district. Data on BP, anthropometry, and mental health scores were collected by using structured questionnaires during house visits. Mental health was examined by using the General Health Questionnaire with 12 items (GHQ-12). Using Stata software, the mean, standard deviation, Pearson's correlation coefficient, and multivariable binary logistic regression model were used for statistical analyses. The overall prevalence of prehypertension was found to be 22%. Blood pressure was found to be positively correlated with different anthropometric measurements, such as weight (SBP = 0.45; DBP = 0.29), height (SBP = 0.38; DBP = 0.20), sitting height (SBP = 0.28; DBP = 0.15), waist circumference (SBP = 0.38; DBP = 0.26), and body mass index (BMI) (SBP = 0.34; DBP = 0.28), which were statistically significant. The study participants with low mental health scores had high mean SBP and DBP values compared to girls with high mental health scores. The early detection of prehypertension and the application of lifestyle modifications among adolescents will help lower the risks of having high BP in adult life.

Keywords Blood pressure · Anthropometry · GHQ · BMI · Mental health · English Bazar Municipality

---

J. Saha (✉) · A. Agarwalla · P. Chouhan
Department of Geography, University of Gour Banga, Malda, West Bengal, India

© The Author(s), under exclusive license to Springer Nature Singapore Pte Ltd. 2024
P. Chouhan et al. (eds.), *Sexual and Reproductive Health of Women*,
https://doi.org/10.1007/978-981-97-8418-9_1

1.1 Introduction

Globally, hypertension is one of the most prevalent public health problems among adults and often develops during childhood and adolescence (Song et al. 2019; Riley et al. 2018; Nag et al. 2018). Hypertension or elevated blood pressure (BP) significantly increases the risk of cardiovascular diseases, chronic kidney diseases, and many other diseases worldwide (World Health Organization 2021; Zhou et al. 2021). Indeed, raised BP or hypertension is a significant risk factor accounting for 10.8 million deaths (19.2% of all deaths in 2019) and 9.3% of disability-adjusted life years (DALYs) lost all over the world (Schutte et al. 2021). Hypertension or elevated blood pressure significantly contributes to premature death and disability. Globally, more than 1.2 billion adults had hypertension in 2021, where two-thirds were living in low- and middle-income countries (World Health Organization 2021).

The Indian economy is undergoing rapid development and modernization, and changing lifestyles have been associated with an increasing tendency toward high blood pressure or hypertension, especially among the urban population (Gupta 2004). India has seen a wide range of hypertension prevalence among children and adolescents, ranging from 0.46% to 15%, respectively (Nag et al. 2018). Recently, studies have found that the overall prevalence of hypertension in children aged 4–19 years was 7%, indicating that it is a significant health problem in India (Meena et al. 2021).

The rising trend of high blood pressure generally occurs due to many environmental and genetic factors, such as age, gender, body size, physical inactivity, diet, stress level during adolescence, obesity, metabolic syndrome, changes in lifestyle, a paucity of employment, and family dynamics remain the primary determinant for developing hypertension later in adult life (Singh and Verma 2021; Kumar et al. 2015; Banerjee et al. 2021; Durrani and Fatima 2012; Das et al. 2005). Due to obesity, children and adolescents today are more likely to experience raised blood pressure or hypertension problems. The asymptomatic nature of the early stages of raised blood pressure during adolescence increases the risk of complications during adulthood (Banerjee et al. 2021; Khan et al. 2010). The inclusion of blood pressure measurements in regular pediatric tests has led to the discovery of asymptomatic high blood pressure in children (Bagga et al. 2007). Some of the consequences associated with high blood pressure, which were previously thought to be limited to adults, are now affecting adolescents as well (Singh and Verma 2021). Therefore, high BP can no longer be considered an adult-onset disease.

The increasing incidence of high blood pressure or hypertension has become a common health problem among children and adolescents, leading to an epidemic of childhood overweight and obesity and to the growing awareness of this disease (Juonala et al. 2011; Nag et al. 2018). Asian populations have been well documented to have a positive association between body mass index (BMI) and high blood pressure. Numerous studies have reported that being overweight or obese increases the risk of insulin resistance in children with an elevated level of systolic blood pressure

(SBP) and diastolic blood pressure (DPB), dyslipidemia, diabetes, etc. (Nag et al. 2018; Hansen et al. 2007; Yusuf et al. 2005).

A significant proportion of India's urban population lives in slums, which are characterized by poor socioeconomic conditions and poverty. Slum dwellers tend to neglect the importance of health and social progress, which increases their chances of developing livelihood diseases. The availability of healthcare services in these regions has been hampered by, for example, a lack of regular employment, the threat of eviction, overcrowding, alcoholism, and other social problems. Hence, the prevalence of high blood pressure and its associated risk factors are more relevant among adolescents living in urban areas due to their sociocultural vulnerabilities, such as literacy, poverty, and poor living conditions.

Field-based research on the prevalence of elevated blood pressure or hypertension in different parts of India is alarming (Banerjee et al. 2016; Todkar et al. 2009). Furthermore, much research in urban slums has focused primarily on child health (Huey et al. 2019), domestic violence against women (Jungari et al. 2022; Jungari and Chinchore 2022; Das et al. 2022), and reproductive and infectious diseases (Lumagbas et al. 2018; Acharyya et al. 2014), among others. Only a few studies that have shown the prevalence of lifestyle diseases such as high blood pressure or hypertension in slums are available (Banerjee et al. 2016). Different patterns of blood pressure (BP) have been found in Indian children and adolescents, especially those related to anthropometric characteristics (Banerjee et al. 2021; Nag et al. 2018; Durrani and Fatima 2012; Sharma et al. 2010). Nevertheless, to the best of our knowledge, no study has yet exemplified the vivid association between blood pressure on one hand and anthropometric measurement and mental well-being on the other among adolescent girls in slum areas. Therefore, the present study attempts to determine the relationship of blood pressure with anthropometric measurements and mental well-being among adolescent girls aged 12–18 years in the slum areas of the English Bazar Municipality of Maldah district in West Bengal. Equipped with this determination, policymakers can make effective strategies for preventing and controlling hypertension among adolescent girls in slum areas.

1.2 Data Sources and Methods

1.2.1 Study Type and Design

This was a cross-sectional study based on epidemiology conducted on adolescent girls aged 12–18 years in the slum areas of English Bazar Municipality (EBM) in Maldah district.

1.2.2 Sample Size and Sampling

For the present study, 388 girls aged 12–18 years in the slum areas of EBM were selected with the help of the simple random sampling technique.

1.2.3 Methods of Sample Collection and Operational Definition

After standardizing and validating all the types of equipment and before visiting any slums, all the measurements were taken by an observer. At the end of the interview, blood pressure was recorded with the help of the auscultatory method in the sitting position and a relaxing manner in a peaceful room. For measuring the BP, with the acromion process, the olecranon process, and circumambience about two-thirds of the upper arm, the cuff's age-specific width was applied. Three readings were taken from each participant at intervals of 5 min, and the average of these readings was considered the final reading. Those girls who were ≥ the 95th percentile of the predicted value of age-specific DBP, SBP, or both were considered to have diastolic hypertension, systolic hypertension, or both, respectively. After the the girls put on light clothes and removed their shoes, their respective weights were measured (nearest 0.1 kg). And after they removed their shoes and were standing straight with their heads positioned so that their eyes and ears were horizontal and their buttocks, shoulders, and heels were touching a vertical surface (wall) with their heads facing forward, the respective heights of the participants were measured (nearest 0.1 cm), and with the help of a trained person, their respective waist circumferences were measured by using nonstretchable tape (with measurements taken to the nearest 0.1 cm) between the iliac crest and the lower ribcage in a standing position. By dividing the weight (kg) and the height (m^2) of the participants, their respective BMI values were calculated, and the overweight and obesity of participants were measured with the help of WHO standard values (≥the 85th and 95th percentiles of body weight).

1.2.4 Statistical Analyses

After each day's data collection, using the Kolmogorov–Smirnov test for normality distribution, continuous data were checked. A nonsignificant *p*-value indicated the normal distribution of the dataset. Thus, mean and standard deviation (SD) were used as the measures of central tendency and dispersion, respectively. The correlation between the two variables was measured with the help of Pearson's correlation coefficient (*r*). A multivariable binary logistic regression model is used to identify anthropometric variables, which were responsible for the increasing blood pressure (SBP and DBP) of adolescent girls aged 10–18 years. To evaluate the sample data, the Statistical Package and Data Science software Stata version 17 (StataCorp LP, College Station, TX) was used.

1.3 Results

1.3.1 Association Between Hypertension and Anthropometric Variables

Table 1.1 displays the mean systolic blood pressure and diastolic blood pressure, which increased gradually with an increase in anthropometric variables such as weight, height, sitting height, waist circumference, and body mass index (BMI).

Table 1.1 Distribution of systolic blood pressure and diastolic blood pressure in relation to anthropometric variables among adolescent girls living in the slum areas of EBM, 2019–20 ($n = 388$)

Variables	n (%)	Mean ± SD SBP	DBP
Weight (kg)			
10–19	45 (11.60)	94.40 ± 5.90	60.80 ± 9.04
20–29	68 (17.53)	97.21 ± 8.43	65.00 ± 11.83
30–39	106 (27.32)	102.54 ± 8.43	68.37 ± 9.09
40–49	89 (22.94)	109.13 ± 9.57	70.11 ± 7.16
50–59	41 (10.57)	109.75 ± 10.60	75.08 ± 7.91
60–69	25 (6.44)	115.25 ± 3.54	81.08 ± 9.90
≥70	14 (3.61)	132.00 ± 5.66	83.00 ± 2.83
r, p-value	388 (100.00)	0.45 < 0.001[a]	0.29 < 0.001[a]
Height (cm)			
110–119	50 (12.89)	94.10 ± 8.66	64.25 ± 15.04
120–129	45 (11.60)	94.36 ± 5.26	64.73 ± 6.13
130–139	62 (15.98)	100.45 ± 8.84	66.39 ± 11.51
140–149	108 (27.84)	103.73 ± 8.70	69.27 ± 8.17
150–159	97 (25.00)	108.24 ± 10.44	70.13 ± 8.62
≥160	26 (6.70)	111.00 ± 13.76	71.35 ± 11.95
r, p-value	388 (100.00)	0.38 < 0.001[a]	0.20 < 0.002[a]
Sitting height (cm)			
60–69	104 (26.80)	100.96 ± 8.24	66.40 ± 10.37
70–79	210 (54.12)	104.41 ± 10.03	69.22 ± 9.18
≥80	74 (19.07)	109.00 ± 10.46	69.37 ± 7.68
r, p-value	388 (100.00)	0.28 < 0.001[a]	0.15 < 0.01[a]
Waist circumferences (cm)			
<50	55 (14.18)	93.56 ± 9.19	59.50 ± 16.26
50–59	75 (19.33)	93.72 ± 9.17	64.89 ± 12.94
60–69	103 (26.55)	102.78 ± 8.90	67.96 ± 9.46
70–79	95 (24.48)	107.05 ± 9.55	69.40 ± 7.33
80–89	41 (10.57)	107.54 ± 10.04	72.32 ± 9.29
≥90	19 (4.90)	120.25 ± 13.96	78.00 ± 6.48
r, p-value	388 (100.00)	0.38 < 0.001[a]	0.26 < 0.001[a]

(continued)

Table 1.1 (continued)

Variables	n (%)	Mean ± SD SBP	DBP
BMI (kg/m^2)			
<18.50	194 (50.00)	102.41 ± 9.72	67.40 ± 9.78
18.50–24.99	149 (38.40)	108.63 ± 9.49	71.59 ± 7.21
≥25	45 (11.60)	114.80 ± 16.27	76.20 ± 8.70
r, p-value	388 (100.00)	0.34 < 0.001[a]	0.28 < 0.001[a]

SD standard deviation, *SBP* systolic blood pressure, *DBP* diastolic blood pressure, *BMI* body mass index

[a] Pearson's correlation coefficients were statistically significant

The mean SBP and mean DBP of the study participants increased with an increase in height range. Significant positive correlations were obtained between SBP and height ($r = 0.38$; $p < 0.001$) and between DBP and height ($r = 0.20$; $p < 0.002$). Mean SBP and DBP also increased uniformly with an increase in weight range and appeared to show significant positive correlations between SBP and weight ($r = 0.45$; $p < 0.001$) and between DBP and weight ($r = 0.29$; $p < 0.001$). Mean SBP and DBP also increased uniformly with an increase in sitting height range and appeared to show significant positive correlations between SBP and sitting height ($r = 0.28$; $p < 0.001$) and between DBP and sitting height ($r = 0.15$; $p < 0.001$). Similar observations were also noted between BP and waist circumference (SBP: $r = 0.38$; $p < 0.001$) (DBP: $r = 0.26$; $p < 0.001$) and between BP and BMI (SBP: $r = 0.34$; $p < 0.001$) (DBP: $r = 0.28$; $p < 0.001$). Waist circumference and BMI also had a significant positive correlation with SBP and one with DBP, separately.

1.3.2 SBP and Anthropometric Variables

Table 1.2 displays the significant variations in the likelihood of high SBP with the selected explanatory variables, where adolescent girls who had weights of 25–39 kg and ≥40 kg (AOR: 6.61; 95% CI: 1.09–39.90; $p < 0.01$) were more likely to have high SBP than were adolescent girls who had low weights (<25 kg). The prevalence of high systolic blood pressure was more likely to be higher among girls with heights ≥155 cm (AOR: 4.23; 95% CI: 1.09–16.46; $p < 0.01$), with a height of 135–154 cm (AOR: 2.71; 95% CI: 0.98–7.48; $p < 0.05$) than the girls with heights of 115–134 cm. A higher likelihood of high SBP was found among the girls who had a sitting height ≥80 cm (AOR: 2.97; 95% CI: 1.19–7.41; $p < 0.01$) or a sitting height of 70–79 cm (AOR: 1.86; 95% CI: 0.97–3.60; $p < 0.001$) than the girls in the reference category. The odds of developing high SBP was 1.46 (AOR: 1.46; 95% CI: 0.26–8.32; $p < 0.01$) and 1.82 times (AOR: 1.82; 95% CI: 0.49–6.74; $p < 0.001$) more likely to be higher among girls with 60–79 cm and ≥80 cm waist

Table 1.2 Multivariable logistic regression for risk of high systolic blood pressure (risk of prehypertension), adjusting for other variables, among adolescent girls in the slum areas of EBM, 2019–2020 ($n = 388$)

Variables	Systolic blood pressure (model 1)	
	AOR	95% CI
Weight (kg)		
<25[a]	1.00	
25–39	1.70**	(0.37–7.85)
≥40	6.61**	(1.09–39.90)
Height (cm)		
115–134[a]	1.00	
135–154	2.71*	(0.98–7.48)
≥155	4.23**	(1.09–16.46)
Sitting height (cm)		
60–69[a]	1.00	
70–79	1.86***	(0.97–3.60)
≥80	2.97**	(1.19–7.41)
Waist circumferences (cm)		
<60[a]	1.00	
60–79	1.46**	(0.26–8.32)
≥80	1.82***	(0.49–6.74)
BMI (kg/m^2)		
Thin[a]	1.00	
Normal	1.12**	(0.08–15.52)
Overweight	1.69***	(0.64–4.50)
Constant	0.23**	(0.06–0.83)
Log likelihood	−136.60	
Pseudo-R^2	0.053	

AOR adjusted odds ratio, *BMI* body mass index, *CI* confidence interval in parentheses
***$p < 0.001$, **$p < 0.01$, *$p < 0.05$
[a] Reference category

circumferences than girls with 60–69 cm waist circumferences. The prevalence of high SBP was significantly more likely to develop among adolescent girls in the overweight (AOR: 1.69; 95% CI: 0.64–4.50; $p < 0.001$) category of the body mass index.

1.3.3 DBP and Anthropometric Variables

Table 1.3 displays the significant variations in the likelihood of high DBP with the selected explanatory variables, where the odds of developing high DBP were 1.32 (AOR: 1.32; 95% CI: 0.40–4.33; $p < 0.001$) and 3.36 times (AOR: 3.36; 95% CI: 1.02–11.09; $p < 0.01$) more likely to be higher among girls who had weights of 25–39 kg and ≥40 kg weight than girls who had weights <25 kg. The prevalence of

Table 1.3 Multivariable logistic regression for risk of high diastolic blood pressure (risk of prehypertension), adjusting for other variables, among adolescent girls in the slum areas of EBM, 2019–2020

Variables	Diastolic blood pressure (model 2)	
	AOR	95% CI
Weight (kg)		
<25[a]	1.00	
25–39	1.32***	(0.40–4.33)
≥40	3.36**	(1.02–11.09)
Height (cm)		
115–134[a]	1.00	
135–154	1.89***	(0.80–4.49)
≥155	3.00**	(1.16–7.77)
Sitting height (cm)		
60–69[a]	1.00	
70–79	1.12***	(0.47–2.69)
≥80	1.40**	(0.71–2.76)
Waist circumferences (cm)		
<60[a]	1.00	
60–79	1.22***	(0.47–3.17)
≥80	2.11***	(0.70–6.35)
BMI (kg/m^2)		
Thin[a]	1.00	
Normal	2.71***	(1.56–4.70)
Overweight	6.65**	(0.68–65.46)
Constant	0.32**	(0.10–1.04)
Log likelihood	−153.87	
Pseudo-R^2	0.08	

AOR adjusted odds ratio, *BMI* body mass index, *CI* confidence interval in parentheses
***$p < 0.001$, **$p < 0.01$, *$p < 0.05$
[a] Reference category

DBP increases with increasing height; girls who had heights of 135–154 cm (AOR: 1.89; 95% CI: 0.80–4.49; $p < 0.001$) and ≥155 cm (AOR: 3.00; 95% CI: 1.16–7.77; $p < 0.01$) were 1.89 times and three times more likely to have DBP than did girls whose heights were 115–134 cm. The prevalence of high diastolic blood pressure was likely to be higher among girls with a sitting height ≥80 cm (AOR: 1.40; 95% CI: 0.71–2.76; $p < 0.001$), followed by those with a sitting height of 70–79 cm (AOR: 1.12; 95% CI: 0.47–2.96; $p < 0.001$), than the girls with a height 60–69cm. A higher likelihood of high SBP was found among the girls who had a waist circumference ≥80 cm (AOR: 2.11; 95% CI: 0.70–6.35; $p < 0.001$) and had a sitting height of 60–79 cm (AOR: 1.22; 95% CI: 0.47–3.17; $p < 0.001$) than the girls in the reference category. The prevalence of DBP was higher among overweight girls (AOR: 6.65; 95% CI: 0.68–65.46; $p < 0.01$) than thin girls, followed by girls who had normal BMI values (AOR: 2.71; 95% CI: 1.56–4.70; $p < 0.001$).

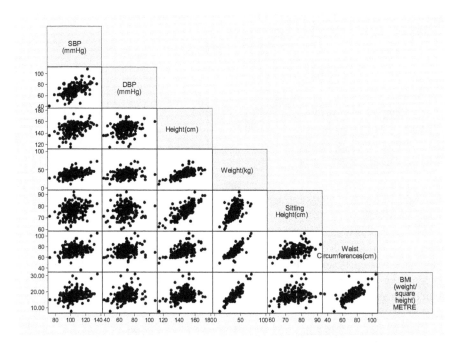

Fig. 1.1 Correlation matrix of blood pressure (SBP and DBP) with different anthropometric measurement variables

1.3.4 Correlation Matrix of Blood Pressure (SBP and DBP) with Different Anthropometric Measurement Variables

Figure 1.1 shows the correlation between SBP and DBP on one hand and different anthropometric variables on the other. According to Fig. 1.1, most of the anthropometric variables (e.g., height, weight, waist circumference, and BMI) are positively related to hypertension (SBP, DBP, or both SBP and DBP), whereas only the sitting height has no or a significantly smaller relation with SBP and DBP.

1.3.5 Blood Pressure and Mental Well-Being

According to Table 1.4, mean SBP and DBP values decreased as the mental well-being score increased, and the occurrence of prehypertension was the lowest among adolescent girls in the range of high mental well-being scores. The total occurrence of prehypertension among adolescent girls was 22%, representing the principle that blood pressure and mental well-being are inversely correlated with each other. With increasing blood pressure, mental well-being decreased. The results show an inverse relationship between blood pressure and mental well-being. Among surveyed girls,

Table 1.4 Relation of blood pressure with mental well-being score among adolescent girls in the slum areas of EBM

Variables	Total	Mental well-being score using GHQ-12		
		Low (≤7)	Moderate (8–10)	High (≥11)
Blood pressure				
Systolic blood pressure (mmHg)	108.61	109.5	108.6	107.7
Diastolic blood pressure (mmHg)	71.90	73.1	72.6	70.1
Prehypertension (%)	22	24	22	21

GHQ general health questionnaire

those girls who had a high average SBP (109.5 mmHg) also had a low mental well-being score (<7).

As soon as average systolic blood pressure increased, the mental well-being score automatically decreased. Moderate and high mental well-being scores correlated with average systolic blood pressure values of 108.6 mmHg and 107.7 mmHg, respectively. Low systolic blood pressure values (107.7 mmHg) correlated more with comparatively high (>11) mental well-being scores than with other scores. The same observation was found in the case of average diastolic blood pressure and an average mental well-being score. A mean diastolic blood pressure of 73.1 mmHg correlated with a lower score on mental well-being. These data indicate that the girls who had higher blood pressure tended to have low mental well-being, and this was due to the effect of their having anxiety or depression. As blood pressure decreased, girls' scores on mental well-being increased; for instance, a mean diastolic blood pressure of 72.6 mmHg correlated with a moderate mental well-being score (8–10), and a mean diastolic blood pressure of 70.1 mmHg correlated with a higher score on mental well-being (>11). For the moderate mental well-being score, the prehypertension percentage was 24%, which is comparatively higher than the others. Participants with a low mental well-being score have 22% more likely to prehypertension, and those with a high mental well-being score have 21% more likely to prehypertension, respectively.

1.4 Discussion

Currently, hypertension is recognized as a significant global public health issue (Lenfant et al. 2003). High blood pressure increases the risk of developing cardiovascular diseases. In developing countries like India, these diseases cause a rise in morbidity and mortality among adults. In India, 57% of all coronary disease deaths are caused by hypertension (Ghosh and Bandyopadhyay 2007). A long, slow, and steady study on hypertension has shown that the childhood and adolescent period is the origin of this. Probably during this period, it goes undetected and manifests later in life. Information related to BP in different communities comes mainly from various cross-sectional studies, which represent an accurate epidemiological picture of prehypertension. This study was carried out on adolescent girls living in the slum areas in English Bazar Municipality and tried to clarify the association between prehypertension and various anthropometric indices.

This study reveals that about 22% of adolescent girls in this study area experience high BP (systolic, diastolic or both). The present research on the SBP and DBP shows a positive relationship between weight (0.45 and 0.29, respectively), height (0.38 and 0.20, respectively), and waist circumference (0.38 and 0.26, respectively), which was also found in the observations of Nag et al. (2018), Moser et al. (2013), Ramalingam and Chacko (2014), Chadha et al. (1999), Durrani and Waseem (2011), Taksande et al. (2008). This study also shows a positive relationship between BP (systolic, diastolic, or both) and BMI values (0.34 and 0.28, respectively), which is similar to the findings in studies by Taksande et al. (2008), Nag et al. (2018), Moser et al. (2013), Dua et al. (2014), Ghosh and Bandyopadhyay (2007).

The prevalence of SBP and DBP increases with increases in the mean weight, height, and BMI value, which is similar to the findings in studies by Ramalingam and Chacko in Tamil Nadu in 2014, Durrani and Waseem in Aligarh in 2011, and Nag et al. in Burdwan Municipal in 2018. According to Verma et al., an increase in the prevalence of hypertension appears among participants who are obese when compared to the nonobese participants (13.7% and 0.4%, respectively), and a similar result was found in the present study. This study indicates that the prevalence of elevated BP (SBP, DBP, or both) is higher with increases in the mean weight and height of the participant, which is similar to the findings in a study by Durrani and Waseem in Aligarh among boys and girls as well as among all their study's other participants.

Some other studies have shown a strong positive relation between obesity and hypertension (Botton et al. 2007), and BMI has been one of the parameters used to identify the risk of developing them (Wang et al. 2008; Ribeiro et al. 2010; Moser et al. 2013). This study reveals that overweight adolescent girls are about 1.6 times more vulnerable to developing high blood pressure than underweight girls are (Moser et al. 2013). The correlation matrix shows a positive relationship between all the anthropometric measures and hypertension (SBP, DBP, or both). Similar findings found in the work of Naflu et al. and Ramoshaba et al. support the results found in this study.

1.4.1 Limitations

This study might have introduced some error in recording the actual BP of a few participants. Multiple factors that affect recordings and that might not have been checked at the time of measuring the BP of participants include diurnal variation (the time of day when the BP was measured), the fasting and nonfasting conditions of participants, and the season of the year, among others.

1.5 Conclusion

The present study revealed that an increase in the measurements of anthropometric variables is a significant factor in hypertension development in that an increase in the prevalence of hypertension corresponds to increases in all the anthropometric variables (weight, height, sitting height, waist circumference, and BMI). Effective policies should be introduced for adolescent girls to decrease the morbidity and long-term complications that arise from hypertension. Children and adolescents must be screened to detect BP; influential variables like overweight should be checked; and regular exercise, proper nutrient intake, and weight control should be encouraged. Adequate health education needs to be introduced at home and in educational institutes so that these risk factors can be eliminated at an early stage.

Declaration

Data Availability The data analyzed in this chapter are available from the corresponding author upon reasonable request. The corresponding author takes responsibility for the integrity and accuracy of the data analysis.

Ethical Approval and Consent to Participate Verbal consent was obtained from all adult study participants, and we also obtained verbal consent from parents and key informants for minor (below 18 years) study participants.

Competing Interest The contributors declare that they have no competing interests.

Funding This research did not receive any specific grants from funding agencies in the public, commercial, or not-for-profit sectors.

References

Acharyya T, Kaur P, Murhekar MV (2014) Prevalence of behavioral risk factors, overweight and hypertension in the urban slums of North 24 Parganas District, West Bengal, India, 2010. Indian J Public Health 58(3):195

Bagga A, Jain R, Vijayakumar M, Kanitkar M, Ali U (2007) Evaluation and management of hypertension. Indian Pediatr 44(2):103–121

Banerjee S, Mukherjee TK, Basu S (2016) Prevalence, awareness, and control of hypertension in the slums of Kolkata. Indian Heart J 68(3):286–294

Banerjee S, Khan MF, Bandyopadhyay K, Selvaraj K, Deshmukh P (2021) Hypertension and its determinants among school going adolescents in selected urban slums of Nagpur city, Maharashtra: a cross-sectional study. Clin Epidemiol Glob Health 12:100832

Botton J, Heude B, Kettaneh A, Borys JM, Lommez A, Bresson JL, FLVS Study Group (2007) Cardiovascular risk factor levels and their relationships with overweight and fat distribution in children: the Fleurbaix Laventie Ville Sante II study. Metabolism 56(5):614–622

Chadha SL, Tandon R, Shekhawat S, Gopinath N (1999) An epidemiological study of blood pressure in school children (5-14 years) in Delhi. Indian Heart J 51(2):178–182

Das SR, Drazner MH, Dries DL, Vega GL, Stanek HG, Abdullah SM, De Lemos JA (2005) Impact of body mass and body composition on circulating levels of natriuretic peptides: results from the Dallas Heart Study. Circulation 112(14):2163–2168

Das T, Das P, Roy TB (2022) Physical violence against women by their partner: a latent class measurement and causal analysis from rural counterparts of Dakshin Dinajpur District, India. Glob Soc Welf 9:229–240

Dua S, Bhuker M, Sharma P, Dhall M, Kapoor S (2014) Body mass index relates to blood pressure among adults. N Am J Med Sci 6(2):89

Durrani AM, Fatima W (2012) Determinants of blood pressure distribution in school children. Eur J Publ Health 22(3):369–373

Durrani AM, Waseem F (2011) Blood pressure distribution and its relation to anthropometric measurements among school children in Aligarh. Indian J Public Health 55(2):121

Ghosh JR, Bandyopadhyay AR (2007) Comparative evaluation of obesity measures: relationship with blood pressures and hypertension. Singapore Med J 48(3):232

Gupta R (2004) Trends in hypertension epidemiology in India. J Hum Hypertens 18(2):73–78

Hansen ML, Gunn PW, Kaelber DC (2007) Underdiagnosis of hypertension in children and adolescents. JAMA 298(8):874–879

Huey SL, Finkelstein JL, Venkatramanan S, Udipi SA, Ghugre P, Thakker V, Mehta S (2019) Prevalence and correlates of undernutrition in young children living in urban slums of Mumbai, India: a cross sectional study. Front Public Health 7:191

Jungari S, Chinchore S (2022) Perception, prevalence, and determinants of intimate partner violence during pregnancy in urban slums of Pune, Maharashtra, India. J Interpers Violence 37(1-2):239–263

Jungari S, Pardhi A, Bomble P (2022) Violence against women during pregnancy in india: a literature review. Violence Against Women 2(1):113–136

Juonala M, Magnussen CG, Berenson GS, Venn A, Burns TL, Sabin MA, Raitakari OT (2011) Childhood adiposity, adult adiposity, and cardiovascular risk factors. N Engl J Med 365:1876–1885

Khan MI, Lala MK, Patil R, Mathur HN, Chauhan NT (2010) A study of the risk factors and the prevalence of hypertension in the adolescent school boys of Ahmedabad City. J Clin Diagn Res 4:3348–3354

Kumar H, Priyanka YA, Arora T, Attri SK, Khandelwal A (2015) Prevalence of hypertension in high school students of a rural area–a pilot study. Indian J Res Rep Med Sci 5:13–18

Lenfant C, Chobanian AV, Jones DW, Roccella EJ (2003) Seventh report of the Joint National Committee on the prevention, detection, evaluation, and treatment of high blood pressure (JNC 7) resetting the hypertension sails. Hypertension 41(6):1178–1179

Lumagbas LB, Coleman HLS, Bunders J, Pariente A, Belonje A, de Cock Buning T (2018) Non-communicable diseases in Indian slums: re-framing the Social Determinants of Health. Glob Health Action 11(1):1438840

Meena J, Singh M, Agarwal A, Chauhan A, Jaiswal N (2021) Prevalence of hypertension among children and adolescents in India: a systematic review and meta-analysis. Indian J Pediatr 88(11):1107–1114

Moser DC, Giuliano IDCB, Titski ACK, Gaya AR, Coelho-e-Silva MJ, Leite N (2013) Anthropometric measures and blood pressure in school children. J Pediatr 89(3):243–249

Nag K, Karmakar N, Saha I, Dasgupta S, Mukhopadhyay BP, Mondal MRI (2018) An epidemiological study of blood pressure and its relation with anthropometric measurements among schoolboys of Burdwan Municipal Area, West Bengal. Indian J Community Med 43(3):157

Ramalingam S, Chacko T (2014) Blood pressure distribution and its association with anthropometric measurements among Asian Indian adolescents in an urban area of Tamil Nadu. Int J Med Sci Public Health 3(9):1100–1104

Ribeiro RC, Coutinho M, Bramorski MA, Giuliano IC, Pavan J (2010) Association of the waist-to-height ratio with cardiovascular risk factors in children and adolescents: the three cities heart study. Int J Prev Med 1(1):39

Riley M, Hernandez AK, Kuznia AL (2018) High blood pressure in children and adolescents. Am Fam Physician 98(8):486–494

Schutte AE, Srinivasapura Venkateshmurthy N, Mohan S, Prabhakaran D (2021) Hypertension in low-and middle-income countries. Circ Res 128(7):808–826

Sharma A, Grover N, Kaushik S, Bhardwaj R, Sankhyan N (2010) Prevalence of hypertension among schoolchildren in Shimla. Indian Pediatr 47(10):873–876

Singh SK, Verma A (2021) Prevalence of hypertension among school going adolescent boys in Najafgarh, Delhi, India. Int J Adolesc Med Health 33:5

Song P, Zhang Y, Yu J, Zha M, Zhu Y, Rahimi K, Rudan I (2019) Global prevalence of hypertension in children: a systematic review and meta-analysis. JAMA Pediatr 173(12):1154–1163

Taksande A, Chaturvedi P, Vilhekar K, Jain M (2008) Distribution of blood pressure in school going children in rural area of Wardha district, Maharashatra, India. Ann Pediatr Cardiol 1(2):101

Todkar SS, Gujarathi VV, Tapare VS (2009) Period prevalence and sociodemographic factors of hypertension in rural Maharashtra: a cross-sectional study. Indian J Community Med 34(3):183

Wang H, Necheles J, Carnethon M, Wang B, Li Z, Wang L, Wang X (2008) Adiposity measures and blood pressure in Chinese children and adolescents. Arch Dis Child 93(9):738–744

World Health Organization (2021) Hypertension. World Health Organization. https://www.who.int/news-room/fact-sheets/detail/hypertension. Accessed 27 November 2022

Yusuf S, Hawken S, Ounpuu S, Bautista L, Franzosi MG, Commerford P, Interheart Study Investigators (2005) Obesity and the risk of myocardial infarction in 27,000 participants from 52 countries: a case-control study. Lancet 366(9497):1640–1649

Zhou B, Perel P, Mensah GA, Ezzati M (2021) Global epidemiology, health burden and effective interventions for elevated blood pressure and hypertension. Nat Rev Cardiol 18(11):785–802

Chapter 2
Homeless Women's Multifaceted Vulnerabilities in India: A Research Roadmap Delineation

Margubur Rahaman, Komal Sureshrao Gajbhiyeand, and Kailash Chandra Das

Abstract Despite the estimated population of homeless women standing at 0.7 million, research dedicated to understanding women's homelessness in India remains lacking. This chapter endeavors to contextualize the multifaceted vulnerabilities among homeless women in India and delineate future research directions. By utilizing a systematic literature review methodology, a total of 30 relevant studies were selected and screened to derive key findings. The study findings underscore the complexity of pathways leading to homelessness among women, driven by socioeconomic poverty and gender-based injustices. Homelessness renders women susceptible to sexual violence and myriad livelihood challenges, consequently impinging upon their mental and physical health and well-being. The prevalence of multiple morbidities among this demographic is notable, compounded by negative attitudes toward healthcare utilization and various structural and individual-level barriers. Moreover, a lack of health awareness further impedes their access to essential healthcare services. Elevated sexual and reproductive health risks persist among homeless women, juxtaposed with inadequate access to relevant services, thereby presenting additional hurdles. In conclusion, while research interest in homeless women is expanding, the dearth of studies focusing on sexual and reproductive health underscores the imperative for further inquiry in this domain. Likewise, policy and research attention are warranted to address the multidimensional poverty

---

M. Rahaman (✉)
Department of Migration and Urban Studies, International Institute for Population Sciences, Mumbai, India

Govind Ballabh Pant Social Science Institute (GBPSSI), Prayagraj, India

K. C. Das
Department of Migration and Urban Studies, International Institute for Population Sciences, Mumbai, India
e-mail: kailash.das@iipsindia.ac.in

K. S. Gajbhiyeand
Department of Population and Development, International Institute for Population Sciences, Mumbai, India

© The Author(s), under exclusive license to Springer Nature Singapore Pte Ltd. 2024
P. Chouhan et al. (eds.), *Sexual and Reproductive Health of Women*, https://doi.org/10.1007/978-981-97-8418-9_2

experienced by homeless women in India and to foster their mental and physical health and well-being, thereby enabling them to live with dignity.

Keywords Factors of female homelessness · Homeless health vulnerability, homeless livelihood vulnerability · India

2.1 Introduction

India ranks 16th in the world on homeless population size: about 1.7 million individuals (World Population Review 2024). The temporal context of homelessness in India reveals a decline in the overall homeless population, from 2.34 million to 1.77 million from 1981 to 2011 (Sahoo and Jeermison 2018). Similarly, spatial variation highlights that Uttar Pradesh has the highest homeless population at 329,125 persons, followed by Maharashtra (210,908 persons), Rajasthan (181,544 persons), and Madhya Pradesh (146,435 persons). The concentration of homelessness is more pronounced in urban areas (Registrar General and Census Commissioner 2011). The gender dimensions of homelessness indicate that about 49% of people experiencing homelessness are women, with children under 5 years old constituting 16% of this population. Furthermore, urban female homelessness increased slightly from 34.4% to 35.8% between 1981 and 2011 (Registrar General and Census Commissioner 2011). The simultaneous increase in homelessness in urban areas may be a result of rural-to-urban labor migration and the limited availability of affordable housing options. Among the urban areas, Kolkata district reports the highest number, followed by Surat, Kanpur Nagar, Ranga Reddy, and Jaipur (Registrar General and Census Commissioner 2011).

Existing literature highlights a complex pathway leading to homelessness, with distinct gender-based variations in India (Krishnadas et al. 2021; Patra and Anand 2008; Singh et al. 2018). Domestic or spousal violence, gender-based violence, and limited societal recognition of women's rights are key drivers of homelessness among women in India (Koul 2022). In contrast, homelessness among men is significantly associated with factors such as poverty, rural-to-urban migration, and socioeconomic deprivation (Singh et al. 2018). In urban areas, homeless women find securing sustained employment to be challenging—for instance, distinct patterns in income sources show that a higher percentage of women (70.6%) and transgender respondents (71.3%) access entitlement-based income, while men are more likely to secure income through formal employment (26.2%) (Chaudhry et al. 2014; Jha and Kumar 2016). Existing studies in Delhi and Bangalore reveal inadequate access to water for sanitation and affordable, quality sanitation facilities for homeless individuals (Chaudhry et al. 2014; Walters 2014). Livelihood vulnerability disparities highlight that homeless women are ten times more at risk than their male counterparts, with adolescent girls particularly vulnerable to sexual abuse and trafficking (Chaudhry et al. 2014). Similarly, women bear additional burdens, including gender-selective limited work participation and exposure to sexual and reproductive violence. This chapter emphasizes that the vulnerability of homeless women is due to the lack of a secure place for undressing and changing clothes. Additionally, the challenge of bathing in public spaces increases the risk of gender-based violence (Chaudhry et al. 2014).

Various forms of violence afflict homeless women on the streets, including sexual harassment, molestation, rape by strangers or fellow homeless individuals, and even gang rape. This pervasive danger persists whether homeless women live alone or with their families, during the day or at night (Bhattacharya 2022). The victims span all age groups, with homeless girls and women with mental illnesses facing heightened vulnerability (Bhattacharya 2022). While the sociodemographic and spatial background of homeless women is well documented in existing literature (Aishwarya 2021; Chaudhry et al. 2014; Jha and Kumar 2016; Sahoo and Jeermison 2018; Singh et al. 2018), only a few studies have addressed reproductive health matters in the Indian context ((Farooq and Srivastava 2023; Menon et al. 2023; Negi 2023; Patra and Anand 2008). Therefore, a descriptive presentation of the multifaceted vulnerabilities of homeless women is relevant to understanding this aspect of their well-being. Moreover, the poor environmental, structural, and sociocultural background of homeless women contributes to increased reproductive health risks among them. Despite the high livelihood and health vulnerabilities among homeless women, no other study has comprehensively contextualized the context of women's homelessness and associated vulnerabilities. From this research perspective, the present chapter aims to determine the factors of homelessness, the health vulnerabilities, and the healthcare needs and practices of homeless women in India. Additionally, this chapter also determines the roadmap of existing research on homeless women and identifies further research needs and directions.

2.2 Methodology

This systematic review was conducted according to the Preferred Reporting Items for Systematic Reviews and Meta-Analyses (PRISMA) guidelines. A comprehensive search strategy was developed to search the following bibliographic databases: PubMed, Embase, MEDLINE, JSTOR, Google Scholar, and Shodhganga. The search strategy combined relevant controlled vocabulary terms (e.g., Mesh terms in PubMed) and keywords related to homelessness, homeless women, reproductive health, contraception, mental health, barriers and challenges for accessing the health, livelihoods, and India.

2.2.1 Search Strategy

The specific search strategy for each database was created by combining terms related to the following: (1) homelessness (e.g. "homeless women," "vagrancy," and "street women"), (2) reproductive health (e.g. "reproductive health," "maternal health," "pregnancy health," "contraceptive agents," "family planning," and "menstrual"), (3) health (e.g. "mental health," "diseases," and "mortality"), and (4) India (e.g. "India" and "Indian"). The search was limited to English-language articles published between 2000 and 2023.

2.2.2 Inclusion and Exclusion Criteria

Eligibility criteria were developed a priori. Inclusion criteria were as follows: (1) original peer-reviewed research articles, books, and thesis; (2) studies conducted in India; (3) and studies that examined reproductive health or contraception use among homeless women. Exclusion criteria were as follows: (1) abstracts only, (2) languages other than English, (3) works that did not focus on the homeless population.

Title/abstract screening was independently conducted by two reviewers to identify potentially relevant articles. Full-text review was then carried out to confirm eligibility on the basis of the inclusion/exclusion criteria. Disagreements at both stages were resolved through discussion. Data extraction from the final set of included studies was performed by two independent reviewers using a standardized form collecting information on study design, sample population, demographics, key findings related to reproductive health, and contraception use among homeless women in India.

2.2.3 Data Extraction

Descriptive synthesis was used to narratively summarize the key features and findings of the included studies. Extracted data such as author, publication year, study location, and results are presented in summary tables. The PRISMA flowchart outlines the chapter selection process. A total of 30 studies met the eligibility criteria and were included in the systematic review. The process for selecting literature for this chapter's systematic review is presented in the Fig. 2.1. The details of the selected literature for this chapter's systematic review are laid out in Table 2.1.

2.3 Results

2.3.1 Prevailing Research Dimensions of Women's Homelessness

Out of a total of 30 selected articles reviewed in the current chapter, 33% of them had examined the factors of homelessness and livelihood vulnerabilities, and 30% had contextualized overall health and well-being (Fig. 2.2). Additionally, 17% had presented purely mental health vulnerabilities, and 10% had explored

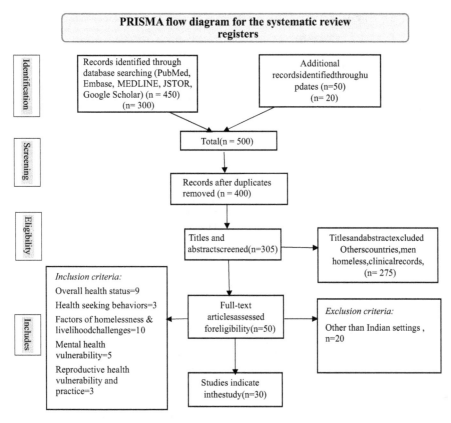

Fig. 2.1 PRISMA flowchart detailing the background criteria for selecting scientific literature for the systematic review in this chapter

health-seeking behavior among homeless women in the Indian context. In addition, only 10% of the selected papers had explored the reproductive health vulnerabilities and practices of homeless women (Fig. 2.2).

2.3.2 Temporal Variability in Female Homelessness Research

All the selected literature included in the chapter was published during 2000–2023. As of 2000, few studies had highlighted the livelihood vulnerabilities, health issues, and health-seeking behaviors of homeless women (Fig. 2.3). However, since 2019, a substantial number of studies have focused on such issues in the Indian context. In summary, the results show that a growing trend of research related to nexus between homeless women's livelihood and health has emerged recently (Fig. 2.3). Although research on homeless women's health has increased over time, a limited research has focused on reproductive health vulnerabilities and practices in Indian settings (Fig. 2.2).

Table 2.1 Description of selected literature for the systematic review in this chapter

Authors	Publication year	Title of the study
Anand and Tiwari (2006)	2006	A gendered perspective of the shelter–transport–livelihood link: the case of poor women in Delhi
Patra and Anand (2008)	2008	Homelessness: a hidden public health problem
Sarikhani (2010)	2010	Status of homeless women and children in Karnataka state based on census of 2001
Suman and Sesha (2010)	2010	Psychosocial Rehabilitation of Young Homeless Women
Sowmya and Suman (2013)	2013	Pathways to homelessness, psychological distress and perceived social support among married women in a shelter: Implications for Trauma Informed Care
Pandey (2016)	2016	Health issues of the homeless population in the NCT of Delhi
Garg et al. (2016)	2016	Mortality among homeless women who remain unclaimed after death: an insight
Prashad et al. (2016)	2016	Treatment seeking behaviour among homeless people: evidences from Mumbai city
Gowda et al. (2017)	2017	Clinical outcome and rehabilitation of homeless mentally ill patients admitted in mental health institute of South India: "know the unknown" project
Moorkath et al. (2018)	2018	Lives without roots: institutionalized homeless women with chronic mental illness
Chourase (2019)	2019	Living conditions health status and security of homeless women: a study in Delhi city
Padgett and Priyam (2019)	2019	Gender, everyday resistance and bodily integrity: women's lives on Delhi streets
Narasimhan et al. (2019)	2019	Responsive mental health systems to address the poverty, homelessness and mental illness nexus: the Banyan experience from India
Nambiar (2020)	2020	Social determinants of health among urban homeless in Delhi, India
Narasimhan et al. (2020)	2020	Homelessness and women living with mental health issues: lessons from the Banyan's experience in Chennai, Tamil Nadu
Veeraiah (2021)	2020	Homeless women in Telangana State, Southern Part of India: a cross-sectional study
Nambiar (2020)	2020	Interventions addressing maternal and child health among the urban poor and homeless: an overview of systematic reviews
Krishnadas et al. (2021)	2021	Factors associated with homelessness among women: a cross-sectional survey of outpatient mental health service users at the Banyan, India

(continued)

Table 2.1 (continued)

Authors	Publication year	Title of the study
Aishwarya (2021)	2021	Urban homelessness of women and urban marginality: sociological perspectives
Dasgupta and Chatterjee (n.d.)	2021	Quality of life of the homeless and restored women with psychosis
Coleman et al. (2022)	2022	Addressing health needs of the homeless in Delhi: standardising on the issues of street medicine practice
Bhattacharya (2022)	2022	Stakeholders facilitating hope and empowerment amidst social suffering: a qualitative documentary analysis exploring lives of homeless women with mental illness
Nambiar et al. (2023)	2022	Roles played by civil society organisations in supporting homeless people with health care-seeking and accessing the social determinants of health in Delhi, India: perspectives of support providers and receivers
Kumari and Sekher (2022)	2022	Situation analysis of "institutionalized" and "homeless" elderly widows abandoned in India's pilgrimage centres: insights into their living conditions and available infrastructural facilities
Richards and Kuhn (2023)	2023	Unsheltered homelessness and health: a literature review
Chakraborty and Garg (2023)	2023	Finding a home in or through mobile phones: access and usage patterns among homeless women in shelter-homes of India
Kalyanasundara et al.	2023	Psychosocial preparedness among homeless people: a study from an urban rehabilitation center in South India
Menon et al. (2023)	2023	Characterization of an extreme phenotype of schizophrenia among women with homelessness
Farooq and Srivastava (2023)	2023	A psychological study of reproductive health awareness and practices among homeless adolescent girls in Nizamuddin, Delhi
Negi (2023)	2023	Fertility and reproductive health: a qualitative study of homeless migrants in Delhi

2.3.3 *Livelihood Vulnerabilities Among Homeless Women*

Research on the livelihood vulnerabilities of homeless women underscores a distressing reality: a significant portion of this demographic grapples with illiteracy, relegating them to informal, low-paying jobs in the unorganized sector or resorting to begging for survival (Sarikhani 2010; Padgett and Priyam 2019). The starkly lower literacy rates among homeless women, as compared to the general female population, exacerbate their marginalization and limit their access to education (Sarikhani 2010). Often, socioeconomic deprivation precipitates their homelessness in urban settings. Tragically, the intersection of homelessness and socioeconomic

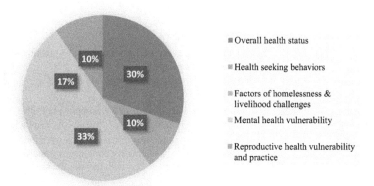

Fig. 2.2 Pie chart displaying the percentage distribution of articles from the literature selected on the basis of their key themes, 2000–2023

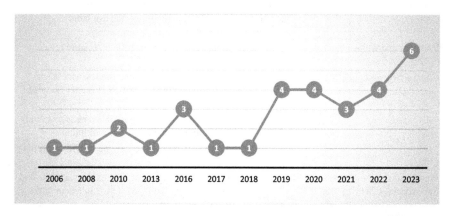

Fig. 2.3 Temporal variability in frequency of the studies on homeless people selected for this chapter, 2000–2023

deprivation heightens the risk of gender-based violence and social discrimination, depriving homeless women of their basic human rights (Veeraiah 2021), whereas the gender divide in accessing and using mobile phones in women's shelters has caused women to miss job opportunities and lose promising futures (Chakraborty and Garg 2023). In the initial period of homelessness, women suffered the most due to their not having a secure place on the street and in shelters. They had to adjust more. The literature has shown that women aged 15–47 years stay at rehabilitation centers where they receive counseling to reduce distress and build stronger bonds with other residents (Suman and Sesha 2010), and domestic violence, sexual abuse, and trafficking are distressingly common experiences for these vulnerable women (Veeraiah 2021). The bodies of homeless women exist within a framework of social vulnerability that maintains their secondary status to men, as seen through factors like marital status, which confines women's labor to the domestic sphere and occupational gender pay gaps in unorganized sectors; this highlights the multiple forms of discrimination that homeless women face from an intersectional perspective (Aishwarya 2021). Studies have revealed that homeless women often lack emotional, social, practical, financial, and guidance support from family members, which is associated with greater psychological distress; despite inadequate subjective well-being, 85% of homeless women expressed optimism about their future (Sowmya and Suman 2013). Although government welfare initiatives for urban poor aim to address homelessness, the capacity of shelters falls woefully short of accommodating the actual homeless population, leaving many without refuge (Veeraiah 2021). Moreover, although government-run elder-care homes and shelters for widows offer basic amenities such as cots, mattresses, clothing, hygiene facilities, visiting areas, on-call medical assistance, and proper lighting, approximately 39% of surveyed residents expressed dissatisfaction, rating the quality of services and facilities as poor (Kumari and Sekher 2022). Consequently, the plight of homeless women persists as a pressing societal issue in urban India, highlighting the urgent need for comprehensive solutions to safeguard their safety, dignity, and access to opportunities.

2.3.4 Multifaceted Health Vulnerabilities Among Homeless Women

Homeless women face a dual burden of health vulnerabilities, encompassing both physical and mental health issues. Among these, acute and chronic respiratory illnesses, such as tuberculosis and chronic lung diseases, are prevalent. Additionally, HIV, infectious diseases, oral infections, dry cough, burning in the chest, joints, and bones, difficulty in recognizing problems, and skin diseases are highly prevalent within this population (Chourase 2019; Pandey 2016). Moreover, mental health problems compound the challenges faced by homeless women, among whom conditions like schizophrenia are particularly prevalent. In particular, homeless women often experience severer psychopathology than do housed women with similar mental health issues, highlighting the exacerbating effect of homelessness on mental well-being. In addition, stress, panic attracts, difficulty sleeping, self-harm, suicidal thoughts, and aggressive behavior are also common mental health problems among homeless women (Pandey 2016). Recent statistics from a cross-sectional study on outpatient homeless women have revealed that 80% of them are more likely to experience mental health issues (Krishnadas et al. 2021). Additionally, existing literature has also highlighted that homeless woman with schizophrenia experience severer psychiatric symptoms, significantly poorer cognitive functioning, and higher levels of disability and require higher doses of antipsychotic medication than do housed women with schizophrenia (Menon et al. 2023).

The prevalence of unhygienic menstrual health practices has been found to be high among homeless women and girls in India. The unhygienic menstrual practices coupled with their lack of secure housing, clean water, and access to sanitation facilities increase vulnerable homeless women's risk of reproductive tract infections, pelvic inflammatory disease, and associated morbidity (Garikipati and Boudot 2017). In addition, painful periods, irregular periods, frequently short periods, blood clots or excess bleeding, prolonged and little bleeding, and intermenstrual bleeding are common menstrual health problems among homeless women (Chourase 2019). The mean age of death of homeless women is 45 years, and their most common causes of death are natural events, followed by acute/chronic lung diseases (Garg et al. 2016).

2.3.5 Healthcare Behaviors and Barriers Among Homeless Women

Despite facing disproportionate disease burdens due to extreme poverty, vulnerability to violence, a lack of shelter, food insecurity, and social marginalization, homeless women underutilize existing healthcare services. The absence of specialized healthcare services and outreach targeted specifically at homeless women exacerbates this situation (Patra and Anand 2008). Homeless women primarily seek healthcare at government hospitals rather than private clinics, regardless of whether they are dealing with acute or chronic health issues. However, the primary obstacle that they face in accessing healthcare is a lack of awareness of available services and entitlements (Prashad et al. 2016). For instance, a study of 300 homeless women found that 64% were unfamiliar with HIV/AIDS, just 5.3% had a lot of knowledge, 18% average knowledge, and 12.7% little knowledge about it, where most were unable to correctly answer transmission questions and where only 7% had a positive attitude compared to 29% who had a negative attitude toward HIV/AIDS (Chourase 2019). Their healthcare-seeking behavior is further influenced by marital status, where widowed women are more inclined to seek treatment for acute conditions, whereas unmarried women tend to prioritize care for chronic illnesses. Additionally, migratory status plays a role in that nonmigrant homeless women have higher treatment rates than migrants do. Treatment-seeking behavior declines with lower income, indicating affordability barriers (Prashad et al. 2016).

In the realm of maternal health, homeless women encounter significant barriers to accessing essential care, stemming from their limited knowledge about and awareness of family planning, safe motherhood practices, and their maternal health rights (Nambiar et al. 2023). The underutilization of maternal and child health services persists, where factors such as the low usage of antenatal care, skilled birth attendant deliveries, and postnatal care contribute to this disparity (Negi 2023). Additionally, a prevalent unmet need for family planning persists within this demographic (Farooq and Srivastava 2023). Barriers such as transportation issues, financial constraints, a lack of necessary documents, discrimination, and fears of losing custody of their children further impede access to maternal healthcare services (Negi 2023). Moreover, homeless women often resort to using unhygienic materials like dirty rags, plastic, sand, and ash during menstruation due to their lack of access to and the affordability of sanitary napkins (Garikipati and Boudot 2017), where the sharing of absorbents is common among them. Despite a high prevalence of mental health issues among homeless women, the utilization of mental healthcare services remains low due to their limited awareness of mental health disorders and available services (Nambiar et al. 2023). Additionally, the scarcity of public mental health services and the absence of shelter-based or homeless-focused mental healthcare camps present major barriers to fulfilling the mental healthcare needs of homeless women. Homeless women with mental illnesses in India face gender-based disadvantages, poverty, and critical incidents, leading to an invisible, disenfranchised existence. The complex nexus between mental illness and homelessness requires tailored health and social care responses, yet few social care interventions exist. This chapter describes the Banyan's continuum of care model for homeless women with mental illness in India – specifically the Emergency Care and Recovery Centre, which offers crisis intervention and reintegration. It discusses implications for mental health policies and practices for this extremely marginalized population (Narasimhan et al. 2020).

2.3.6 Discussion

The present chapter significantly contributes to the existing literature by delineating various dimensions of women's homelessness within Indian settings. First, it provides a comprehensive summary of the pathways leading to women's homelessness and the vulnerabilities in livelihood associated with those pathways. Second, it contextualizes the multifaceted health vulnerabilities faced by homeless women and examines existing healthcare practices and their associated barriers. Lastly, it outlines a roadmap for future research on women's homelessness and identifies areas that require further exploration.

The foremost findings of this chapter underscore that homeless women in India are predominantly illiterate and socioeconomically disadvantaged (Sarikhani 2010). Moreover, they bear the burden of multiple health issues due to their impoverished circumstances. Consequently, their overall well-being is markedly poor (Chourase 2019; Pandey 2016). The pathways leading to women's homelessness highlight a nexus of factors, such as a history of domestic violence, poverty, social discrimination, and migration, along with intergenerational homelessness (Chourase 2019; Krishnadas et al. 2021). Living in homelessness exposes women to additional burdens, particularly various forms of domestic violence, including sexual violence. Despite engaging in work activities for survival, their employment options are severely limited, and they often face discrimination and violence in the workplace

(Monteiro and Nalini 2021). Homeless women endure significant challenges and injustices, and they persist in their efforts to survive while compromising their basic human and socioeconomic rights and dignity. Although the Indian Constitution guarantees equality in rights (article 14–18), the pervasive discrimination and violence experienced by homeless women underscore the reality that socioeconomically underprivileged individuals are surviving without basic rights. Although the government of India has implemented various programs aimed at ensuring the right to live with dignity, such as the PM Awas Yojana and homeless shelters, a substantial gap remains between government initiatives, implementation, and the actual needs of the homeless population (Goel et al. 2017; Gohil and Gandhi 2019). In the context of shelter provision for homeless people, adopting a gender-centric approach is crucial to effectively address the accommodation needs of homeless women. Prioritizing gender-sensitive shelters can help alleviate issues such as the lack of shelter options tailored to women's needs and external violence against homeless women, thereby enhancing both their livelihoods and mental health and well-being. The majority of homeless cases stem from socioeconomic poverty and displacement induced by natural disasters (Devakumar 2008). Therefore, the current chapter suggests the need for existing policy revision, focusing on target-based approaches such as emergency shelter services and economic support services in disaster-prone areas. Diverse economic sustainability opportunities and support for underprivileged populations are recommended to reduce forced migration and homelessness. Simultaneously, urban homelessness presents a more significant challenge than rural homelessness due to rapid rural-to-urban migration, complex urban employment opportunities, wage disparities, and living costs. In this regard, the government should prioritize equity-based housing facilities for informal migrant laborers, especially those migrating with families, female migrants, and single female migrants with children. Recently, the Indian government's Union Cabinet (IGUC), under the leadership of PM Narendra Modi, approved the development of Affordable Rental Housing Complexes (ARHCs) with the aim of providing decent and affordable accommodation for lakhs of migrant workers residing in cities (Bhate and Samuel 2023). According to sources in the Ministry of Housing and Urban Affairs, the rent for these complexes will range between INR 1000 and INR 3000 per month. Municipalities will have the authority to determine the allocation of these rental houses. Initially, around three lakh migrants, comprising construction workers and service providers in sectors such as hospitality, health, domestic work, commercial establishments, and students, will benefit from this initiative by being able to access affordable rental housing. The decision by the IGUC is highly commendable, and hopefully, it will effectively address the issue of affordable housing among migrants, including the homeless population. Additionally, efforts should be directed toward encouraging informal sectors to provide housing allowances for their employees. By adopting such an approach, policymakers can take significant strides toward addressing the systemic challenges faced by homeless women in India.

The secondary findings of this chapter highlight that homeless women suffer the dual burden of health vulnerabilities, encompassing both physical and mental health issues. They are disproportionately affected by acute and chronic respiratory illnesses, such as tuberculosis and chronic lung diseases, mental health problems (Chourase 2019; Pandey 2016). Additionally, they are susceptible to various other health challenges including HIV, infectious diseases, oral infections, disabilities, and injuries (Chourase 2019; Pandey 2016). Living in unsheltered conditions exposes homeless women to various risks, including environmental pollution, unsafe sexual practices, physical and sexual violence, and precarious employment situations (Chourase 2019; Nambiar 2020). Despite the presence of government and nonprofit shelter services, the deteriorated shelter conditions often leave homeless women vulnerable to infectious diseases like tuberculosis (Nambiar 2020). A lack of sanitation facilities in temporary shelters further increases their risk of contracting infectious diseases, and physical and sexual violence remains a constant threat (Nambiar 2020). Moreover, homeless women often lack knowledge about HIV/AIDS transmission pathways and harbor negative attitudes toward these diseases, further exacerbating their vulnerability (Chourase 2019). Homeless women with mental illnesses in India face a myriad of challenges stemming from familial, economic, societal, and cultural factors (Moorkath et al. 2018). They often experience rejection, a lack of family support, and the denial of their rights, leading to severe psychopathology and a lower quality of life than that of mentally ill women living with families (Dasgupta and Chatterjee n.d.; Gowda et al. 2017; Menon et al. 2023). Substance abuse as a coping mechanism further aggravates their health vulnerability (Richards and Kuhn 2023). However, interventions by nongovernmental organizations (NGOs) and community-based care models offer hope by providing tailored mental health services, crisis support, and vocational rehabilitation (Bhattacharya 2022; Narasimhan et al. 2019). The prevalence of unhygienic menstrual health practices among homeless women in India exacerbates their vulnerability to reproductive tract infections and associated morbidities (Garikipati and Boudot 2017). This, coupled with livelihood vulnerability and multiple disease burdens, results in significantly a lower life expectancy for homeless women compared to housed women (Garg et al. 2016). Addressing both immediate health concerns and underlying socioeconomic factors is crucial to improve the well-being and quality of life of this marginalized population.

The tertiary findings of this chapter contextualize the healthcare needs, practices, and associated barriers among homeless women. The results indicate that despite homeless women's facing complex health challenges, they often underutilize health services due to various barriers, such as difficulty navigating systems, a lack of tailored services, concerns over stigma, misconceptions about illnesses, and technological obstacles in care systems (Coleman et al. 2022). A pressing need persists for interventions that address the multidimensional health needs of homeless women, including providing access to shelter, addressing food insecurity, providing mental healthcare, treating substance abuse cases, and sensitizing health systems to their unique needs. Furthermore, homeless women face high risks related to fertility behavior, maternal health, unmet needs for family planning, and unsafe sexual practices. However, their utilization of sexual and reproductive health services remains low, highlighting a critical issue that requires attention. Promoting safe motherhood and sexual and reproductive well-being among homeless women is essential. The recent introduction of the Ayushman Bharat–Health and Wellness Centres (AB-HWCs) program by the government of India is a positive step toward promoting health and well-being, including sexual and reproductive wellness, among socioeconomically disadvantaged populations (Lahariya 2020). By including migrants and the homeless population as beneficiaries, this program aims to provide quality and affordable healthcare services to those in need. This initiative aims to benefit homeless women in the near future. Although such initiatives are commendable, the reach of AB-HWCs needs to be extended by introducing mobile healthcare camps targeting informal labor migrants and clusters of homeless residents. This expansion would ensure that these vulnerable populations receive essential health surveillance and access to healthcare services, thus improving their well-being and health outcomes.

Finally, the present chapter outlines a roadmap for research on homeless women in Indian settings. The present chapter concludes that although a noticeable increase in research on this topic has taken place over time, particularly in recent years, concerns persist about the neglect of sexual and reproductive health issues, specifically maternal and child health, and associated healthcare utilization. Despite the international recognition of high-risk fertility behavior among homeless women (Nambiar et al. 2023; McGeough et al. 2020), research in this area remains limited in the Indian context. This lack of focus has failed to adequately address maternal and child health issues, healthcare behaviors, and the challenges and opportunities associated with them to improve health services for homeless mothers in India. Therefore, this chapter suggests that further research is needed to explore maternal and child health among homeless women in Indian settings. By understanding these issues more comprehensively, researchers can delineate a clear policy roadmap aimed at addressing the unique healthcare needs of homeless mothers in India. Such research endeavors hold the potential to inform targeted interventions and policies that will ultimately enhance the health and well-being of this vulnerable population.

2.3.6.1 Limitations and Strengths of this Chapter

The findings of this chapter are based on an analysis of electronically available research databases and selective search engine tools. Importantly, significant literature on homeless women might have been overlooked due to the limitations inherent in these search methods. Despite this potential limitation, this chapter ensures transparency and declares no conflicts of interest. Despite these limitations, this chapter serves as a valuable resource for researchers, policymakers, and readers seeking to understand the context of women's homelessness in India. By providing insights into the existing research landscape, it offers a foundation for further exploration and discussion on this important societal issue.

2.3.7 Conclusion

The plight of homeless women in India is a multifaceted issue deeply entrenched in socioeconomic disparities and systemic challenges. The journey toward homelessness for these women is marked by a tangled web of adversities, including experiences of domestic violence, poverty, social marginalization, and the complexities of migration. Intergenerational homelessness further exacerbates their vulnerability, perpetuating a cycle of deprivation. Moreover, the burden of poor health adds another layer of complexity to their already-precarious existence. Struggling with both physical and mental health challenges, homeless women face significant barriers to accessing essential healthcare services. Despite the recent surge in research attention, critical gaps persist, particularly in addressing their sexual and reproductive health needs. Efforts to alleviate the plight of homeless women must go beyond the mere acknowledgment of their struggles. Comprehensive interventions that address the root causes of homelessness, provide tailored healthcare services, and tackle societal stigma are imperative. Empowering homeless women through targeted support programs and amplifying their voices in policy discourse are essential steps toward fostering a more inclusive and equitable society. Ultimately, the journey toward meaningful change demands collective action and unwavering commitment from all sectors of society. By prioritizing the needs of homeless women and ensuring that their rights and dignity are upheld, we can work toward building a more just and compassionate society for all.

Declaration

Availability of Data and Materials All data related to this study are reported in this document.

Ethics Approval and Consent to Participate Approval and consent are not applicable.

Competing Interests The authors declare that they have no competing interests.

Funding This chapter did not receive any specific grant from funding agencies in the public, commercial, or not-for-profit sectors.

References

Aishwarya B (2021) Urban homelessness of women and urban marginality: sociological perspectives. Int J Adv Res Innov Ideas Educ 7:2395

Anand A, Tiwari G (2006) A gendered perspective of the shelter–transport–livelihood link: the case of poor women in Delhi. Transp Rev 26(1):63–80

Bhate A, Samuel M (2023) Affordable housing in India: a beneficiary perspective. Indian J Publ Admin 69(1):188–203

Bhattacharya P (2022) "Nowhere to sleep safe": impact of sexual violence on homeless women in India. J Psychosexual Health 4(4):223–226

Chakraborty D, Garg C (2023) Finding a home in or through mobile phones: access and usage patterns among homeless women in shelter-homes of India. Mobile Media Commun 12:20501579231191925

Chaudhry S, Joseph A, Singh IP (2014) Violence and violations: the reality of homeless women in India. Indian J Integr Res Law 2:4

Chourase M (2019) Living conditions health status and security of homeless women A study in Delhi city

Coleman HLS, Levy-Philipp L, Balt E, Zuiderent-Jerak T, Mander H, Bunders J, Syurina E (2022) Addressing health needs of the homeless in Delhi: standardising on the issues of Street Medicine practice. Glob Public Health 17(11):2991–3004

Dasgupta U, Chatterjee A (n.d.) Quality of life of the homeless and restored women with psychosis

Devakumar J (2008) Internal displacement in contemporary india: homeless in their own state. Proc Indian History Congress 69:1211–1225

Farooq A, Srivastava R (2023) A psychological study of reproductive health awareness and practices among homeless adolescent girls in Nizamuddin, Delhi. J ReAttach Ther Dev Diver 6(5):395–405

Garg A, Behera C, Chopra S, Bhardwaj DN (2016) Mortality among homeless women who remain unclaimed after death: an insight. Natl Med J India 29(4):207

Garikipati S, Boudot C (2017) To pad or not to pad: towards better sanitary care for women in Indian slums. J Int Dev 29(1):32–51

Goel G, Ghosh P, Ojha MK, Shukla A (2017) Urban homeless shelters in India: miseries untold and promises unmet. Cities 71:88–96

Gohil J, Gandhi ZH (2019) Pradhan Mantri Awas Yojana (PMAY) scheme—an emerging prospect of affordable housing in India. Int Res J Eng Technol 6(12):2546–2550

Gowda GS, Gopika G, Kumar CN, Manjunatha N, Yadav R, Srinivas D, Dawn BR, Math SB (2017) Clinical outcome and rehabilitation of homeless mentally ill patients admitted in mental health institute of South India: "know the unknown" project. Asian J Psychiatr 30:49–53

Jha MK, Kumar P (2016) Homeless migrants in Mumbai: life and labour in urban space. Econ Pol Wkly 51:69–77

Koul P (2022) Violence, homelessness and gender: a socio-legal issue in India. Part 2 Indian Journal of Integrated Research in Law

Krishnadas P, Narasimhan L, Joseph T, Bunders J, Regeer B (2021) Factors associated with homelessness among women: a cross-sectional survey of outpatient mental health service users at The Banyan, India. J Public Health 43(2):17–25

Kumari A, Sekher TV (2022) Situation analysis of 'institutionalized' and 'homeless' elderly widows abandoned in India's pilgrimage centres: insights into their living conditions and available infrastructural facilities. Int J Commun Med Public Health 9(4):1831

Lahariya C (2020) Health & wellness centers to strengthen primary health care in India: concept, progress and ways forward. Indian J Pediat 87(11):916–929

McGeough C, Walsh A, Clyne B (2020) Barriers and facilitators perceived by women while homeless and pregnant in accessing antenatal and or postnatal healthcare: a qualitative evidence synthesis. Health Soc Care Community 28(5):1380–1393

Menon J, Kantipudi SJ, Mani A, Radhakrishnan R (2023) Characterization of an extreme phenotype of schizophrenia among women with homelessness. medRxiv, 2023–2027

Monteiro TS, Nalini R (2021) Mental health at the intersections of marginalization: a conceptual model to explore the mental health concerns of women sanitation workers in India. Asian Soc Work Policy Rev 15(2):102–111

Moorkath F, Vranda MN, Naveenkumar C (2018) Lives without roots: institutionalized homeless women with chronic mental illness. Indian J Psychol Med 40(5):476–481

Nambiar D (2020) Social determinants of health among urban homeless in Delhi, India. Eur J Pub Health 30(5):166–329

Nambiar D, Mathew B, Dubey S, Moola S (2023) Interventions addressing maternal and child health among the urban poor and homeless: an overview of systematic reviews. BMC Public Health 23(1):1–11

Narasimhan L, Gopikumar V, Jayakumar V, Bunders J, Regeer B (2019) Responsive mental health systems to address the poverty, homelessness and mental illness nexus: the Banyan experience from India. Int J Ment Heal Syst 13(1):1–10

Narasimhan L, Kishore Kumar KV, Regeer B, Gopikumar V (2020) Homelessness and women living with mental health issues: lessons from the Banyan's experience in Chennai, Tamil Nadu. In: Gender and mental health: combining theory and practice. Springer, Cham, pp 173–191

Negi S (2023) Fertility and reproductive health: a qualitative study of homeless migrants in Delhi. Oriental Anthropol 23(2):349–363

Padgett DK, Priyam P (2019) Gender, everyday resistance and bodily integrity: women's lives on Delhi streets. Affilia 34(2):170–185

Pandey VK (2016) Health issues of the homeless population in the Nct of Delhi

Patra S, Anand K (2008) Homelessness: a hidden public health problem. Indian J Public Health 52:164–170

Prashad L, Lhugdim H, Dutta M (2016) Treatment seeking behaviour among homeless people: evidences from Mumbai City. S Asian J Participative Dev 16(1):81

Registrar General & Census Commissioner (2011) PCA HS: primary census abstract data for houseless, India & States/UTs - District level – 2011. PC11_PCA-HS. Ministry of Home Affairs, Government of India, New Delhi

Richards J, Kuhn R (2023) Unsheltered homelessness and health: a literature review. AJPM Focus 2(1):100043

Sahoo H, Jeermison R (2018) Houseless population in India: trends, patterns and characteristics

Sarikhani N (2010) Status of homeless women and children in Karnataka state based on census of 2001. Anthropologist 12(2):119–125

Singh N, Koiri P, Shukla SK (2018) Signposting invisibles: a study of the homeless population in India. Chin Soc Dialog 3:179–196

Sowmya HS, Suman LN (2013) Pathways to homelessness, psychological distress and perceived social support among married women in a shelter: implications for trauma informed care. Indian J Clin Psychol 40:109–115

Suman LN, Sesha BV (2010) Psychosocial rehabilitation of young homeless women. J Psychosoc Res 5:47–53

Veeraiah K (2021) Homeless women in Telangana State, Southern Part of India: a cross - sectional study. Int J Sci Res 10:1477

Walters V (2014) Urban homelessness and the right to water and sanitation: experiences from India's cities. Water Policy 16(4):755–772

World Population Review (2024) Homelessness by country 2024

Chapter 3
Menstrual Irregularities Among Women: A Literature Review

Mahashweta Chakrabarty, Subhojit Let, Sourav Chowdhury, and Vineet Kumar

Abstract Menstrual cycles are considered irregular when their duration is less than 21 days or more than 35 days, and they are characterized by unusually light or heavy bleeding. These irregularities are typically caused by hormonal imbalances, which alter the menstrual pattern and are associated with various health conditions. Given these implications, irregular menstruation is a significant indicator of women's overall health. This review aims to clarify the definitions and types of menstrual irregularities, discuss their prevalence, identify risk factors, and explore their broader impact on women's health.

A thorough search of the PubMed, Medline, and Google Scholar databases was performed. The study included articles published in English from 2015 to 2023, focusing on the epidemiology and health impacts of menstrual irregularities. Articles that were reviews or duplicates were excluded to ensure data accuracy and integrity. This review highlighted that irregular menstrual cycles are linked to various health conditions, such as metabolic syndrome, type 2 diabetes, coronary heart disease, and rheumatoid arthritis. These irregularities can also lead to complications like anemia, osteoporosis, psychological challenges, diminished quality of life, and infertility. Additionally, menstrual irregularities increase the risk of hypertensive disorders during pregnancy and adverse obstetric and neonatal outcomes. Understanding the factors contributing to menstrual irregularities is crucial for developing preventive measures and treatment strategies.

Keywords Irregular menstruation · Factors · Women · India

M. Chakrabarty · S. Let (✉) · V. Kumar
Department of Geography, Banaras Hindu University, Varanasi, Uttar Pradesh, India
e-mail: subhojitlet123@gmail.com

S. Chowdhury
Department of Geography, Raiganj University, Raiganj, West Bengal, India

3.1 Introduction

Menstruation is a critical biological process that occurs in women, transgender men, and some nonbinary individuals during their reproductive year (Babbar et al. 2023). Typically commencing between the ages of 12 and 15, menstruation continues until menopause, which generally occurs between the ages of 45 and 50 (Ahuja 2016; Meher and Sahoo 2024). The menstrual cycle involves a complex interplay of hormones that readies the body for a possible pregnancy every month. While the average menstrual cycle is approximately 28 days, it can vary from 20 to 40 days, and a "normal" cycle is typically defined as lasting between 21 and 35 days (Cleveland Clinic 2022).

A normal menstrual period lasts between 2 and 7 days and occurs in a predictable pattern (Omidvar et al. 2018). However, a significant number of women experience menstrual irregularities, which can manifest as variations in cycle length, bleeding duration, and flow intensity (Monga and Gokhale 2023). These irregularities are often defined as cycles that are shorter than 21 days or longer than 35 days and feature periods that are unusually heavy or light (Mittiku et al. 2022). Symptoms can include irregular spotting, skipped periods, and severe abdominal cramps.

The prevalence of menstrual irregularities varies widely, affecting approximately 5% to 35.6% of women, depending on the population studied and the criteria used (Kwak et al. 2019). Factors such as age, geographical location, lifestyle, and occupation can influence the prevalence rates (Kwak et al. 2019; Negi et al. 2018). For instance, adolescents and women approaching menopause (perimenopausal women) are more likely to experience irregular cycles due to hormonal fluctuations (Delamater and Santoro 2018). Similarly, lifestyle factors such as high levels of physical activity, stress, and body weight can impact menstrual regularity (Chauhan et al. 2021).

Several underlying conditions can contribute to menstrual irregularities. Polycystic ovary syndrome (PCOS) is a prevalent hormonal disorder that can lead to irregularities in menstrual cycles (Louwers and Laven 2020). Other contributing factors include the use of contraceptives, breastfeeding, and thyroid disorders. Additionally, the insertion of intrauterine devices (IUDs) and intense physical activity can also lead to irregular periods (Dural et al. 2020; Negi et al. 2018). Modifiable risk factors, such as obesity, stress, and smoking, play significant roles in influencing menstrual patterns (Attia et al. 2023).

The implications of menstrual irregularities extend beyond mere inconvenience. They can be indicative of more-serious health issues, such as metabolic syndrome, cardiovascular diseases, type 2 diabetes, and autoimmune disorders like rheumatoid arthritis (Attia et al. 2023; Santos-Moreno et al. 2022).

Given the widespread prevalence and the potential health implications of menstrual irregularities, understanding them is crucial for healthcare providers. This comprehensive review aims to explore the definitions, types, prevalence, risk factors, and causes of menstrual irregularities. By examining the broader health impacts of menstrual irregularities, this review seeks to provide insights that can inform prevention and treatment strategies. Effectively addressing menstrual irregularities requires taking a multidisciplinary approach that considers the physiological, psychological, and socioeconomic factors influencing menstrual health.

3.2 Procedures and Techniques

An extensive literature review was carried out utilizing PubMed, Medline, and Google Scholar and using keywords such as "normal menstrual cycle," "irregular menstruation," and "health impact of menstrual irregularities." The review encompassed articles written in English, published from 2015 to 2023, and focused on the epidemiology and health impacts of menstrual irregularities. Reviews and duplicate articles were excluded to maintain data accuracy.

3.3 Results

3.3.1 Definitions and Prevalence

Irregular menstruation is characterized by changes in the time between cycles, variations in blood loss during a period (either more or less than normal), or significant deviations in the duration of menstruation from the established norm (Mittiku et al. 2022). The average age of individuals presenting with menstrual irregularities has been reported as 33 years (Mahreen and Nadia 2013).

Menstrual irregularities encompass a broad spectrum of deviations from the typical menstrual cycle, including variations in cycle length, duration, and flow intensity. These irregularities may manifest as cycles shorter than 21 days or longer than 35 days, along with unpredictable bleeding patterns and abnormal blood flow, either heavier or lighter than usual (Habiba and Benagiano 2023; Itriyeva 2022). Adolescents and perimenopausal women are particularly prone to these irregularities due to hormonal fluctuations (Beevi et al. 2017; Somwanshi et al. 2017). However, structural issues, such as fibroids or endometrial polyps, and risks of malignancies increase with age (Bhardwaj et al. 2022). The global prevalence of menstrual irregularities varies significantly, influenced by socioeconomic, environmental, and lifestyle factors, with reports ranging from 5% to 35.6% (Kwak et al. 2019).

3.3.2 Risk Factors

The risk factors for menstrual irregularities are multifaceted, including both intrinsic elements and extrinsic elements. Hormonal imbalances are among the primary causes, often linked to conditions such as PCOS and thyroid disorders (Christodoulopoulou et al. 2016). Lifestyle factors such as obesity, high stress levels, and smoking are also significant contributors (Nagma et al. 2015; Sakai and Ohashi 2020). Additionally, environmental factors, including age, body weight, physical activity, and dietary habits, play crucial roles in influencing menstrual regularity (Negi et al. 2018; Singh et al. 2019). Exposure to organic solvents and other environmental toxins has been associated with disruptions in menstrual cycles. An early or late onset of menarche further predisposes women to experience menstrual irregularities throughout their reproductive years.

3.3.3 Health Impacts

Irregular menstrual cycles are linked to various health impacts.

Metabolic syndrome: Women experiencing menstrual irregularities often exhibit characteristics of metabolic syndrome, such as a high body mass index (BMI), hypertension, dyslipidemia, and impaired glucose tolerance (Ali and Guidozzi 2020; Katsimardou et al. 2020).

Type 2 diabetes mellitus: A notable correlation exists between irregular menstrual cycles and insulin resistance, which serves as a precursor to type 2 diabetes (Wang et al. 2020).

Cardiovascular diseases: Irregular menstrual cycles are associated with a higher risk of coronary heart disease and other cardiovascular issues than are regular cycles (Gast et al. 2010). The link is partly attributed to the relationship between menstrual irregularities and metabolic disorders, including PCOS, which contributes to cardiovascular risk factors (Shufelt et al. 2017).

Rheumatoid arthritis: Autoimmune diseases, such as rheumatoid arthritis, are more prevalent among women with irregular menstrual cycles. This relationship indicates that the interactions between hormonal and immune systems contribute to the development of autoimmune disorders.

3.3.4 Psychological and Quality of Life Impacts

Menstrual irregularities have profound effects on mental health and overall quality of life. Women with irregular cycles frequently report higher levels of stress, anxiety, and depression than do those with regular cycles (Bhardwaj et al. 2022). The unpredictability and discomfort associated with irregular periods can disrupt daily activities, professional responsibilities, and social interactions, leading to a diminished quality of life. Additionally, the stigma and lack of awareness surrounding menstrual health can exacerbate psychological distress.

3.4 Conclusion

Menstrual irregularities are significant public health concerns that affect various aspects of women's lives. They are indicative of broader health issues and can lead to serious conditions if left unaddressed. Understanding the definitions, types, prevalence, risk factors, causes, and health impacts of menstrual irregularities is crucial for developing effective prevention and treatment strategies. This review underscores the need for a comprehensive approach to managing menstrual health, encompassing medical, psychological, and lifestyle interventions to improve overall well-being and quality of life for affected individuals.

References

Ahuja M (2016) Age of menopause and determinants of menopause age: a PAN India survey by IMS. J Mid-Life Health 7(3):126–131. https://doi.org/10.4103/0976-7800.191012
Ali AT, Guidozzi F (2020) Midlife women's health consequences associated with polycystic ovary syndrome. Climacteric 23(2):116–122
Attia GM, Alharbi OA, Aljohani RM (2023) The impact of irregular menstruation on health: a review of the literature. Cureus 15(11):e49146. https://doi.org/10.7759/cureus.49146
Babbar K, Martin J, Varanasi P, Avendaño I (2023) Inclusion means everyone: standing up for transgender and non-binary individuals who menstruate worldwide. Lancet Reg Health 13:100177. https://doi.org/10.1016/j.lansea.2023.100177
Beevi NP, Bindhu AS, Haran JC, Jose R (2017) Menstrual problems among adolescent girls in Thiruvananthapuram district. Int J Commun Med Public Health 4(8):2995–2998. https://doi.org/10.18203/2394-6040.ijcmph20173360
Bhardwaj P, Yadav SK, Taneja J (2022) Magnitude and associated factors of menstrual irregularity among young girls: a cross-sectional study during COVID-19 second wave in India. J Family Med Prim Care 11(12):7769. https://doi.org/10.4103/JFMPC.JFMPC_1201_22
Chauhan S, Kumar P, Patel R, Srivastava S, Jean Simon D, Muhammad T (2021) Association of lifestyle factors with menstrual problems and its treatment-seeking behavior among adolescent girls. Clin Epidemiol Global Health 12:100905. https://doi.org/10.1016/j.cegh.2021.100905
Christodoulopoulou V, Trakakis E, Pergialiotis V, Peppa M, Chrelias C, Kassanos D, Papantoniou N (2016) Clinical and biochemical characteristics in pcos women with menstrual abnormalities. J Family Reprod Health 10(4):184–190
Cleveland Clinic (2022) Menstrual cycle (normal menstruation): overview & phases. Cleveland. https://my.clevelandclinic.org/health/articles/10132-menstrual-cycle
Delamater L, Santoro N (2018) Management of the perimenopause. Clin Obstet Gynecol 61(3):419–432. https://doi.org/10.1097/GRF.0000000000000389
Dural Ö, Taş İS, Akhan SE (2020) Management of menstrual and gynecologic concerns in girls with special needs. J Clin Res Pediatr Endocrinol 12(Suppl 1):41–45. https://doi.org/10.4274/jcrpe.galenos.2019.2019.S0174

Gast G-CM, Grobbee DE, Smit HA, Bueno-de-Mesquita HB, Samsioe GN, van der Schouw YT (2010) Menstrual cycle characteristics and risk of coronary heart disease and type 2 diabetes. Fertil Steril 94(6):2379–2381

Habiba M, Benagiano G (2023) The duration of menstrual blood loss: historical to current understanding. Reprod Med 4(3):145–165

Itriyeva K (2022) The normal menstrual cycle. Curr Probl Pediatr Adolesc Health Care 52(5):101183

Katsimardou A, Imprialos K, Stavropoulos K, Sachinidis A, Doumas M, Athyros V (2020) Hypertension in metabolic syndrome: novel insights. Curr Hypertens Rev 16(1):12–18

Kwak Y, Kim Y, Baek KA (2019) Prevalence of irregular menstruation according to socioeconomic status: a population-based nationwide cross-sectional study. PLoS ONE 14(3):e0214071. https://doi.org/10.1371/JOURNAL.PONE.0214071

Louwers YV, Laven JSE (2020) Characteristics of polycystic ovary syndrome throughout life. Ther Adv Reprod Health 14:263349412091103. https://doi.org/10.1177/2633494120911038

Mahreen M, Nadia J (2013) Pattern of menstrual irregularities amongst women presenting to gynecological outpatient department. JIMDC 2:9–12

Meher T, Sahoo H (2024) Secular trend in age at menarche among Indian women. Sci Rep 14(1):1–11. https://doi.org/10.1038/s41598-024-55657-7

Mittiku YM, Mekonen H, Wogie G, Tizazu MA, Wake GE (2022) Menstrual irregularity and its associated factors among college students in Ethiopia, 2021. Front Global Women's Health 3:917643. https://doi.org/10.3389/fgwh.2022.917643

Monga R, Gokhale D (2023) Menstrual irregularities: understanding the role of influential factors. Cardiometry 25:378–386. https://doi.org/10.18137/CARDIOMETRY.2022.25.378386

Nagma S, Kapoor G, Bharti R, Batra A, Batra A, Aggarwal A, Sablok A (2015) To evaluate the effect of perceived stress on menstrual function. J Clin Diagn Res 9(3):QC01. https://doi.org/10.7860/JCDR/2015/6906.5611

Negi P, Mishra A, Lakhera P (2018) Menstrual abnormalities and their association with lifestyle pattern in adolescent girls of Garhwal, India. J Family Med Prim Care 7(4):804. https://doi.org/10.4103/jfmpc.jfmpc_159_17

Omidvar S, Amiri FN, Bakhtiari A, Begum K (2018) A study on menstruation of Indian adolescent girls in an urban area of South India. J Family Med Prim Care 7(4):698–702. https://doi.org/10.4103/jfmpc.jfmpc_258_17

Sakai H, Ohashi K (2020) Effects of past environmental tobacco smoke exposure on the menstrual cycle and menstrual phase-related symptoms: a cross-sectional study. Obst Gynaecol Res 47(1):243–253. https://doi.org/10.1111/jog.14496

Santos-Moreno P, Rodríguez-Vargas G-S, Martínez S, Ibatá L, Rojas-Villarraga A (2022) Metabolic abnormalities, cardiovascular disease, and metabolic syndrome in adult rheumatoid arthritis patients: current perspectives and clinical implications. Open Access Rheumatol 14:255–267. https://doi.org/10.2147/OARRR.S285407

Shufelt CL, Torbati T, Dutra E (2017) Hypothalamic amenorrhea and the long-term health consequences. Semin Reprod Med 35(3):256

Singh M, Rajoura O, Honnakamble R (2019) Menstrual patterns and problems in association with body mass index among adolescent school girls. J Family Med Prim Care 8(9):2855. https://doi.org/10.4103/jfmpc.jfmpc_474_19

Somwanshi SB, Gaikwad VM, Dhamak KB, Gaware VM, Scholar UG (2017) Women's health issue: a brief overview on irregulatities in menstruation. Int J Novel Res Dev 2(5):140

Wang Y-X, Shan Z, Arvizu M, Pan A, Manson JE, Missmer SA, Sun Q, Chavarro JE (2020) Associations of menstrual cycle characteristics across the reproductive life span and lifestyle factors with risk of type 2 diabetes. JAMA Netw Open 3(12):e2027928

Chapter 4
Contextualising Anaemia Among Reproductive Women in West Bengal: Trends, Patterns, and Predictors

Subhojit Let , Seema Tiwari , and Aditya Singh

Abstract Anaemia poses a public health challenge, impacting numerous individuals and posing significant health risks. This study examines the prevalence and trends of anaemia among women of reproductive age (WRA) in West Bengal, as well as the factors associated with it from 2015 to 2021. This study analysed 14,032 and 15,870 WRA aged 15–49 from the fourth and fifth National Family Health Surveys (NFHS-4 and NFHS-5), respectively, using descriptive statistics and multivariable logistic regression. The findings revealed that, anaemia in West Bengal has increased from 62.5% to 71.4%, marking a 9-percentage-point (PP) rise from NFHS-4. District-wise analysis revealed a notable increase in anaemia across all districts, where Murshidabad experienced the highest increase, at 20 pp. Other districts with significant increases include Nadia (16 PP), Malda (14 PP), and Paschim Medinipur (14 PP). However, South 24 Parganas and Purulia were the only districts where anaemia rates witnessed a decline between the survey periods. In both surveys, Kolkata exhibited the lowest prevalence rate. Regression analysis revealed that the odds of having anaemia were higher among older women compared to younger women, women with more children compared to those with no children, women who breastfed compared to those who did not, and Scheduled Tribe (ST) women compared to women from other social groups.

Keywords Anaemia · NFHS · Women's health · Women of reproductive age · West Bengal

4.1 Introduction

Approximately 1.6 billion people worldwide have anaemia, including one in three women aged 15–49, which amounts to roughly half a billion individuals in this age group (Jamnok et al. 2020; World Health Organisation 2015). According to 2011

S. Let · S. Tiwari (✉) · A. Singh (✉)
Department of Geography, Banaras Hindu University, Varanasi, Uttar Pradesh, India
e-mail: adityasingh@bhu.ac.in

© The Author(s), under exclusive license to Springer Nature Singapore Pte Ltd. 2024
P. Chouhan et al. (eds.), *Sexual and Reproductive Health of Women*,
https://doi.org/10.1007/978-981-97-8418-9_4

estimates from the World Health Organisation (WHO), a significant proportion of pregnant women, nonpregnant women, and women globally were affected by anaemia (World Health Organisation 2015).

Women of reproductive age (WRA) are considered more vulnerable to anaemia, with an increased likelihood of complications during pregnancy and childbirth, including antepartum haemorrhage, and postpartum haemorrhage (Balarajan et al. 2011; Gautam et al. 2019, 2002; World Health Organisation 2014). Earlier research on anaemia has identified associations with married women (Gautam et al. 2019; Teshale et al. 2020), pregnant people, body mass index (BMI), high parity (Win and Ko 2018), residence type (Kibret et al. 2019), sources of drinking water (Gautam et al. 2019), breastfeeding (Harding et al. 2018; Lee et al. 2014), wealth, education, caste (Balarajan et al. 2013; Sharif et al. 2023), and food insecurity (Corsi et al. 2012; Onyeneho et al. 2019).

Anaemia is estimated to impact 43% of women in developing countries, with a notably higher prevalence in India. Recent findings from the Indian National Family Health Survey (NFHS) series reveal that 57% of WRA are affected by anaemia (Mog and Ghosh 2021). Anaemia is even more alarming among especially states in West Bengal, where more than 70% of women are anaemic in NFHS-5.

Although numerous national-level studies have been conducted on anaemia with a focus on children and men, research at the intrastate level, particularly in West Bengal, specifically addressing anaemia among WRA remains lacking. Our study has two objectives: to analyse the prevalence of and changes in anaemia and to identify determinants associated with anaemia during NFHS-4 and NFHS-5 (2015–2021). By achieving these objectives, the study aims to offer valuable insights for public health researchers and healthcare professionals, enabling them to comprehensively grasp the dynamic patterns of anaemia in West Bengal.

4.2 Database and Methodology

4.2.1 Database

This study utilised data from NFHS-4 conducted during 2015–2016 and NFHS-5 conducted during 2019–2021. Specifically, it included information from 14,032 and 15,870 women of reproductive age in West Bengal taken from a 2015 survey and a 2019 survey. It's important to clarify that in this study, the terms "women of reproductive age" (WRA) and "women" are used interchangeably.

4.2.2 Dependent Variable

The dependent variable is binary, coded as '1' for women who are anaemic and '0' for women who are not anaemic.

4.2.3 Predictor Covariates

The predictor covariates were the age of women, marital status, the number of children women have, breastfeeding and pregnancy status, education, social groups, religion, household wealth status, women's places of residence, mass media exposure, the dietary habits of women, contraceptive use by women, alcohol consumption by women, tobacco consumption by women, body mass index, diabetes, and the amenorrhea status of women. The selection of these independent variables was based on previous research on anaemia (Bharati et al. 2015; Ghosh et al. 2020; Jamnok et al. 2020; Jana et al. 2022; Kibret et al. 2019; Let et al. 2023, 2024; Loy et al. 2019; Mistry et al. 2018; Nankinga and Aguta 2019; Rohisha et al. 2019; Singh et al. 2023; Teshale et al. 2020; Win and Ko 2018).

4.2.4 Statistical Analysis

The study used descriptive and multivariable logistics regression to analyse the prevalence of and changes in anaemia among WRA in West Bengal (Chen and Chen 2011). Logistic regression results were represented by adjusted odds ratios (AORs), *p*-values less than 0.05, and 95% confidence intervals (CIs). Multicollinearity was checked by using the variance inflation factor (VIF). Stata 16 was used for statistical analysis, and ArcMap 10.5 was utilised to create maps. The 'Svyset' command in Stata was employed to manage the survey design of the NFHS data.

4.3 Results

4.3.1 Prevalence of Anaemia Among Respondents, According to Various Characteristics

Table 4.1 shows that in 2015, 62.5% of the WRA in West Bengal were identified as being anaemic, whereas it was 71.4% in NFHS-5. This indicates a 9-percentage-point (PP) increase in anaemia during 2015–2021.

Additionally, anaemia was high among WRA who married before 18 years. Among social groups, ST women exhibited the highest anaemia (75.5% and 82.2%), followed by Scheduled Caste (SC) women (65.8% and 74.9%). A steady decrease in anaemia was observed with increasing household wealth, the wealthiest women showing the lowest rates of anaemia in both survey rounds. Women residing in rural areas had higher anaemia prevalence than those living in urban areas. Additionally, anaemia was more common among women following a vegetarian diet than among nonvegetarian women. Women who abstained from alcohol had a higher prevalence

Table 4.1 Prevalence of anaemia among WRA in West Bengal, according to respondents' characteristics in NFHS-4 and NFHS-5

Respondent's characteristics	NFHS 4 (2015–2016)		NFHS 5 (2019–2021)	
	Anaemia (%)	95% CI (lower, upper)	Anaemia (%)	95% CI (lower, upper)
Biodemographic and socioeconomic variables				
Age (in years)	$\chi^2 = 24.5453$, p-value <0.001		$\chi^2 = 30.8856$, p-value <0.001	
15–19	63.1	[60.55, 65.51]	72.0	[69.74, 74.16]
20–29	61.0	[59.22, 62.82]	70.1	[68.24, 71.91]
30–39	63.0	[60.99, 64.86]	71.8	[69.91, 73.69]
40–49	66.5	[64.42, 68.55]	75.4	[73.52, 77.16]
Marital status	$\chi^2 = 9.2188$, p-value 0.042		$\chi^2 = 36.3004$, p-value <0.001	
Not married	60.7	[58.02, 63.39]	68.7	[66.04, 71.19]
Married before age 18 years	64.3	[62.69, 65.84]	74.5	[72.86, 75.99]
Married at age 18 years or later	63.0	[61.28, 64.63]	71.3	[69.53, 73.03]
Parity	$\chi^2 = 42.3476$, p-value <0.001		$\chi^2 = 48.0056$, p-value <0.001	
No children	59.7	[57.43, 61.83]	69.1	[66.91, 71.32]
1–2 children	62.9	[61.51, 64.33]	72.1	[70.47, 73.57]
3–4 children	67.3	[65.25, 69.36]	76.9	[75.06, 78.79]
5 and above	66.7	[62.39, 70.80]	72.9	[68.39, 77.10]
Breastfeeding and pregnancy	$\chi^2 = 36.8617$, p-value <0.001		$\chi^2 = 30.7710$, p-value <0.001	
Pregnant	54.2	[49.06, 59.15]	62.2	[57.23, 66.96]
Breastfeeding (not pregnant)	67.2	[65.10, 69.31]	74.7	[72.50, 76.71]
No breastfeeding/not pregnant	62.6	[61.25, 63.97]	72.0	[70.56, 73.44]
Level of education	$\chi^2 = 86.0253$, p-value <0.001		$\chi^2 = 85.9963$, p-value <0.001	
Without education	68.4	[66.53, 70.29]	77.9	[75.98, 79.69]
Primary	65.8	[63.65, 67.98]	71.8	[69.48, 73.98]
Secondary	60.9	[59.35, 62.43]	71.6	[70.11, 73.07]
Higher	55.6	[50.59, 60.43]	65.3	[61.91, 68.51]
Social groups	$\chi^2 = 129.8572$, p-value <0.001		$\chi^2 = 132.3565$, p-value <0.001	
SC	65.8	[63.95, 67.66]	74.9	[73.07, 76.72]
ST	75.7	[72.06, 79.06]	82.3	[78.81, 85.30]
OBC	57.7	[54.58, 60.67]	69.5	[66.59, 72.31]
Others	60.7	[58.90, 62.44]	68.5	[66.57, 70.31]
Religion	$\chi^2 = 81.8265$, p-value <0.001		$\chi^2 = 50.4474$, p-value <0.001	

(continued)

Table 4.1 (continued)

Respondent's characteristics	NFHS 4 (2015–2016) Anaemia (%)	95% CI (lower, upper)	NFHS 5 (2019–2021) Anaemia (%)	95% CI (lower, upper)
Hindu	64.9	[63.60, 66.27]	73.5	[72.08, 74.90]
Muslim	56.2	[53.51, 58.82]	67.3	[64.61, 69.91]
Christian	77.5	[67.82, 84.85]	73.3	[60.80, 82.86]
Others	58.1	[50.45, 65.29]	71.4	[57.46, 82.23]
Household wealth	$\chi^2 = 150.5198$, p-value <0.001		$\chi^2 = 178.4250$, p-value <0.001	
Poorest	71.9	[69.79, 73.87]	79.7	[77.72, 81.60]
Poorer	65.4	[63.04, 67.71]	74.7	[72.63, 76.68]
Middle	61.3	[59.14, 63.39]	72.6	[70.53, 74.59]
Richer	59.1	[56.86, 61.23]	68.1	[65.70, 70.49]
Richest	57.8	[54.74, 60.87]	66.0	[63.24, 68.60]
Residence	$\chi^2 = 56.2201$, p-value <0.001		$\chi^2 = 134.7105$, p-value <0.001	
Urban	58.5	[55.96, 60.98]	66.2	[63.80, 68.49]
Rural	65.2	[63.76, 66.55]	75.1	[73.51, 76.55]
Behavioural variables				
Mass media	$\chi^2 = 57.8365$, p-value <0.001		$\chi^2 = 56.6503$, p-value <0.001	
No	67.4	[64.88, 69.80]	74.8	[72.82, 76.72]
Low	64.2	[62.80, 65.51]	72.3	[70.81, 73.69]
Medium	58.1	[55.64, 60.51]	64.6	[60.90, 68.08]
High	61.4	[55.25, 67.29]	0.00	[0.00]
Dietary	$\chi^2 = 2.1753$, p-value 0.1242		$\chi^2 = 0.1713$, p-value 0.7405	
Vegetarian	71.5	[60.52, 80.46]	73.7	[63.94, 81.54]
Nonvegetarian	63.1	[61.85, 64.33]	72.2	[70.81, 73.46]
Current contraceptive use	$\chi^2 = 4.6109$, p-value 0.0692		$\chi^2 = 0.0023$, p-value 0.9702	
No use or traditional use	62.3	[60.68, 63.91]	72.2	[70.53, 73.72]
Modern use	64.1	[62.56, 65.55]	72.2	[70.55, 73.76]
Alcohol consumption	$\chi^2 = 1.4334$, p-value 0.2341		$\chi^2 = 1.1220$, p-value 0.3157	
No	63.2	[61.94, 64.42]	72.2	[70.86, 73.50]
Yes	58.0	[48.98, 66.45]	68.0	[58.84, 75.93]
Tobacco consumption in any form	$\chi^2 = 21.8713$, p-value <0.001		$\chi^2 = 16.3052$, p-value 0.0002	
No tobacco use	62.5	[61.25, 63.81]	71.8	[70.40, 73.13]
Tobacco use: smoke or smokeless	69.3	[66.36, 72.02]	77.7	[74.83, 80.26]

(continued)

Table 4.1 (continued)

Respondent's characteristics	NFHS 4 (2015–2016)		NFHS 5 (2019–2021)	
	Anaemia (%)	95% CI (lower, upper)	Anaemia (%)	95% CI (lower, upper)
Health-related variables				
Body mass index	$\chi^2 = 93.8636$, p-value <0.001		$\chi^2 = 66.9193$, p-value <0.001	
Underweight	69.2	[67.04, 71.32]	77.5	[75.32, 79.47]
Normal weight	63.0	[61.46, 64.47]	72.4	[70.87, 73.91]
Overweight	56.9	[54.16, 59.53]	68.2	[65.82, 70.49]
Obese	56.5	[50.78, 62.05]	66.5	[61.93, 70.72]
Currently having diabetes	$\chi^2 = 1.4078$, p-value 0.5667		$\chi^2 = 18.2286$, p-value 0.0030	
No	63.2	[61.93, 64.45]	71.9	[70.54, 73.24]
Yes	59.2	[51.16, 66.76]	69.4	[63.09, 74.99]
Don't know	63.3	[58.41, 67.89]	78.7	[75.27, 81.81]
Currently amenorrhoeic	$\chi^2 = 10.0693$, p-value 0.0097		$\chi^2 = 5.1282$, p-value 0.0572	
No	62.9	[61.65, 64.13]	72.1	[70.71, 73.35]
Yes	70.1	[64.59, 75.01]	77.5	[71.72, 82.43]
Year	62.5	[61.90, 64.37]	71.4	[70.83, 73.47]

Note: All percentages are weighted; p-value <0.05; *CI* confidence interval

of anaemia, whereas those who used tobacco in any form were more likely to be anaemic. Anaemia rates also rose among overweight women and diabetic women.

4.3.2 Illustration of Anaemia in West Bengal During 2015–2016 and 2019–2021

Figure 4.1a shows that nine out of 18 districts had anaemia rates exceeding 50%, two districts (Dakshin Dinajpur and Purulia) surpassing a 75% prevalence. Notably, Kolkata had the lowest anaemia rate, at 46.4%, and Purulia had the highest rate, at 80%.

According to Fig. 4.1b, in NFHS-5, only three districts recorded anaemia rates below 65%, and none reported a rate below 50%. Notably, seven districts had an anaemia prevalence rate exceeding 75%. Kolkata retained its status as the district with the lowest anaemia rate, even in NFHS-5. Conversely, Dakshin Dinajpur had the highest anaemia rate, at 82.04%.

Figure 4.2 illustrates the district-level change in anaemia among WRA in West Bengal between 2015 and 2021. The results revealed a notable—i.e. 9 PP—increase in anaemia among WRA in West Bengal. Furthermore, anaemia has seen a significant increase in almost every districts, comprising nearly 90% of all districts. Particularly noteworthy is Murshidabad, which experienced the most pronounced

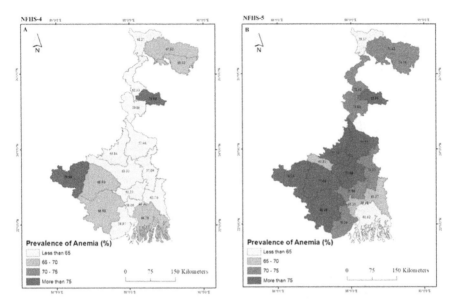

Fig. 4.1 (**a**) Anaemia prevalence during NFHS-4 among WRA in West Bengal and (**b**) anaemia prevalence during NFHS-5 among WRA in West Bengal

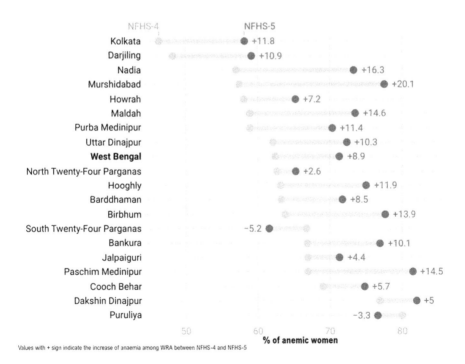

Fig. 4.2 Changes in anaemia among WRA across districts in West Bengal from 2015 to 2021

increase in anaemia: 20 PP. Additionally, Nadia (16 PP), Malda (14 PP), and Paschim Medinipur (14 PP) closely followed with their significant increments in anaemia rates. Notably, South 24 Parganas and Purulia were the only districts that showed a reduction in anaemia.

4.3.3 Logistic Regression Results

The results of logistic regression revealed that women aged 40–49 years had a 19% higher odds of being anaemic. Anaemia was 30% more odds (1.30, 1.16–1.46) among women with three to four children compared to women without children. Additionally, breastfeeding women had a 50% greater odds of anaemia (1.50, 1.29–1.76) than pregnant women. Furthermore, women belonging to the ST category had a 34% higher odds of having anaemia (1.34, 1.20–1.49). Women in higher wealth quintiles had a 30% lower odds of anaemia (0.68, 0.62–0.75) compared to those in the lowest quintile. Women residing in rural area had a 24% greater odds of being anaemic (1.24, 1.16–1.32) compared to their urban counterparts. Conversely, women who consumed alcohol had a 50% lower odds of anaemia (0.55, 0.44–0.69) and women who were obese had over a 30% lower odds (0.66, 0.57–0.77) (See table 4.2).

Table 4.2 Determinants of anaemia among WRA in West Bengal between 2015 and 2021

Background characteristics	Model I 95% CI				Model II 95% CI				Model III 95% CI			
	AOR	Lower	Upper	p-Value	AOR	Lower	Upper	p-Value	AOR	Lower	Upper	p-Value
Biodemographic and socioeconomic variables												
Age (in years)												
15–19®	1.00				1.00				1.00			
20–29	0.87	0.79	0.96	0.007	0.89	0.82	0.98	0.013	0.92	0.84	1.01	0.076
30–39	0.92	0.82	1.03	0.152	0.94	0.85	1.05	0.29	1	0.9	1.11	0.99
40–49	1.11	0.98	1.26	0.102	1.12	1	1.26	0.048	1.19	1.06	1.34	0.003
Marital status												
Not married®	1.00											
Married before 18	1.03	0.91	1.16	0.688								
Married on 18 and above	1.02	0.91	1.15	0.72								
Parity												
No children®	1.00				1.00				1.00			
1–2 children	1.07	0.96	1.2	0.227	1.11	1.02	1.22	0.021	1.17	1.07	1.28	0.001
3–4 children	1.14	1.00	1.3	0.043	1.19	1.06	1.34	0.002	1.3	1.16	1.46	<0.001
5 and above	1.03	0.85	1.23	0.779	1.07	0.9	1.27	0.459	1.18	1	1.41	0.055
Breastfeeding and pregnancy												
Pregnant®					1.00				1.00			
Breastfeeding (not pregnant)	1.59	1.36	1.85	<0.001	1.66	1.43	1.93	0	1.51	1.29	1.76	<0.001
No breastfeeding/not pregnant	1.35	1.16	1.56	<0.001	1.41	1.23	1.62	0	1.34	1.16	1.54	<0.001
Level of education												
No education®	1.00											
Primary	0.94	0.86	1.02	0.14								
Secondary	0.96	0.89	1.04	0.322								

(continued)

Table 4.2 (continued)

Background characteristics	Model I 95% CI AOR	Lower	Upper	p-Value	Model II 95% CI AOR	Lower	Upper	p-Value	Model III 95% CI AOR	Lower	Upper	p-Value
Higher	0.96	0.85	1.09	0.501								
Social groups												
SC®	1.00				1.00				1.00			
ST	1.31	1.18	1.45	<0.001	1.34	1.21	1.49	<0.001	1.34	1.2	1.49	<0.001
OBC	0.84	0.77	0.91	<0.001	0.84	0.77	0.91	<0.001	0.84	0.77	0.91	<0.001
Others	0.84	0.79	0.9	<0.001	0.85	0.79	0.9	<0.001	0.86	0.81	0.92	<0.001
Religion												
Hindu®	1.00				1.00				1.00			
Muslim	0.81	0.75	0.87	<0.001	0.79	0.74	0.85	<0.001	0.79	0.73	0.85	<0.001
Christian	0.9	0.69	1.16	0.41	0.91	0.7	1.18	0.463	0.9	0.69	1.17	0.431
Other	0.53	0.45	0.63	<0.001	0.55	0.46	0.65	<0.001	0.62	0.52	0.74	<0.001
Household wealth												
Poorest®	1.00				1.00				1.00			
Poorer	0.8	0.73	0.87	<0.001	0.8	0.74	0.87	<0.001	0.81	0.74	0.88	<0.001
Middle	0.72	0.66	0.78	<0.001	0.74	0.68	0.8	<0.001	0.74	0.68	0.81	<0.001
Richer	0.64	0.59	0.7	<0.001	0.67	0.61	0.73	<0.001	0.68	.062	0.75	<0.001
Richest	0.64	0.58	0.71	<0.001	0.7	0.63	0.78	<0.001	0.71	0.63	0.78	<0.001
Type of place of residence												
Urban®	1.00				1.00				1.00			
Rural	1.23	1.15	1.31	<0.001	1.22	1.15	1.31	<0.001	1.24	1.16	1.32	<0.001
Behavioural variables												
Mass media												
None®					1.00				1.00			

Low	0.99	0.92	1.06	0.765	1.04	0.97	1.12	0.236
Medium	0.75	0.68	0.82	<0.001	0.91	0.82	1	0.046
High	0.82	0.67	1.01	0.067	1.14	0.92	1.41	0.226
Dietary habit								
Vegetarian®	1.00							
Nonvegetarian	0.82	0.63	1.08	0.155				
Current contraceptive use								
No use or traditional® use	1.00				1.00			
Modern use	0.89	0.84	0.94	<0.001	0.88	0.83	0.94	<0.001
Alcohol consumption								
No®	1.00				1.00			
Yes	0.53	0.42	0.66	<0.001	0.55	0.44	0.69	<0.001
Tobacco consumption in any form								
No tobacco®	1.00							
Tobacco use: smoke or smokeless	1.1	1	1.21	0.055				
Health-related variables								
Body mass index								
Underweight®					1.00			
Normal weight					0.8	0.74	0.85	<0.001
Overweight					0.68	0.62	0.74	<0.001
Obese					0.66	0.57	0.77	<0.001
Currently having diabetes								
No®					1.00			
Yes					0.87	0.73	1.04	0.12
Don't know					1.09	0.96	1.24	0.173
Currently amenorrhoeic								

(continued)

Table 4.2 (continued)

Background characteristics	Model I				Model II				Model III			
	AOR	95% CI		p-Value	AOR	95% CI		p-Value	AOR	95% CI		p-Value
		Lower	Upper			Lower	Upper			Lower	Upper	
No®									1.00			
Yes									1.22	1.03	1.44	0.02
Year												
NFHS 4®									1.00			
NFHS 5									1.52	1.44	1.6	<0.001

AOR adjusted odds ration, *CI* confidence interval, ® reference category

4.4 Discussion

In West Bengal, 71% of women had anaemia in NFHS-5, marking a 9 PP rise from NFHS-4. District-level analysis revealed a significant increase in anaemia across 18 districts, where Murshidabad experienced the highest increase, at 20 PP. However, South 24 Parganas and Purulia were the only districts where anaemia declined between NFHS-4 and NFHS-5. Additionally, anaemia was associated with women aged 40 to 49 years, those with 3 to 4 children, women belonging to ST, women from poorer households, those living in rural areas, underweight women, and women experiencing amenorrhea.

Older women had a higher chance of being anaemic. However, the results contrast with those of some earlier Indian studies, which have suggested that younger women are susceptible to anaemia (Bharati et al. 2015; Jana et al. 2022). This may be due to factors such as chronic diseases and iron anaemia, which are more common in older women (Corona et al. 2014; Krishnapillai et al. 2022). Higher parity and anaemia had a positive correlation (Al-farsi et al. 2011; Imai 2020; Jana et al. 2022). One possible explanation for this is that women with high parity might experience increased blood loss during childbirth, leading to lower haemoglobin levels (Al-farsi et al. 2011; Armah-Ansah 2023; Imai 2020; Jana et al. 2022; Shah et al. 2020; Win and Ko 2018). ST women were also more likely to be anaemic. ST women are poorly connected with the rest of Indian society and belong to the poor wealth quintile, which can lead to nutritional deficiencies and inadequate medical care, all of which might affect anaemia among ST WRA (Balarajan et al. 2013; Jungari and Chauhan 2017; Kamath et al. 2013; Sharif et al. 2023). Additionally, the results also revealed that poor women were more prone to having anaemia (Balarajan et al. 2011). The potential reason for this result could be that women of higher socioeconomic status tend to incorporate more iron-rich foods into their diets and maintain proper nutrition, whereas those with lower incomes encounter challenges in achieving these, which might affect the level of anaemia among WRA (Bharati et al. 2019; Lee et al. 2014; Rammohan et al. 2012).

Consistent with earlier studies, this research also found that rural women were more susceptible to anaemia (Ghosh et al. 2020; Jana et al. 2022). This may be because women in rural areas often face greater challenges related to eating balanced meals, securing adequate food resources, and accessing healthcare services (Abate et al. 2021; Bharati et al. 2019; Dean and Sharkey 2011). Underweight women were more prone to being anaemic, and similar results have been found in India and other countries (Bentley and Griffiths 2003; Bharati et al. 2008; Ghose et al. 2016; Qin et al. 2013; Win and Ko 2018). The potential reason for this could be that underweight women have inadequate diets and experience a deficiency in essential nutrient intake, particularly the intake of iron and folate, serving as the primary contributing factor to anaemia among WRA (Chakrabarty et al. 2023; Win and Ko 2018). The Indian government has launched some programmes to increase access to iron and folic acid supplements and to increase awareness of anaemia like the national iron+ initiative and the Anaemia Mukt Bharat (AMB). Despite these efforts, more-comprehensive policies are needed to effectively lower anaemia rates among WRA. In particular, state-specific strategies are crucial, especially in West Bengal, where anaemia rates have significantly increased since 2015. It's important to create specific solutions that tackle the different factors contributing to anaemia in West Bengal, making sure to include all relevant factors in the process of making policies.

This is the first study to examine intrastate anaemia changes in West Bengal during 2015–2021. This approach enables policymakers to gain in-depth insights into anaemia in West Bengal. This study has some limitations, such as the absence of some variables related to vitamins, which could play important roles in the determination of anaemia.

4.5 Conclusion

Older age women, women with high parity, ST women, poor women, rural women, and underweight women were identified as those most likely to have anaemia. Although existing initiatives like the national iron+ initiative and the AMB programme are already in place, these findings suggest that targeted district-specific policies are urgently needed to effectively address rising anaemia rates.

Declaration

Data Availability The data and materials for this chapter are sourced from publicly available secondary sources accessible on the DHS's official website. Interested individuals can register at the provided link to freely download the necessary data.

Ethics Approval and Consent to Participate This chapter is based on secondary data; therefore, ethical approval is not required to conduct this study.

Competing Interests The authors declare that they have no competing interests.

Funding No funding was received.

References

Abate TW, Getahun B, Birhan MM, Aknaw GM, Belay SA, Demeke D, Abie DD, Alemu AM, Mengiste Y (2021) The urban–rural differential in the association between household wealth index and anemia among women in reproductive age in Ethiopia, 2016. BMC Womens Health 21(1):1–8. https://doi.org/10.1186/s12905-021-01461-8

Al-farsi YM, Brooks DR, Werler MM, Cabral HJ, Al-shafei MA (2011) Effect of high parity on occurrence of anemia in pregnancy: a cohort study. BMC Pregnancy Childbirth 11:1471–2393. https://doi.org/10.1186/1471-2393-11-7

Armah-Ansah EK (2023) Determinants of anemia among women of childbearing age: analysis of the 2018 Mali demographic and health survey. Arch Public Health 81(1):1–13. https://doi.org/10.1186/s13690-023-01023-4

Balarajan Y, Ramakrishnan U, Özaltin E, Shankar AH, Subramanian SV (2011) Anaemia in low-income and middle-income countries. Lancet 378(9809):2123–2135. https://doi.org/10.1016/S0140-6736(10)62304-5

Balarajan YS, Fawzi WW, Subramanian SV (2013) Changing patterns of social inequalities in anaemia among women in India: cross-sectional study using nationally representative data. BMJ Open 3(3):1–11. https://doi.org/10.1136/bmjopen-2012-002233

Bentley ME, Griffiths PL (2003) The burden of anemia among women in India. Eur J Clin Nutr 57(1):52–60. https://doi.org/10.1038/sj.ejcn.1601504

Bharati P, Som S, Chakrabarty S, Bharti S, Pal M (2008) Prevalence of anemia and its determinants among nonpregnant and pregnant women in India. Asia Pac J Public Health 20:347–359. https://doi.org/10.1177/1010539508322762

Bharati S, Pal M, Som S, Bharati P (2015) Temporal trend of anemia among reproductive-aged women in India. Asia Pac J Public Health 27(2):NP1193–NP1207. https://doi.org/10.1177/1010539512442567

Bharati S, Pal M, Sen S, Bharati P (2019) Malnutrition and anaemia among adult women in India. J Biosoc Sci 51(5):1–11. https://doi.org/10.1017/S002193201800041X

Chakrabarty M, Singh A, Singh S, Chowdhury S (2023) Is the burden of anaemia among Indian adolescent women increasing? Evidence from Indian Demographic and Health Surveys (2015–21). PLOS Glob Publ Health 3(9):e0002117. https://doi.org/10.1371/journal.pgph.0002117

Chen Y-T, Chen MC (2011) Using Chi square statistics to measure similarities for text categorization. Expert Syst Appl 38:3085–3090. https://doi.org/10.1016/j.eswa.2010.08.100

Corona LP, de Duarte YAO, Lebrão ML (2014) Prevalence of anemia and associated factors in older adults: evidence from the SABE Study. Rev Saude Publica 48(5):723–731. https://doi.org/10.1590/S0034-8910.2014048005039

Corsi DJ, Neuman M, Finlay JE, Subramanian SV (2012) Demographic and health surveys: a profile. November, 1602–1613. https://doi.org/10.1093/ije/dys184

Dean WR, Sharkey JR (2011) Rural and urban differences in the associations between characteristics of the community food environment and fruit and vegetable intake. J Nutr Educ Behav 43(6):426–433. https://doi.org/10.1016/j.jneb.2010.07.001

Gautam VP, Bansal Y, Taneja DK, Saha R, Shah B, Marg Z, Khurd P (2002) Prevalence of anaemia amongst pregnant women and its socio-demographic associates in a rural area of Delhi. Indian J Community Med 27(4):157–160

Gautam S, Min H, Kim H, Jeong H (2019) Determining factors for the prevalence of anemia in women of reproductive age in Nepal: evidence from recent national survey data. PLoS One 14(6):e0218288. https://doi.org/10.1371/journal.pone.0218288

Ghose B, Yaya S, Tang S (2016) Anemia status in relation to body mass index among women of childbearing age in Bangladesh. Asia Pac J Public Health 28(7):611–619. https://doi.org/10.1177/1010539516660374

Ghosh P, Dasgupta A, Paul B, Roy S, Biswas A, Yadav A (2020) A cross-sectional study on prevalence and determinants of anemia among women of reproductive age in a rural community of West Bengal. J Family Med Prim Care 9(11):5547. https://doi.org/10.4103/jfmpc.jfmpc_1209_20

Harding KL, Namirembe G, Webb P (2018) Determinants of anemia among women and children in Nepal and Pakistan: an analysis of recent national survey data. Matern Child Nutr 14:1–13. https://doi.org/10.1111/mcn.12478

Imai K (2020) Parity-based assessment of anemia and iron deficiency in pregnant women. Taiwan J Obstet Gynecol 59(6):838–841. https://doi.org/10.1016/j.tjog.2020.09.010

Jamnok J, Sanchaisuriya K, Sanchaisuriya P, Fucharoen G, Fucharoen S, Ahmed F (2020) Factors associated with anaemia and iron deficiency among women of reproductive age in Northeast Thailand: a cross-sectional study. BMC Public Health 20(1):1–8. https://doi.org/10.1186/s12889-020-8248-1

Jana A, Chattopadhyay A, Saha UR (2022) Identifying risk factors in explaining women's anaemia in limited resource areas: evidence from West Bengal of India and Bangladesh. BMC Public Health 22(1):1–16. https://doi.org/10.1186/s12889-022-13806-5

Jungari S, Chauhan BG (2017) Caste, wealth and regional inequalities in health status of women and children in India. Contemporary Voice Dalit 9(1):87–100. https://doi.org/10.1177/2455328X17690644

Kamath R, Majeed J, Chandrasekaran V, Pattanshetty S (2013) Prevalence of anemia among tribal women of reproductive age in Udupi Taluk, Karnataka. J Family Med Prim Care 2(4):345. https://doi.org/10.4103/2249-4863.123881

Kibret KT, Chojenta C, D'Arcy E, Loxton D (2019) Spatial distribution and determinant factors of anaemia among women of reproductive age in Ethiopia: a multilevel and spatial analysis. BMJ Open 9:1–14. https://doi.org/10.1136/bmjopen-2018-027276

Krishnapillai A, Omar MA, Ariaratnam S, Awaluddin S, Sooryanarayana R, Kiau HB, Tauhid NM, Ghazali SS (2022) The prevalence of anemia and its associated factors among older persons: findings from the national health and morbidity survey (NHMS) 2015. Int J Environ Res Public Health 19(9):4983. https://doi.org/10.3390/ijerph19094983

Lee J, Lee JH, Ahn S, Kim JW, Chang H, Kim YJ, Lee K, Kim JH, Bang S, Lee JS (2014) Prevalence and risk factors for iron deficiency anemia in the Korean population : results of the Fifth Korea National Health and Nutrition Examination Survey, pp 224–229

Let S, Tiwari S, Singh A, Chakrabarty M (2023) Spatiotemporal change in wealth-based inequalities in overweight/obesity among women of reproductive age in India, 2015–2021. Clin Epidemiol Glob Health 24:101458. https://doi.org/10.1016/j.cegh.2023.101458

Let S, Tiwari S, Singh A, Chakrabarty M (2024) Prevalence and determinants of anaemia among women of reproductive age in aspirational districts of India: an analysis of NFHS 4 and NFHS 5 data. BMC Public Health 24(1):437. https://doi.org/10.1186/s12889-024-17789-3

Loy SL, Lim LM, Chan S-Y, Tan PT, Chee YL, Quah PL, Chan JKY, Tan KH, Yap F, Godfrey KM, Shek LP, Chong MF-F, Kramer MS, Chong Y-S, Chi C (2019) Iron status and risk factors of iron deficiency among pregnant women in Singapore: a cross-sectional study. BMC Public Health 19(1):397. https://doi.org/10.1186/s12889-019-6736-y

Mistry R, Jones AD, Pednekar MS, Dhumal G, Dasika A, Kulkarni U, Gomare M, Gupta PC (2018) Antenatal tobacco use and iron deficiency anemia: integrating tobacco control into antenatal care in urban India. Reprod Health 15(1):1–8. https://doi.org/10.1186/s12978-018-0516-5

Mog M, Ghosh K (2021) Prevalence of anaemia among women of reproductive age (15–49): a spatial-temporal comprehensive study of Maharashtra districts. Clin Epidemiol Glob Health 11:100712. https://doi.org/10.1016/j.cegh.2021.100712

Nankinga O, Aguta D (2019) Determinants of Anemia among women in Uganda: further analysis of the Uganda demographic and health surveys. BMC Public Health 19(1):1–9. https://doi.org/10.1186/s12889-019-8114-1

Onyeneho NG, Ozumba BC, Subramanian SV (2019) Determinants of childhood anemia in India. Sci Rep 9(1):1–7. https://doi.org/10.1038/s41598-019-52793-3

Qin Y, Melse-Boonstra A, Pan X, Yuan B, Dai Y, Zhao J, Zimmermann MB, Kok FJ, Zhou M, Shi Z (2013) Anemia in relation to body mass index and waist circumference among chinese women. Nutr J 12(1):10–12. https://doi.org/10.1186/1475-2891-12-10

Rammohan A, Awofeso N, Robitaille M-C (2012) Addressing female iron-deficiency anaemia in India: is vegetarianism the major obstacle? ISRN Publ Health 2012:1–8. https://doi.org/10.5402/2012/765476

Rohisha IK, Jose TT, Chakrabarty J (2019) Prevalence of anemia among tribal women. J Family Med Prim Care 6(2):145–147. https://doi.org/10.4103/jfmpc.jfmpc

Shah T, Warsi J, Laghari Z (2020) Anemia and its association with parity. Professional Med J 27(5):968–972. https://doi.org/10.29309/tpmj/2020.27.05.3959

Sharif N, Das B, Alam A (2023) Prevalence of anemia among reproductive women in different social group in India: cross-sectional study using nationally representative data. PLoS ONE 18(2):1–22. https://doi.org/10.1371/journal.pone.0281015

Singh A, Let S, Tiwari S, Chakrabarty M (2023) Spatiotemporal variations and determinants of overweight/obesity among women of reproductive age in urban India during 2005-2021. BMC Public Health 23(1):1–19. https://doi.org/10.1186/s12889-023-16842-x

Teshale AB, Tesema GA, Worku MG, Yeshaw Y, Tessema ZT (2020) Anemia and its associated factors among women of reproductive age in eastern Africa: a multilevel mixed-effects generalized linear model. PLoS ONE 15(9):1–16. https://doi.org/10.1371/journal.pone.0238957

Win HH, Ko MK (2018) Geographical disparities and determinants of anaemia among women of reproductive age in Myanmar: analysis of the 2015-2016 Myanmar Demographic and Health Survey. WHO South-East Asia J Publ Health 7(2):107–113. https://doi.org/10.4103/2224-3151.239422

World Health Organisation (2014) Global nutrition target 2025: anaemia policy brief (Issue 6). World Health Organisation, Geneva

World Health Organisation (2015) The global prevalence of anaemia in 2011. World Health Organisation, Geneva

Chapter 5
Tracking the Changes in Socioeconomic Disparities in Menstrual Hygienic Product Use Among Young Women in Urban India: A Repeated Cross-Sectional Analysis

Mahashweta Chakrabarty and **Aditya Singh**

Abstract During menstruation, the use of hygienic products (HPs), including sanitary napkins, locally prepared napkins, tampons, and menstrual cups, is known to minimize the risk of gynecological diseases. The use of HPs is more unequal in urban India than in rural India. Scant literature is available on socioeconomic disparities in HP usage over time. This study examined socioeconomic disparities in HP use in urban India and its states from 2015–16 to 2019–21 by using the Erreygers concentration index (CI) and rate ratios. Additionally, the study sought to break down the observed inequality into contributing factors. Information of 68,459 and 54,561 urban women (aged 15–24 years) from the fourth and fifth National Family Health Surveys (NFHS-4 and NFHS-5), respectively, were used. The findings revealed a 15% increase in HP use among women in urban India between 2015–16 and 2019–21. The CI for the use of HPs stood at 0.382 in 2015–16 and decreased to 0.302 in 2019–21, highlighting the persistent concentration of HP use among women belonging to wealthier households. Although a decline in socioeconomic disparity has taken place over time, this decline has widely varied across different Indian states. The study revealed that socioeconomic disparity, as measured by CI, has decreased in 21 Indian states out of 28. Notably, Arunachal Pradesh, Telangana, and Andhra Pradesh have successfully reduced socioeconomic disparity by more than 50%. That disparity has noticeably increased in Gujarat and Meghalaya. The results of inequality decomposition highlighted that education and exposure to mass media account for over 80% of the socioeconomic disparity observed in HP use. Targeted interventions are needed to promote equitable access to these products. State-specific policies and addressing factors like education and mass-media exposure can contribute to reducing socioeconomic disparities in HP use.

M. Chakrabarty (✉) · A. Singh (✉)
Department of Geography, Banaras Hindu University, Varanasi, Uttar Pradesh, India
e-mail: adityasingh@bhu.ac.in; mahashweta.c1997@gmail.com

© The Author(s), under exclusive license to Springer Nature Singapore Pte Ltd. 2024
P. Chouhan et al. (eds.), *Sexual and Reproductive Health of Women*, https://doi.org/10.1007/978-981-97-8418-9_5

Keywords Menstrual hygiene · Urban women · Hygienic products · Socioeconomic inequality · The Erreygers concentration index · NFHS

5.1 Introduction

Menstruation, a natural bodily phenomena, affects a significant portion of the global population, including women and girls, transgender men and boys, and many nonbinary individuals of reproductive age (Roeckel et al. 2019). However, many menstruators face unjust restrictions on managing their menstrual cycle, compromising their dignity and well-being (Roeckel et al. 2019). The promotion of proper menstrual hygiene is crucial because it aligns with various United Nations Sustainable Development Goals (SDGs). Although no standalone SDG is dedicated to menstrual hygiene, it intersects with SDGs 3, 4, 5, 8, and 12, all of which rely on providing women and girls with adequate sanitation and hygiene for safe and dignified menstruation (Guterres 2020).

The tools used to manage menstruation vary, including sanitary napkins, tampons, menstrual cups, and other materials, which offer discretion and prevent visible bloodstains (Singh et al. 2022a, b). However, in several developing countries, like India, young girls often resort to using worn-out rags as absorbents due to limited resources, resulting in unhygienic practices that pose significant health risks. This unhygienic practice can result in several infections (Anand et al. 2015). Consequently, the pressing needs of women, including access to safe menstrual management, the widespread dissemination of information, and increased awareness of healthy menstrual practices, are imperative to address (Balakrishnan et al. 2022).

Determining the factors that influence the utilization of hygienic products (HPs) in India is a complex undertaking. Previous research has indicated that factors such as wealth, education, and the place of residence are among the strongest predictors of HP usage (Babbar et al. 2021; Chauhan et al. 2021; Singh et al. 2022c). Additionally, awareness of HPs and interactions with healthcare workers have been found to significantly impact their usage (Ram et al. 2020). Studies conducted in India have documented socioeconomic disparities in the adoption of HPs, with a preference for such products among the affluent (Roy et al. 2021; Singh et al. 2013). However, existing studies have predominantly concentrated on investigating the correlation between these variables, without conducting a quantitative evaluation of socioeconomic disparities in HP use within urban India. Moreover, no examination of how these disparities evolve over time has been carried out in Urban India.

This chapter focuses specifically on the urban context of India in that it presents a unique setting for investigating menstrual hygiene practices. Urban areas generally provide better access to resources such as healthcare facilities, educational institutions, and markets than rural areas do (Chen et al. 2019). However, urban settings also impose challenges, such as overcrowding, inadequate sanitation infrastructure, and socioeconomic disparities (Chakravarthy et al. 2019). These factors significantly influence menstrual hygiene among women in urban areas, underscoring the importance of examining the socioeconomic disparities related to the use of HPs within this specific context.

Furthermore, urban India has witnessed rapid growth and demographic shifts due to increasing urbanization and rural-to-urban migration (Chakravarthy et al. 2019; Kumar and Mohanty 2011). This transition has brought about changes in lifestyle, cultural norms, and resource access, all of which can profoundly impact menstrual hygiene practices. By investigating socioeconomic disparities in HP use among young urban women, this chapter aims to uncover the unique dynamics and patterns of disparity within urban settings.

Therefore, the objective of this chapter is threefold: first, to quantify the socioeconomic disparities associated with HP use among young urban women in India; second, to analyze the changing patterns of these disparities across different Indian states over time; and third, to identify the factors contributing to these disparities.

5.2 Methods

5.2.1 Data Source

This chapter utilizes the datasets from the fourth National Family Health Survey (NFHS-4) and the fifth National Family Health Survey (NFHS-5). In both survey rounds, data on menstrual product use were collected specifically from women aged 15–24 years. For this analysis, the focus was specifically on young women (15–24 years) of urban India. Out of the 699,686 interviewed women aged 15–49 years in NFHS-4, 68,459 were selected, who were then asked questions related to their use of menstrual products. Similarly, from the NFHS-5, out of the 724,115 interviewed women, 54,561 were selected.

5.2.2 Variables

5.2.2.1 Dependent Variable

In both rounds of NFHS, women were asked a multiple-response question on the absorbents they used during their menstruation to prevent visible blood stains. The question provided six response options: (a) cloth, (b) locally prepared napkins, (c) sanitary napkins, (d) tampons, (e) nothing, and (f) others.

To analyze the data and understand the use of HPs, we constructed a dichotomous outcome variable. Women who used products such as sanitary napkins, locally made napkins, and tampons were considered as "exclusive users of HPs" (coded as "0"). Contrary to this, women who used non-HPs such as clothes, used a combination of HPs and non-HPs, or did not use any product were coded as "1."

5.2.2.2 Independent Variables

In this chapter, household wealth status served as the main predictor, and we utilized the household wealth factor score as a proxy of the household's socioeconomic status. The wealth factor scores are derived through the application of principal component analysis (PCA) on various financial proxies, such as housing standards, amenities within households, durable goods ownership, and the extent of land ownership (Kumar et al. 2015).

Sociodemographic predictors such as age at menarche, child marriage, respondent's level of education, religion, social groups, respondent's type of home, and mass-media exposure were considered to identify various contributors to the existing socioeconomic disparity. The selection of variables is informed by prior research on the management of menstrual hygiene (Anand et al. 2015; Chauhan et al. 2021; Kathuria and Raj 2018; Ram et al. 2020; Roy et al. 2021; Vishwakarma et al. 2020).

5.2.3 Statistical Analysis

To identify disparity in the use of HPs between women from the richest and poorest wealth quintiles in India and its states, the richest–poorest ratio was computed. This ratio compares the prevalence of HP use (as a percentage) among women in the wealthiest households with that among women in the poorest households. In this calculation, the numerator represents the prevalence in the richest wealth quintiles, whereas the denominator represents the prevalence in the poorest households. A ratio of more than 1.0 indicates a higher advantage for the numerator group (richest wealth quintiles), whereas a ratio of less than 1.0 suggests a higher risk for the numerator group (Chowdhury et al. 2022).

The Erreygers concentration index (CI) and concentration curve (CC) were used to assess socioeconomic disparity in the use of HPs among young women in urban India and its states over time. The CI measures this disparity, whose values range from -1 to $+1$. A negative CI with a CC above the equality line indicates the health phenomena (in this study the use of HPs) is concentrated among poor, whereas a positive CI with a CC below the line indicates the phenomena is concentrated among the rich. Additionally, to identify the contributors of socioeconomic disparity in HP use among young women in India, Erreygers's CI was likewise broken down or decomposed for both rounds of NFHS.

5.3 Results

5.3.1 Change in the Use of HPs by Wealth Quintiles

The utilization of HPs among young urban women in India has shown an overall increase from 2015–16 to 2019–21. In 2015–16, the use of HPs was recorded at 56.7%, whereas in 2019–2021, it rose to 68.1% in urban India. This upward trend was consistent across different wealth quintiles, indicating an improvement in the adoption of HPs among various socioeconomic groups over time.

According to an examination of the use of HPs in different wealth quintiles, even among the poorest wealth quintiles a significant increase has been taken place. In 2015–16, the use of HPs among the poorest quintile was 31.3%, which rose to 50.3% in 2019–21. Similarly, among the richest wealth quintiles, the utilization increased from 79.7% in 2015–16 to 85.1% in 2019–21. The trends in the utilization of HPs among other wealth quintiles followed a similar pattern (see Fig. 5.1).

Although an increase in the use of HPs across all wealth quintiles took place from 2015–16 to 2019–21, the rise was higher among higher-income groups than among poor groups. Additionally, despite an overall upward trend in the adoption of

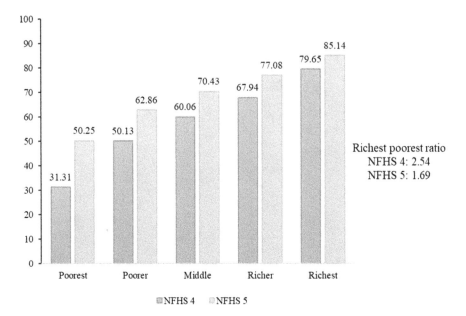

Fig. 5.1 HP use (in %) across household wealth quintiles in urban India, in NFHS-4 and NFHS-5

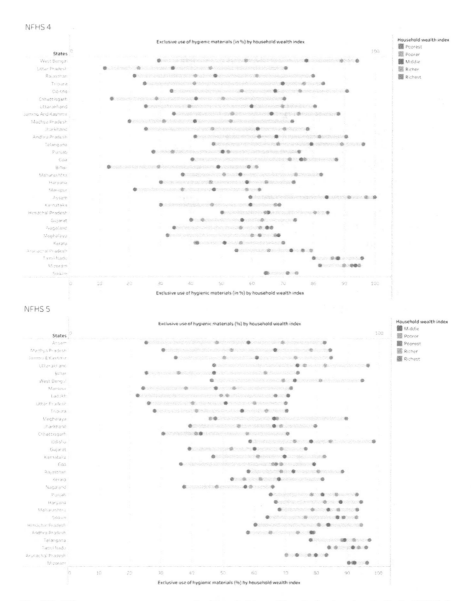

Fig. 5.2 HP use among young women by household wealth quintiles in urban India, in NFHS-4 and NFHS-5

HPs across all states figure 5.2 indicates persistent economic disparities in their usage, showing a significant rich–poor gap in every state of India.

To take a holistic picture of the disparities in the use of HPs between the most economically privileged and the least privileged groups, we computed the ratios of the richest to those of the poorest for India and its states.

5.3.2 Richest–Poorest Ratios in the Use of HPs Across Indian States from 2015–16 to 2019–21

The richest–poorest ratio provided insights into the relative disparity in the use of HPs among women from the poorest and richest wealth categories. In this analysis, the richest economic group served as the primary interest group (numerator). Overall, the ratio was consistently greater than 1.0 across all states and over time, indicating that urban women from the richest households in India were more prone to use HPs during menstruation than women from the poorest households (Table 5.1). However, the ratios exhibited substantial variation among the states of India.

For instance, during 2015–16, the ratio exceeded 3.0 and 6.0 in nine states: Bihar, Chhattisgarh, Jharkhand, Madhya Pradesh, Rajasthan, Tripura, Uttar Pradesh, Uttarakhand, and West Bengal. This indicated that urban women from the wealthiest households in these states were using HPs at a rate three to six times higher than that of the poorest women within the same states. However, the ratios decreased to less than 3.0 during 2019–21 in these aforementioned states. Nevertheless, during 2019–21, women from the richest wealth categories in ten states reported a rate of HP use during menstruation that was two times higher than that of the poorest women in the same states.

Given that the richest–poorest ratios offer a relative indication of disparity in the use of HPs across two wealth quintiles, this chapter undertook additional calculations of CIs for India and its states over time. The purpose was to assess socioeconomic disparities in the use of HPs during menstruation. By employing CIs, a more comprehensive measure of disparity was obtained.

5.3.3 Geographical Variation in Socioeconomic Disparity in HP Use Over Time

Figure 5.3 displays the level of socioeconomic disparity in HP use from 2015–16 to 2019–21, as measured by Erreygers's CI and CC. Overall, the results from Erreygers's CI indicate a pro-rich concentration in HP use among young women during menstruation over time. The analysis reveals a decline in disparity across household wealth over the studied period. Specifically, the value of the CI decreased from 0.382 in 2015–16 to 0.302 in 2019–21.

In India, socioeconomic disparity in HP use has witnessed a reduction of 20% between 2015–16 and 2019–21. However, the magnitude of change in the disparity of access to HPs varies across states.

Table 5.2 shows that socioeconomic disparity in the use of HPs has reduced in 21 out of 28 states in India. The greatest reduction in disparity is observed in Arunachal Pradesh (56.6%), followed by Telangana, Andhra Pradesh, Rajasthan, Maharashtra, Punjab, Haryana, Odisha, West Bengal, Chhattisgarh, Jharkhand, Uttar Pradesh, Uttarakhand, Tripura, Nagaland, Kerala, and Assam over time. Conversely,

Table 5.1 State-wise richest–poorest ratios in HP use among young urban women, during 2015–2016 and 2019–2021

States	NFHS-4			NFHS-5		
	Use of HPs among poorest (%)	Use of HPs among richest (%)	Rate ratio	Use of HPs among poorest (%)	Use of HPs among richest (%)	Rate ratio
Andaman and Nicobar Islands	59.40	100.00	1.68	88.79	96.85	1.09
Andhra Pradesh	41.40	90.58	2.19	58.12	79.09	1.36
Arunachal Pradesh	54.91	76.46	1.39	73.79	83.16	1.13
Assam	59.40	100.00	1.68	25.21	82.38	3.27
Bihar	13.08	58.94	4.51	25.29	73.83	2.92
Chandigarh	27.46	89.02	3.24	77.65	100.00	1.29
Chhattisgarh	13.99	70.38	5.03	30.82	70.67	2.29
DNH	49.05	70.02	1.43	66.87	80.74	1.21
DD	16.17	97.29	6.02	69.70	96.11	1.38
Goa	40.60	87.47	2.15	36.39	66.99	1.84
Gujarat	40.23	73.92	1.84	39.26	76.48	1.95
Haryana	30.30	73.47	2.42	66.87	94.41	1.41
Himachal Pradesh	50.26	84.61	1.68	60.48	83.71	1.38
Jammu and Kashmir	34.36	88.01	2.56	34.66	84.48	2.44
Jharkhand	25.41	78.02	3.07	39.38	79.57	2.02
Karnataka	30.23	68.77	2.27	46.86	82.55	1.76
Kerala	42.20	70.11	1.66	52.84	81.96	1.55
Lakshadweep	100.00	96.35	0.96	22.52	66.70	2.96
Madhya Pradesh	19.83	73.03	3.68	88.02	71.81	0.82
Maharashtra	37.47	82.47	2.20	30.59	84.25	2.75
Manipur	21.69	62.44	2.88	68.13	93.12	1.37
Meghalaya	32.39	62.49	1.93	24.36	71.75	2.95
Mizoram	82.16	92.42	1.12	47.41	89.43	1.89
Nagaland	34.50	66.26	1.92	90.41	96.42	1.07
Delhi	47.53	91.13	1.92	37.51	65.83	1.75
Odisha	33.70	90.79	2.69	58.65	98.38	1.68
Puducherry	78.05	98.19	1.26	86.94	91.51	1.05
Punjab	27.78	75.26	2.71	65.27	93.08	1.43
Rajasthan	21.48	79.78	3.71	58.14	88.27	1.52
Sikkim	64.44	71.53	1.11	64.25	88.77	1.38
Tamil Nadu	80.13	95.94	1.20	84.08	96.05	1.14
Tripura	24.81	83.00	3.35	78.15	97.08	1.24
Uttar Pradesh	11.62	70.80	6.09	27.91	70.33	2.52
Uttarakhand	25.29	80.36	3.18	26.07	70.05	2.69
West Bengal	29.47	94.07	3.19	47.06	96.48	2.05
Telangana	47.46	96.18	2.03	46.31	94.66	2.04

HPs hygienic products, *DNH* Dadra and Nagar Haveli, *DD* Daman and Diu

5 Tracking the Changes in Socioeconomic Disparities in Menstrual Hygienic Product... 67

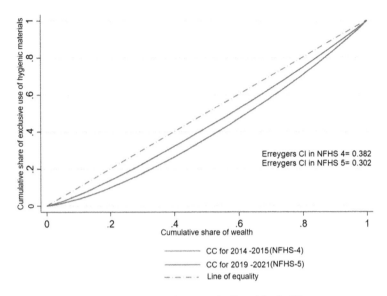

Fig. 5.3 Concentration curves showing socioeconomic disparities in HP use among young urban women in India during 2015–2016 and 2019–2021

Table 5.2 Socioeconomic disparity (measured by Erreygers CI) in HP use among young urban women during 2015–2016 and 2019–2021

States	NFHS-5			NFHS-4			CI gap
	Erreygers's CI	SE	p-Value	Erreygers's CI	SE	p-Value	
Arunachal Pradesh	0.084	0.026	<0.001	0.194	0.033	<0.001	−0.110
Telangana	0.148	0.016	<0.001	0.339	0.031	<0.001	−0.191
Chandigarh	0.203	0.048	<0.001	0.454	0.059	<0.001	−0.251
Andhra Pradesh	0.148	0.036	<0.001	0.322	0.033	<0.001	−0.175
Rajasthan	0.241	0.018	<0.001	0.460	0.016	<0.001	−0.219
Maharashtra	0.203	0.015	<0.001	0.363	0.018	<0.001	−0.160
Punjab	0.227	0.021	<0.001	0.392	0.024	<0.001	−0.165
Haryana	0.201	0.019	<0.001	0.321	0.022	<0.001	−0.119
Odisha	0.300	0.027	<0.001	0.475	0.023	<0.001	−0.176
West Bengal	0.366	0.023	<0.001	0.571	0.026	<0.001	−0.205
Chhattisgarh	0.303	0.027	<0.001	0.454	0.021	<0.001	−0.150
Jharkhand	0.315	0.026	<0.001	0.470	0.020	<0.001	−0.155
Uttar Pradesh	0.346	0.014	<0.001	0.459	0.010	<0.001	−0.113
Uttarakhand	0.322	0.033	<0.001	0.427	0.024	<0.001	−0.105
Tripura	0.376	0.059	<0.001	0.483	0.052	<0.001	−0.107
Nagaland	0.213	0.041	<0.001	0.272	0.032	<0.001	−0.059
Kerala	0.198	0.032	<0.001	0.234	0.033	<0.001	−0.036
Assam	0.437	0.031	<0.001	0.513	0.031	<0.001	−0.075
Bihar	0.412	0.025	<0.001	0.423	0.020	<0.001	−0.012

(continued)

Table 5.2 (continued)

States	NFHS-5			NFHS-4			
	Erreygers's CI	SE	p-Value	Erreygers's CI	SE	p-Value	CI gap
Jammu and Kashmir	0.425	0.031	<0.001	0.434	0.029	<0.001	−0.009
Goa	0.255	0.060	<0.001	0.255	0.064	<0.001	−0.001
Karnataka	0.311	0.020	<0.001	0.311	0.021	<0.001	0.000
Manipur	0.322	0.045	<0.001	0.316	0.027	<0.001	0.005
Madhya Pradesh	0.452	0.018	<0.001	0.440	0.013	<0.001	0.012
Tamil Nadu	0.103	0.013	<0.001	0.098	0.013	<0.001	0.005
Himachal Pradesh	0.249	0.062	<0.001	0.232	0.072	0.002	0.017
Delhi	0.210	0.014	<0.001	0.194	0.019	<0.001	0.016
Meghalaya	0.359	0.045	<0.001	0.310	0.041	<0.001	0.049
Gujarat	0.294	0.020	<0.001	0.249	0.022	<0.001	0.045
India	0.302	0.004	<0.001	0.382	0.004	<0.001	−0.080

CI concentration index, *SE* standard error

socioeconomic disparities in HP use have increased the most in Gujarat, followed by Meghalaya (by more than 15%).

5.3.4 Breaking Down the Socioeconomic Disparity in the Use of HPs Over Time

Table 5.3 shows the results from Erreygers's decomposition analysis. Education, exposure to mass media, religion, and social groups significantly contribute to the observed disparities, with education and media explaining over 80% of the disparities, in both rounds. Regional residents and social groups contribute the remaining 10%, consistently observed over time.

Table 5.3 Breakdown of socioeconomic disparity in HP use among young urban women in India during 2015–2016 and 2019–2021

Variable	NFHS-4				NFHS-5			
	Elasticity	CI	Contribution	Contribution (%)	Elasticity	CI	Contribution	Contribution (%)
Age at menarche	−0.063	0.029	−0.002	−0.50	0.029	0.017	0.000	0.23
Education	1.016	0.231	0.235	64.79	0.721	0.139	0.100	47.66
Religion	0.243	0.061	0.015	4.09	0.217	0.019	0.004	1.98
SC/ST	−0.054	−0.166	0.009	2.47	−0.035	−0.186	0.006	3.08
Mass-media exposure	0.828	0.115	0.095	26.23	0.465	0.145	0.068	32.05
Child marriage	−0.031	−0.139	0.004	1.18	−0.025	−0.118	0.003	1.40
Type of home	−0.036	−0.124	0.004	1.24	−0.038	−0.106	0.004	1.92
North	−0.023	−0.055	0.001	0.36	0.113	0.171	0.019	9.22
Central	0.003	0.000	0.000	0.00	−0.060	−0.014	0.001	0.40
East	0.000	−0.008	0.000	0.00	0.034	−0.236	−0.008	−3.76
West	0.064	0.050	0.003	0.88	0.099	0.087	0.009	4.09
South	0.071	−0.045	−0.003	−0.89	0.147	0.025	0.004	1.75
Northeast	0.007	0.082	0.001	0.15	0.000	−0.033	0.000	0.00
CI (explained)			0.363	100			0.211	100
CI (actual)			0.382				0.302	
CI (unexplained)			0.019				0.091	

CI concentration index

5.4 Discussion

This chapter aims to assess the level and pattern of socioeconomic disparity in HP use among young women in urban India over time. In addition to quantifying the degree of disparity, we also explore the factors that contribute to this disparity, making our findings policy relevant and informative for interventions. Our study has revealed several noteworthy findings. First, women from higher socioeconomic backgrounds in urban India exhibit a significantly greater prevalence of using HPs during menstruation. This indicates a disproportionate concentration of the use of HPs among women from wealthier households in urban India. Second, the socioeconomic disparity in HP use was not uniform across the states of India. The highest levels of economic disparity in the utilization of HPs were observed in Madhya Pradesh, a state located in central India. In contrast, Tamil Nadu, in southern India, and Mizoram, in the northeastern region, exhibited the lowest levels of disparity in this respect. Third, our results indicate that the pro-rich disparity in HP use can be attributed to factors such as women's education, exposure to mass media, social groups, and religion.

HP utilization has shown a marked increase with the rise in women's education. Studies conducted in India (Chauhan et al. 2021; Ram et al. 2020) and other countries (Bhusal 2020; Juyal et al. 2014) consistently highlight the significant role that education plays in the adoption of HPs. Educated women tend to be more knowledgeable about the benefits and importance of HPs, understand the risks associated with using unhygienic menstrual products, and often enjoy greater decision-making autonomy and economic independence (Chauhan et al. 2021; Ram et al. 2020; Roy et al. 2021). Our research indicates a noticeable disparity favoring wealthier segments in terms of educational attainment, which in turn significantly influences the use of HPs among urban women.

Urban young women are more likely to utilize HPs when exposed to mass media, which raises awareness of menstrual hygiene initiatives and policies. Mass media acts as a reliable source of spreading information about the benefits and availability of products, thereby potentially influencing attitudes toward disposable sanitary napkins (Chauhan et al. 2021; Dube and Sharma 2012; Ghosh et al. 2021; Mahon and Fernandes 2010; Roy et al. 2021). Our research indicates that mass-media exposure is more prevalent among wealthier urban women, contributing to the disparity in HP usage. Thus, reducing the gap in mass-media exposure could help minimize the socioeconomic disparity in HP utilization in Uran India.

Regional differences also play significant role in the variation in HP use among urban young women. The usage rate is higher among urban women in the southern and northern regions than among those in the central region (Roy et al. 2021; Singh et al. 2013). These findings are consistent with previous studies, which have highlighted the discrepancies in HP usage between the southern and central regions of India (Ram et al. 2020; Sivakami et al. 2019; van Eijk et al. 2016). The higher usage in southern states can be attributed to their advanced socioeconomic development and effective public healthcare systems. In contrast, the central region shows lower utilization, primarily due to underdeveloped economic conditions, widespread poverty, and poorly functioning healthcare infrastructure. Additionally, social taboos may further impede HP use among economically disadvantaged urban women in these areas.

To address socioeconomic disparity in the use of HPs, various government initiatives have been introduced, including the Menstrual Hygiene Scheme. While these efforts aim to promote awareness and accessibility to sanitary napkins, challenges in procurement have hampered effective implementation in certain states, such as Haryana, Madhya Pradesh, Maharashtra, and Uttarakhand (Barua et al. 2020). Our study corroborates these challenges, highlighting the need for improved procurement strategies to ensure the consistent availability of HPs (Singh 2019).

Furthermore, despite the introduction of subsidized sanitary napkins under the *Suvidha* brand in government-subsidized pharmacies, reports indicate recurring instances of supply shortages, echoing concerns raised in our research findings. Additionally, our study underscores the disparities in access to HPs among urban women, particularly in economically disadvantaged households, aligning with the observed socioeconomic disparities in product usage.

Although states like Tamil Nadu have introduced successful initiatives, including the distribution of free sanitary napkins through the *Pudhu Yugam* scheme and the installation of vending machines with the help of local nongovernmental organizations, these efforts are often limited in scope and not widely scalable. Our study highlights the importance of expanding these programs to cover a larger population and to address ongoing socioeconomic disparities in access to hygienic practices.

5.5 Conclusion

This chapter not only revealed the status and progress of economic disparity in HP use across Indian states but also identified the main contributing factors to existing socioeconomic disparity. Therefore, any government strategy must focus on educating and empowering poor urban women through mass media to help them choose from the various safe and affordable options available.

Acknowledgments Support from Banaras Hindu University's Institute of Eminence seed grant no. R/Dev/D/IoE/Equipment/seed grant-II/2022–2023/48726 is acknowledged by Dr. Aditya Singh. Gratitude is also expressed for the Junior Research Fellowship granted to Mahashweta Chakrabarty by the University Grants Commission for her PhD work. This chapter is a part of Mahashweta Chakrabarty's PhD research.

Declarations

Competing Interests The authors declare that they have no competing interests.

Authors' Contributions Mahashweta Chakrabarty conducted data analysis, created Stata codes, implemented methodology, generated visualizations, and drafted the original manuscript. Aditya Singh supervised the project and also reviewed and edited the manuscript.

Funding No funding was received.

Availability of Data and Materials The data and materials for this chapter are sourced from publicly available secondary sources accessible at https://dhsprogram.com/methodology/survey/survey-display-541.cfm. Interested individuals can register at the provided link to freely download the necessary data.

References

Anand E, Singh J, Unisa S (2015) Menstrual hygiene practices and its association with reproductive tract infections and abnormal vaginal discharge among women in India. Sex Reprod Healthc 6(4):249–254. https://doi.org/10.1016/j.srhc.2015.06.001
Babbar K, Saluja D, Sivakami M (2021) How socio-demographic and mass media factors affect sanitary item usage among women in rural and urban India. Waterlines
Balakrishnan S, Carolin A, Sudharsan B, Shivasakthimani R (2022) The prevalence of reproductive tract infections based on the syndromic management approach among ever-married rural women in Kancheepuram District, Tamil Nadu: a community-based cross-sectional study. Cureus 14(3):23314. https://doi.org/10.7759/cureus.23314
Barua A, Watson K, Plesons M, Chandra-Mouli V, Sharma K (2020) Adolescent health programming in India: a rapid review. Reprod Health 17(1):87. https://doi.org/10.1186/s12978-020-00929-4
Bhusal CK (2020) Practice of menstrual hygiene and associated factors among adolescent school girls in Dang district, Nepal. Adv Prev Med 2020:1–7. https://doi.org/10.1155/2020/1292070
Chakravarthy V, Rajagopal S, Joshi B (2019) Does menstrual hygiene management in urban slums need a different lens? Challenges faced by women and girls in Jaipur and Delhi. Indian J Gend Stud 26(1-2):138–159. https://doi.org/10.1177/0971521518811174
Chauhan S, Kumar P, Marbaniang SP, Srivastava S, Patel R, Dhillon P (2021) Examining the predictors of use of sanitary napkins among adolescent girls: a multi-level approach. PLoS ONE 16(4):1–14. https://doi.org/10.1371/journal.pone.0250788
Chen X, Orom H, Hay JL, Waters EA, Schofield E, Li Y, Kiviniemi MT (2019) Differences in rural and urban health information access and use. J Rural Health 35(3):405–417. https://doi.org/10.1111/jrh.12335
Chowdhury S, Singh A, Kasemi N, Chakrabarty M (2022) Economic inequality in intimate partner violence among forward and backward class women in india: a decomposition analysis. Vict Offenders 19:1003–1029. https://doi.org/10.1080/15564886.2022.2080312
Dube S, Sharma K (2012) Knowledge, attitude and practice regarding reproductive health among urban and rural girls: a comparative study. Stud Ethno-Med 6(2):85–94. https://doi.org/10.1080/09735070.2012.11886424
Ghosh R, Mozumdar A, Chattopadhyay A, Acharya R (2021) Mass media exposure and use of reversible modern contraceptives among married women in India: an analysis of the NFHS 2015-16 data. PLoS ONE 16(7):1–23. https://doi.org/10.1371/journal.pone.0254400
Guterres A (2020) The sustainable development goals report 2020. In: United Nations publication issued by the Department of Economic and Social Affairs
Juyal R, Kandpal SD, Semwal J (2014) Menstrual hygiene and reproductive morbidity in adolescent girls in Dehradun, India. Bangladesh J Med Sci 13(2):170–174. https://doi.org/10.3329/bjms.v13i2.14257
Kathuria B, Raj S (2018) Effects of socio-economic conditions on usage of hygienic method of menstrual protection among young women in EAG states of India. Amity J Healthc Manage 3(1):40–52

Kumar A, Mohanty SK (2011) Intra-urban differentials in the utilization of reproductive healthcare in India, 1992-2006. J Urban Health 88(2):311–328. https://doi.org/10.1007/s11524-010-9532-7

Kumar A, Kumari D, Singh A (2015) Increasing socioeconomic inequality in childhood undernutrition in urban India: trends between 1992-93, 1998-99 and 2005-06. Health Policy Plan 30(8):1003–1016. https://doi.org/10.1093/heapol/czu104

Mahon T, Fernandes M (2010) Menstrual hygiene in South Asia: a neglected issue for WASH (water, sanitation and hygiene) programmes. Gend Dev 18(1):99–113. https://doi.org/10.1080/13552071003600083

Ram U, Pradhan MR, Patel S, Ram F (2020) Factors associated with disposable menstrual absorbent use among young women in India. Int Perspect Sex Reprod Health 46:223–234. https://doi.org/10.1363/46e0320

Roeckel S, Cabrera-Clerget A, Yamakoshi B (2019) Guide to menstrual hygiene materials. UNICEF, pp 6–36. https://www.unicef.org/media/91346/file/UNICEF-Guide-menstrual-hygiene-materials-2019.pdf

Roy A, Paul P, Saha J, Barman B, Kapasia N, Chouhan P (2021) Prevalence and correlates of menstrual hygiene practices among young currently married women aged 15–24 years: an analysis from a nationally representative survey of India. Eur J Contracept Reprod Health Care 26(1):1–10. https://doi.org/10.1080/13625187.2020.1810227

Singh N (2019) One-rupee sanitary pads welcome, but govt's Janaushadhi stores often don't have them. The Print, 283474. https://theprint.in/india/one-rupee-sanitary-pads-welcome-but-govts-janaushadhi-stores-often-dont-have-them/283474/

Singh A, Kumar A, Kumar A (2013) Determinants of neonatal mortality in rural India, 2007–2008. PeerJ 1(1):e75. https://doi.org/10.7717/peerj.75

Singh A, Chakrabarty M, Chowdhury S, Singh S (2022a) Exclusive use of hygienic menstrual absorbents among rural adolescent women in India: A geospatial analysis. Clin Epidemiol Global Health 17:101116. https://doi.org/10.1016/j.cegh.2022.101116

Singh A, Chakrabarty M, Singh S, Chandra R, Chowdhury S, Singh A (2022b) Menstrual hygiene practices among adolescent women in rural India: a cross-sectional study. BMC Public Health 22(1):2126. https://doi.org/10.1186/s12889-022-14622-7

Singh A, Chakrabarty M, Singh S, Mohan D, Chandra R, Chowdhury S (2022c) Wealth-based inequality in the exclusive use of hygienic materials during menstruation among young women in urban India. PLoS One 17(11):e0277095. https://doi.org/10.1371/journal.pone.0277095

Sivakami M, van Eijk AM, Thakur H, Kakade N, Patil C, Shinde S, Surani N, Bauman A, Zulaika G, Kabir Y, Dobhal A, Singh P, Tahiliani B, Mason L, Alexander KT, Thakkar MB, Laserson KF, Phillips-Howard PA (2019) Effect of menstruation on girls and their schooling, and facilitators of menstrual hygiene management in schools: surveys in government schools in three states in India, 2015. J Glob Health 9(1):10408. https://doi.org/10.7189/jogh.09.010408

van Eijk AM, Sivakami M, Thakkar MB, Bauman A, Laserson KF, Coates S, Phillips-Howard PA (2016) Menstrual hygiene management among adolescent girls in India: a systematic review and meta-analysis. BMJ Open 6(3):e010290. https://doi.org/10.1136/bmjopen-2015-010290

Vishwakarma D, Puri P, Sharma SK (2020) Interlinking menstrual hygiene with women's empowerment and reproductive tract infections: evidence from India. Clin Epidemiol Global Health 10:100668. https://doi.org/10.1016/j.cegh.2020.11.001

Part II
Women's Reproductive Rights

Chapter 6
Critics on Abortion Rights in India: Issues and Policy Perspectives

Parama Bannerji and Rohit Bannerji

Abstract In medical terms, before the viability of embryos, abortion refers to pregnancy termination via the expulsion or removal of the embryo or fetus. Studies also point out that of the numerous causes of high maternal mortality, abortion is one of the leading causes. The literature, however, has revealed that though abortion has been legalized in India, cases of unsafe abortions continue, wherein lies the risk of high-level morbidity and sometimes mortality. The literature review in this chapter identifies the gap and asks why people turn to unsafe abortive practices when abortion is legalized in India. It also raises the question of whether any loopholes appear in the present policies of abortion, which is a hurdle in the supply-side economics of abortion. This chapter, by reviewing the literature, attempts to answer that question and concludes that in spite of liberalized abortion laws, scientific and accurate study, the inclusion of diverse viewpoints on policies related to abortion, and easing the progression of abortive services are needed to organize awareness campaigns so that unsafe abortion practices are infrequent or so that women opt for safe abortion practices.

Keywords Abortion · Reproductive health · Medical termination of pregnancy · Abortion policies · Unsafe abortion

6.1 Introduction

If one considers several issues on reproductive health, the most controversial one is abortion. Abortion has existed throughout recorded history, yet the controversy has not stopped. This study, exploring the existing literature, focuses on the issues related to abortion in India from history to the present. Laws pertaining to abortions

P. Bannerji (✉)
Nababarrackpur Prafulla Chandra Mahavidyala, Kolkata, India

R. Bannerji
ESI-PGIMSR Medical College and Hospital, Joka, West Bengal, India

© The Author(s), under exclusive license to Springer Nature Singapore Pte Ltd. 2024
P. Chouhan et al. (eds.), *Sexual and Reproductive Health of Women*, https://doi.org/10.1007/978-981-97-8418-9_6

vary from one country or other jurisdiction to another. While some deal with it liberally, others have stringent laws. However, abortion is legalized in India for a broad range of social and medical reasons. In India, induced abortion is legal under the Medical Termination of Pregnancy (MTP) Act 1971. However, in almost 25 countries, it is prohibited by law (Focus 2030). Hirve (2004) points out that despite years of legalization for abortion in India, women still turn to unsafe abortive services, which contributes to morbidity and maternal mortality. According to Visaria et al. (2004), the state does not have verifiable records on abortion cases, and whatever estimates they have contain wide regional differences and a rural–urban differential. For administrators or women's health advocates, such a situation hampers the design of interventions. A number of studies have been conducted on why women still turn to unsafe abortive services, such as the one by the International Institute for Population Sciences (IIPS), that by the Mumbai and Population Council, that in New Delhi, and that at the Guttmacher Institute in New York, USA. All these studies have pointed to a similar pattern. The issues included parental preference for sons and sex-selective abortion, confidentiality, the permission of the spouse for abortion, the expense of and preference for the private sector, etc. The main question here is, even if abortion services are broadly legal, what is prompting people to adopt unsafe and illegal methods of abortion? The absence of actual numerical figures on unlawful abortion complicates this. This chapter critically reviews the situation of abortion incidence in India, factors prompting abortion, barriers to and ideological understandings of the process, and the flaws in the policies related to safe abortion practice, which lead to opting for illegal termination of pregnancy. This study uses the methodology of qualitative literature review to collect research and findings from primarily qualitative studies and surveys.

Abortion has been practiced throughout history and across all countries. However, the practice is diverse in procedures and techniques and varies in legal status. To date, whereas it is prohibited in countries like Aruba and Egypt, it is accepted on request in countries like Greece and Nepal. Associated with this is also the right of women to their reproductive choice, which is upheld differently in different countries. In such a situation, unless the study is contextualized, it will be difficult to understand the problem of abortion practice and chart a way forward. Hence, the context of India is studied as a case study because the case study–based approach allows for more-detailed analysis. This article thus synthesizes the findings of a number of studies with the objective of reviewing India's policy and identifying whether a gap exists between what has been set in policy and what is actually happening while implementing it at the ground level. In general, the present study answered the following questions: (1) How have abortion-related policies changed in India over time; (2) what abortion services are currently available to women; and (3) what are the gaps in obtaining safe and legal abortion services?

6.2 Material and Methodology

This study follows the method of qualitative literature review. This review study tends to interpret and aggregate data from published literature and cohesively present them to answer the research question. The literature review for this study included a survey of scholarly sources on abortion-related topics by using the Google search engine and accessing the Scopus and PubMed databases. It also covered policy reviews, survey output, and qualitative studies. This overview of the existing literature enabled the identification of the gap in the literature and the topics to be covered for this study. The study thus took a descriptive approach due to the marked heterogeneity of studies.

6.3 Results

6.3.1 Historical Perspectives: Practice of and Attitudes Toward Abortion

Early cultures used nonsurgical methods of abortion like climbing, paddling, weightlifting, etc. In India, Vedic laws, however, pointed to the need to preserve male fetuses of the three upper castes. Women were also excommunicated by religious courts if they practiced abortions. Assyrian law mandated punishing women who performed abortions against their husbands' wishes, and historical records have pointed out that people in Japan practiced abortion even in the twelfth century. Early classical texts in Greco-Roman culture pointed out that abortion was not punishable. Attitudes toward abortion were, however, different in different cultures. For example, the Stoics of Greco-Roman culture treated the fetus as a plant and found abortion morally acceptable. Didache, an early Christian work written before 1000 CE, condemned abortion. To date, Eastern Orthodox as well as Roman Catholic churches oppose abortion. At other times in history, records have pointed out that until the late 1800s, no legal restrictions were imposed on female healers to practice abortion in some countries in Western Europe and the United States. By the end of the nineteenth century, abortion was legally restricted in most countries in Europe—the United Kingdom, France, Portugal, Spain, and Italy. These countries extended such restriction to their colonies. According to Berer (2017), historically, abortion was restricted for primarily three reasons: Dangerous abortion practices could kill a lot of women, abortion practices were considered immoral, or antiabortion laws were passed to protect fetuses. In the present era, the definition of *abortion* varies depending on the context. Universally, abortion may be one of two types: spontaneous abortion or induced abortion. *Spontaneous abortion* means abortion that occurs automatically without any external pressure, also known as miscarriage. The other type of abortion, which is under study now, is induced abortion, which is intentional and requires the help of an external force. It also varies from country to country and from institution to institution. To standardize the definition, the definitions of three institutions, namely the National Center for Health Statistics, the US Centers for Disease Control and Prevention (CDC), and the World Health Organization (WHO), are considered. These institutes loosely define *abortion* as pregnancy termination before 20 weeks of gestation or of a fetus born weighing less than 500 g. By taking a philosophical approach, it can be defined as "the act that a woman performs in voluntarily terminating, or allowing another person to terminate, her pregnancy" (Warren 1973).

6.3.2 The Global Context of Abortion Rights and Associated Outcomes

According to the think tank Focus 2030, 41% of women worldwide live under restrictive laws related to abortion, causing 39,000 women and girls to die from unsafe abortion practices. The Centre for Reproductive Rights divided countries into five categories according to their restrictions on abortion. Category I includes 25 countries that prohibit abortion altogether, like Aruba, Egypt, El Salvador, Iraq, and the Philippines. Category II includes 39 countries, like Antigua, Bangladesh, Sri Lanka, Sudan, and Syria, that allow abortion to save women's lives. Category III includes 56 countries, like Argentina, Ecuador, Ghana, Malaysia, and Mauritius), that allow abortion to preserve health. Category IV includes 14 countries, like Ethiopia, the United Kingdom, Hong Kong, and India, that allow abortion for the sake of reaching broad socioeconomic objectives. Finally, Category IV includes 66 countries, like Austria, Korea, Greece, Nepal, and Spain, that allow abortion on request.

6.3.3 Abortion Practices in India

The International Institute for Population Sciences (IIPS), the Mumbai and Population Council, New Delhi, and the Guttmacher Institute in New York, USA, conducted the first study in India to estimate the incidence of abortion. In India, those who deliver abortion services range from traditional birth attendants and midwives to medical doctors. Despite legal provisions, abortion services remain unregulated. That same study pointed out that the state has mostly concentrated more on sterilization services, and abortion services remain predominantly in the domain of clinics in the private sector. Also, unsafe abortions have caused 20% of maternal deaths.

6.3.4 Abortion Incidence in India

The Guttmacher Institute estimated that 15.6 million abortions took place in India in 2015, of which 3.4 million (22%) were conducted in healthcare facilities, whereas 11.5 million (73%) were conducted through medical methods outside such facilities, and 5% used nonmedical methods. According to Mathai (1997), abortion data in India severely lacks validity. The data generally come from one of two sources: clinic/hospital records or individual surveys of women. Abortion may be highly stigmatized or illegal, and hence, such data are difficult to obtain, and induced abortion incidence is often underestimated even when abortion is legal. In 2002, Johnston pointed out that the National Family Health Survey collects abortion data. However, they report a very low incidence of abortion. According to Rahaman et al. (2023), the gap between cases of reported legal abortion and total abortion cases indicates that less than 10% of the abortions that take place in India are conducted legally. According to Johnston, though the exact number is unknown, around one million abortions are legal, out of the total of 6.7 million in India per year.

6.3.5 Mortality and Morbidity in India from Unsafe Abortion

According to Mathai (1997), incomplete abortion, hemorrhage, uterine injury, and cervical injury are some of the complications associated with unsafe abortion, and adolescents are particularly prone to abortion-related morbidity and mortality. Another report, the United Nations Population Fund (UNFPA)'s State of the World Population Report 2022, stated that about 67% of abortions are unsafe.

6.3.6 Methods of Abortion in India

Another study by Mathai (1997) has pointed out that the method of abortion ranges from life-threatening ones at unregistered facilities to relatively safe ones at registered centers. Methods of inducing abortion include vaginal and oral methods. At unregistered centers, abortion may be induced through rudimentary techniques such as inserting sticks, herbs, roots, or other foreign bodies into the uterus. Rural medical providers (RMPs, or "quacks") sell medicines for oral use to induce abortion. Auxiliary nurses/midwives (ANMs) and Indian system medical practitioners (ISMPs) use intra-amniotic injections such as orally ingested abortifacients like chloroquine tablets, among others. A recent groundbreaking study unveiled a stark reality: In India, nearly a third of abortions are conducted under perilous conditions (Rahaman et al. 2023). This eye-opening research sheds light on a myriad of factors influencing this concerning trend. From the age of women to the composition of their families and from where they reside to their access to family-planning services, each element plays a pivotal role. Disturbingly, these unsafe procedures often occur early in pregnancy, with many resorting to self-administered medications. The reasons behind such risky decisions are as diverse as they are troubling, including unintended pregnancies and dire health complications. The urgent need for targeted interventions tailored to the unique regional, demographic, and social dynamics at play across India is clear. This is not just about statistics; it is about the lives and well-being of countless women. Simultaneously, another study by Rahaman et al. (2022) delved more deeply, uncovering a glaring urban–rural disparity. It is not just about geography, though; it is also about education, socioeconomic status, and access to vital resources. In urban areas, the vulnerability of younger women to unsafe abortion practices is alarming, especially when coupled with low spousal education levels. Contrastingly, in rural settings, the lack of education among spouses and the grip of poverty exacerbate the risks. Moreover, the revelation that the unmet need for family planning significantly contributes to this crisis, particularly in rural regions, underscores the importance of comprehensive interventions. These studies serve as a clarion call to action, demanding not just awareness but also tangible solutions that address the multifaceted challenges that women face across India.

6.3.7 The Issue of Gender-Selective Abortion in India

According to Hesketh et al. (2011), though some laws forbid fetal sex determination and sex-selective abortion in China, India, and South Korea, only in South Korea is the law stringent. Further, Arnold et al. (2002) estimates from the 2001 census of India pointed to high sex ratios for young children, which may be due to the growing use of sex-selective abortions to satisfy parental preferences for sons in India. The same author pointed out that according to the 1998–1999 National Family Health Survey (NFHS-2), the sex ratio at birth in India has been abnormally high (107–121 boys per 100 girls) in 16 of India's 26 states. The reason may be the extensive use of sex-selective abortions, particularly in three states: Gujarat, Haryana, and Punjab. According to Nandi and Deolalika (2011), after abortion was legalized in India in 1971, diagnosing the sex of the fetus became easier with improved technologies. With this, the practice of sex-selective abortions became widespread. In response to the crisis, the government of India came up with the National Pre-Conception and Pre-Natal Diagnostics Techniques (PNDT) Act of 1994, which was implemented in 1996 and which banned sex-selective abortions in India. However, a ubiquitous decline in the sex ratio definitely points to its abuse and to the use of sex-selective abortion services.

6.3.8 Barriers to Abortion Service Delivery

According to Hirve (2004), the main barrier to abortion care remains its neglect of this service in the public sector. According to an article by Godbole, an adult woman of "sound mind" is not legally bound to secure the approval of her partner if she wishes to have an abortion. However, in a patriarchal society like India, women find accessing abortion difficult; healthcare providers often ask women to secure partner permission; and the confidentiality of the woman is not protected. Further, marginalized women, such as single women or those from Scheduled Tribe communities, those affected by HIV, and even sex workers, face discrimination in accessing abortion, leading to unsafe abortions.

6.3.9 Abortion Policy Perspectives in India

When India was a British colony, it made abortion punishable in following the British Offences against the Person Act of 1861. However, globally, since the 1960s, abortion laws have been liberalized in Europe and at one time in the United States. In India, under the Indian Penal Code of 1860 (IPC), voluntarily terminating a pregnancy is considered a criminal offense. But here the liberalization of abortion laws began in 1964 to curb the unsafe abortion practices followed by many. The government of India thus appointed the Shah Committee to review all aspects of abortion. In 1966, therefore, abortion laws were liberalized for medical reasons and out of compassion. Following this came the Medical Termination of Pregnancy Act of 1971 and its regulation in 1975, where the required preconditions of approval for an abortion facility were taken into account. The MTP Act was the first step in respecting the reproductive choice of women with a "pro-choice" stance. The act stipulated that the termination of pregnancy can be performed by what it called a registered medical practitioner who has knowledge in the field of gynecology as per the requirements in the *MTP Act* and also has proper medical qualification according to the *Indian Medical Council Act*. India thus enacted its abortion law 2 years before the Supreme Court of the United States' original decision on *Roe v. Wade*, which was a landmark case of abortion law. According to Hirve (2004), although the initial years of MTP, up to the 1990s, showed a marginal increase of 10% in the abortion cases reported at approved abortion facilities, a declining trend took place later, and from the beginning of the 1990s, speculations abounded that for every legal abortion, the corresponding figure for illegal ones ranged from two to ten. Reform in abortion law has again taken place since 2000, and the Medical Termination of Pregnancy Act was enacted in 2002. That act tried to cut red tape, and at the state level, the act allowed district-level committees to approve abortion facilities. In an effort to reduce illegal abortion centers, it assigned 2 to 7 years of imprisonment for individual providers and owners of facilities not approved or maintained by the government. However, new challenges needed better solutions and amendments to the existing act, and more research on illegal abortions and estimates on their impacts on maternal morbidity are needed.

The next reform came after the Medical Termination of Pregnancy (Amendment) Bill, on March 2, 2020, which became the MTP (Amendment) Act of 2021. It was a bid to allow medical legalization. It categorizes three situations: one where the pregnancy lasts for less than 20 weeks, the one where the pregnancy lasts longer than 20 weeks but less than 24 weeks, and the one where the pregnancy lasts longer than 24 weeks. The main difference between the MTP Act of 1971 and the present one is that it covers unmarried women. It also expands the gestational period from 20 weeks to 24 weeks for rape survivors and beyond 24 weeks for fetal anomalies. It also stresses confidentiality, and a breach can lead to 1 year of imprisonment. Thus, with this amendment, now rape survivors and unmarried women can legally undergo medical termination. That amendment in the act includes the following change: If the termination would take place after 24 weeks, the High Court or Supreme Court would not be required to issue a writ. Now, by following the case of *Mahima Yadav v. Government of NCT of Delhi and Others,* the Honourable Court sets up a board to look after the problems that women face after 24 weeks of gestation. Also, this act was an indicator of positive development in society in that the definition changed from "pregnant married woman" to "pregnant woman" and also from "her husband" to "her partner."

6.3.10 Challenges in Abortion and Abortion Care in India

According to Stillman et al. (2014), the Guttmacher study indicated that the number of approved facilities had increased from 1877 in 1976 to 12,510 in 2010, but in rural areas, access to safe abortion services remains inadequate. Although most of the abortion facilities are in urban areas, rural women comprise 70% of the population. The same study points out that in recent times, the most common reasons for abortion are to limit family size and to increase the spacing between births. On top of this, challenges include an inadequate number of medically approved abortion facilities or services like postabortion family-planning counseling. Another project, namely the Abortion Assessment Project–India, which began in August 2000, had huge spatial coverage in India. Hirve (2004) pointed out the regulation of these services in both the public and the private sectors. He also pointed out the limited knowledge of legal provisions and unnecessary spousal consent requirements. Another drawback of abortion services is the lack of coordination between abortion services and other reproductive health services. According to Barge and Rajagopal (1996), several studies conducted in Uttar Pradesh have reported a limited number of abortion service providers, which may contribute to the spread of HIV or even mortality.

6.4 Discussion

The preceding section pointed out that though the literature on abortion laws or procedures is not lacking, a significant limitation persists in accessing estimates on abortion cases in India, the specific procedures that women opted for, and the outcomes of abortion procedures on the reproductive health of women. As mentioned, from time immemorial, women have used several methods of birth control and abortion. Abortion is not only a technical and medical issue. It is also the focal point of a broader ideological conflict that questions women's sexuality, family values, and motherhood. As a result, it has sparked controversy along strong ethical, moral, and political lines. As a part of the discussion, to address the issue of safe motherhood, the issue of safe abortion should be prioritized. The available literature features an identifiable dearth of verifiable abortion data. Data-collection instruments need to be designed to immediately collect abortion incidence data while also respecting local and cultural norms. The services of abortion-providing centers also urgently need to be improved. According to the literature reviewed, a thorough review of MTP policy, such as reviewing the procedures for licensing facilities, is urgently needed. Upgradation of the facilities that currently offer abortion services is needed. The confidentiality of women and abortion services must be prioritized to prevent people from turning to unsafe services (Mathai 1997). Increasing the accessibility of safe abortion services is recommended, with a greater number of facilities based in rural areas. Increasing the affordability of safe abortion services is also needed. According to Johnston, the high cost associated with safe abortion services has prompted women to access abortion services from relatively cheaper and untrained providers. Increasing awareness of the gestation period when an abortion could be considered safe is an important component in awareness campaigns on the dangers of unsafe abortions. Even over the 50 years of since the implementation of the MTP Act, abortion has still not been decriminalized in the Indian Penal Code of 1860 (IPC). The MTP Act only acts as a safeguard for doctors by stating the conditions under which they may terminate a pregnancy.

This review pointed to a number of other areas which need research. Given the dearth of specific abortion data on each state and its urban and rural areas, drafting region-specific policy related to the establishment of new facilities or upgrading the existing ones remains a challenge. Abortion services also need to be understood from the perspective of women. Abortion remains a stigma, and attempts to decriminalize have fallen short of expectations despite the liberalization of laws. Other research needs include understanding women's perspectives when they seek abortion services. These may provide input for the design of abortion-related awareness campaigns. A recent judgment of the Supreme Court (29 September 2022) declared abortion as a right, and the implication has now been treated as a victory for the "pro-choice" abortion school of thought against the "pro-life" school. In India, women can now access safe abortion practices, irrespective of whether they are married, within 24 weeks of the gestational period. An overwhelming trend toward the legalization of abortion rights has taken place globally, and India has been following this trend. Whereas abortion is absolutely restricted in countries like Egypt, El Salvador, and Iraq, India's stance on abortion may serve as a precedent to recognize the realities faced by women and interpret the abortion rights of women as fundamental. The ruling of the Supreme Court of India definitely represents a shift toward recognizing Indian women's reproductive rights, but more remains to be done. Revised laws are required at the state and national levels, and a regular ground survey is needed to assess the health status of pregnant women. Though this judgment is progressive, when looking back at the amended MTP Act, one often fails to understand the logic behind the setting of limits on the gestational week of 20 or 24 weeks. Beyond 24 weeks, women are refrained from their right to reproductive choice, and no concern is given to their mental health beyond 24 weeks. Legal, procedural and social barriers to accessing abortion services in India should be removed. The service needs to be immediately extended to rural primary healthcare centers. The centers providing abortion services must at all costs respect the confidentiality and privacy of women seeking abortions. Stricter laws prohibiting early marriage, greater awareness and information dissemination among women on their reproductive rights, and reducing the number of sex-selective abortions will promote healthier outcomes for women.

6.4.1 Limitations

Two of the significant limitations of this chapter are time constraints and a dearth of verifiable abortion-related data. The topic of abortion is vast, with numerous practices, laws, and rulings that require intensive research over a long time frame. Also, abortion is a taboo topic, and a large number of illegal abortions are never recorded. This too has served as a limitation to the study.

6.5 Conclusion

Although abortion is a vulnerable health concern for women, patriarchal interests are controlling policies related to it. Unsafe abortion can cause morbidity or mortality, and it remains a matter of grave concern for Indian women. Studies have also revealed that current legal abortion services are not meeting the needs of Indian women, more specifically those in rural areas. Improving the services of registered abortion facilities is thus urgently needed to attract patients to safe abortion facilities. A policy change may be needed, but any change in policy should consult with and collectively include members of the health department, public and private abortion providers, and other stakeholders. Available safe abortion services must also be socioeconomically viable. They should not remain underutilized due to factors at the individual or community level, factors such as a lack of awareness of the legality of abortion, unnecessary documentation and paperwork, and understanding the implications of unsafe abortion, among others.

Declaration

Availability of Data and Material All data related to this study are reported in this document.

Ethics Approval and Consent to Participate Ethical approval and consent are not applicable.

Competing Interests The authors declare that they have no competing interests.

Funding This chapter did not receive any specific grant from funding agencies in the public, commercial, or not-for-profit sectors.

References

Arnold F et al (2002) Sex-selective abortions in India. Popul Dev Rev 28(4):759–785. http://www.jstor.org/stable/3092788. Accessed 12 January 2024
Barge S, Rajagopal S (1996) Situation an analysis of MTP facilities in Maharashtra. Soc Change 26:226–244
Berer M (2017) Abortion law and policy around the world: in search of decriminalization. Health Hum Rights 19(1):13–27
Hesketh T, Lu L, Xing ZW (2011) The consequences of son preference and sex-selective abortion in China and other Asian countries. CMAJ 183(12):1374–1377. https://doi.org/10.1503/cmaj.101368. Epub 2011 March 14. PMID: 21402684; PMCID: PMC3168620.
Hirve SS (2004) Abortion law, policy and services in India: a critical review. Reprod Health Matters 12(24):114–121. https://doi.org/10.1016/s0968-8080(04)24017-4. PMID: 15938164
Mathai ST (1997) Making abortion safer. J Fam Welf 43(2):71–80
Nandi A, Deolalika B (2011) Does a legal ban on sex-selective abortions improve child sex ratios? Evidence from a policy change in India. J Dev Econ 103:216–228
Rahaman M, Das P, Chouhan P, Das KC, Roy A, Kapasia N (2022) Examining the rural-urban divide in predisposing, enabling, and need factors of unsafe abortion in India using Andersen's behavioral model. BMC Public Health 22(1):1–14
Rahaman M, Roy A, Chouhan P, Das KC, Rana MJ (2023) Revisiting the predisposing, enabling, and need factors of unsafe abortion in India using the Heckman Probit model. J Biosoc Sci 56(3):459–479. https://doi.org/10.1017/S002193202300024X
Stillman M, Frost J, Singh S, Moore A, Kalyanwala S (2014) Abortion in India: a literature review. Guttmacher Institute, New York
Visaria L et al (2004) Abortion in India: emerging issues from qualitative studies. Econ Polit Wkly 39(46):5044–5052
Warren MA (1973) On the moral and legal status of abortion. Monist 57(1):43–61

Chapter 7
Linkages Between Women's Education and Family Planning

Jay Saha and **Avijit Roy**

Abstract The present chapter aims to examine the influence of women's education, wealth, and mass media exposure on their use of family-planning methods within the Empowered Action Group (EAG) states of India. Data for this study are derived from the fifth National Family Health Survey (NFHS-5), conducted between 2019 and 2021 and encompassing 86,035 married women in the EAG states. The chapter employs descriptive and bivariate analyses, chi-square tests, and unadjusted and adjusted multivariable binary logistic regression analyses to explore the intricate relationships among women's education, wealth quintile, mass media exposure, and other sociodemographic variables and family-planning methods. The results show that women's education positively correlates with family planning, challenging conventional expectations. As wealth quintile increases, a notable rise in family-planning utilization occurs. Mass media exposure emerges as a significant influencer, underscoring the need for targeted campaigns. This chapter also delves into the influence of age, place of residence, social groups, and son preference on the use of family-planning methods. Policy recommendations encompass educational interventions, economic empowerment programs, and targeted media campaigns in the EAG states of India.

Keywords Women's education · Family planning · NFHS-5 · India

7.1 Introduction

India is experiencing significant changes in its dynamic demographic landscape, influenced by intricate socioeconomic factors that play roles in reproductive health decisions (Maleche et al. 2019; Sarkar 2020). Over time, a noteworthy decrease in

---

J. Saha (✉)
Department of Geography, University of Gour Banga, Malda, West Bengal, India

A. Roy
Department of Geography, Malda College, Malda, West Bengal, India

the unmet need for contraception in India has taken place, as indicated by the National Family and Health Survey (NFHS) data, showing a reduction from over 23% in NFHS-3 to 12.9% in NFHS-4. However, this decline is not uniform across states and districts. The latest NFHS-5 data highlight that the unmet needs for spacing and limiting in India were 4% and 5.4%, respectively, whereas the unmet demand for family planning stood at 9.4%. Importantly, 87.9% of the demand for contraception was met (Singh et al. 2023).

Recognizing the persistent challenges, especially in high-fertility districts across seven Empowered Action Group (EAG) states, the government of India launched Mission Parivar Vikas in 2016. Operating under the National Health Mission, this initiative aims to enhance access to family-planning services in districts where the total fertility rate (TFR) remains at three children or above. These high-needs districts are located in the states of Bihar, Uttar Pradesh, Madhya Pradesh, Rajasthan, Chhattisgarh, Jharkhand, and Assam, collectively referred to as the EAG states. The EAG states, including Bihar, Madhya Pradesh, Jharkhand, Chhattisgarh, Uttar Pradesh, Rajasthan, Uttarakhand, and Odisha, are socioeconomically less developed, contributing to 48% of India's population and facing unique challenges (Chowdhury et al. 2023; Kumar and Singh 2016). This research aims to delve into the multifaceted dynamics shaping the use of family-planning methods in the EAG states, utilizing the rich dataset of the National Family Health Survey-5.

In this context, understanding the interplay of education, wealth, and mass media exposure becomes crucial. Although the influence of these factors on family planning has been acknowledged at a national level, the specific nuances within the EAG states require a dedicated investigation. Women's education, often regarded as a global marker of progress, goes beyond empowerment to become a determinant of the choice to use family-planning methods (Haque et al. 2021). Similarly, the intricate relationship between household wealth and reproductive decisions remains understudied, particularly in the unique context of the EAG states (Smith et al. 2020). Additionally, the role of mass media in disseminating information and shaping perceptions cannot be overstated, making it a critical determinant in decision-making processes.

While previous studies have identified socioeconomic and demographic predictors of the use of family-planning methods in India, with specific attention to individual, community, and district levels, a scarcity of research has focused on the influence of women's education, wealth, and mass media exposure on family-planning methods in the EAG states (Agrahari et al. 2016; Bajwa et al. 2012; Singh et al. 2012). This chapter aims to fill this critical gap, providing nuanced insights that can inform tailored interventions and policies.

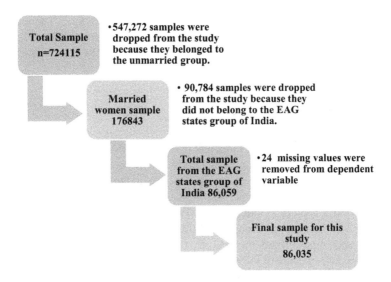

Fig. 7.1 Sample selection procedures from NFHS-5 data

7.2 Data and Methods

7.2.1 Study Design and Sample

This study relies on data from the fifth round of the National Family Health Survey, conducted between 2019 and 2021. NFHS constitutes a series of nationally representative cross-sectional surveys designed to gather data on various socioeconomic, demographic, reproductive health, maternal and child welfare, and family-planning aspects in India. NFHS-5, administered by the Ministry of Health and Family Welfare of the government of India, was overseen by the International Institute of Population Sciences (IIPS) as the nodal surveying agency. Employing a two-stage stratified sampling approach, NFHS-5 successfully interviewed 724,115 women aged 15–49 years from 636,699 households, achieving an impressive 97% response rate. For our study, we specifically focus on a total of 86,035 married women. The sample-selection procedure is shown in Fig. 7.1.

7.2.2 Outcome Variable

In our study, the outcome variable is the use of family-planning methods, including female sterilization, male sterilization, intrauterine device (IUD), injectables, pills, female condoms, male condoms, emergency contraception, diaphragm, foam/jelly, the standard-days method, lactational amenorrhea, rhythm method, withdrawal, traditional methods, and modern methods. In the NFHS survey, respondents were asked the question, "Have you used the abovementioned methods?" The responses are coded as '1' for 'yes' and '0' for 'no'. Subsequently, these variables are merged to create the binary outcome variable "family-planning method" for our study.

7.2.3 Explanatory Variables

Numerous prior studies, both in India and elsewhere, have established connections between the use of family-planning methods and women's education, household wealth quintile, mass media exposure, and other sociodemographic factors (Abreha and Zereyesus 2021; Lesthaeghe 2020; Sharifi and Khavarian-Garmsir 2020). Drawing on various theories and frameworks, such as the theory of planned behavior, social cognitive theory, demographic transition theory, ecological frameworks, and gender and empowerment frameworks, that have been presented in the past, this study incorporates a range of factors, including women's age, social groups, education level, wealth quintile(as a proxy for household income), exposure to mass media, son preference, and residence (Ajzen 2020; Bairoliya and Miller 2021; Ezenwaka et al. 2020; Hutchinson et al. 2021; Thomas and Gupta 2021).

7.2.4 Statistical Analyses

In this study, we employed descriptive and bivariate analyses to delve into the intricate relationships among women's education, wealth, and mass media exposure concerning family-planning methods. The significance of the outcome variable—i.e., family-planning method—is assessed by using a chi-square test in conjunction with women's education, wealth, mass media exposure, and other explanatory variables. Additionally, both unadjusted odds ratio (UOR) and adjusted odds ratio (AOR) multivariate binary logistic regression analyses are conducted to assess the impact of women's education, wealth, and mass media exposure on family-planning methods. The results are presented in odds ratios (ORs) with a 95% confidence interval (CI). To ensure national representativeness, individual weights are applied to the estimates. Stata version 17 is utilized for all the analyses in this study.

Table 7.1 Background characteristics and prevalence of using a family-planning method among married women

Variables	Total	Percentage (%)	Women (n)	Prevalence (%)	p-Value
Age group (years)					<0.001
Less than 30	61,674	71.68	47,993	77.82	
30 and above	24,361	28.32	20,656	84.79	
Social group					<0.001
SC	19,068	22.16	15,220	79.82	
ST	13,130	15.26	10,052	76.56	
OBC	40,151	46.67	32,200	80.20	
GEN	13,686	15.91	11,177	81.67	
Women's education level					<0.001
No education	24,290	28.23	18,980	78.14	
Primary	11,569	13.45	9354	80.85	
Secondary	39,193	45.55	31,166	79.52	
Higher	10,983	12.77	9149	83.30	
Wealth quintile					<0.001
Poorest	28,999	33.71	21,848	75.34	
Poorer	21,149	24.58	16,810	79.48	
Middle	14,953	17.38	12,253	81.94	
Richer	11,771	13.68	9807	83.31	
Richest	9163	10.65	7931	86.55	
Mass media exposure					<0.001
No	34,650	40.27	26,116	75.37	
Yes	51,385	59.73	42,533	82.77	
Son preference					<0.001
0	8037	9.34	6400	79.63	
1	52,320	60.81	41,941	80.16	
>2	25,678	29.85	20,308	79.09	
Place of residence					<0.001
Urban	13,346	15.51	11,184	83.80	
Rural	72,689	84.49	57,465	79.06	

Note: p-values are derived from Pearson's chi-square test

7.3 Results

7.3.1 Background Characteristics of the Respondents

Table 7.1 provides a comprehensive overview of the demographic and socioeconomic characteristics of the respondents in the present study. Notably, 71.68% of the women in this study are below the age of 30, the remaining 28.32% aged 30 years or older. According to the social group distribution, Other Backward Classes (OBC) form the largest group, at 46.67%, followed by Scheduled Caste (SC) at 22.16%, Scheduled Tribe (ST) at 15.26%, and general (GEN) at 15.91%. In the case of women's level of education, a significant proportion of women have secondary education (45.55%), followed by no education (28.23%), primary education (13.45%), and higher education (12.77%). According to the wealth distribution, the middle-class category has the highest percentage (17.38%), followed by the richest (10.65%), richer (13.68%), poorer (24.58%), and poorest (33.71%). On the basis of mass-media exposure, the majority of women (59.73%) have it, emphasizing its prevalence within the study population. The distribution of son preference reveals that 60.81% have one son, 29.85% have more than two sons, and 9.34% have no sons. Lastly, in terms of residence, 84.49% of respondents live in rural areas, whereas 15.51% reside in urban areas.

7.3.2 Prevalence of the Use of Family-Planning Methods Among Married Women in EAG States of India

Table 7.1 sheds light on the prevalence of the use of family-planning methods across diverse characteristics of female respondents in the study. According to an examination of the age dynamics, women aged 30 years or older demonstrate a notably higher prevalence of family-planning methods (84.79%) compared to their younger counterparts (77.82%). This discernible pattern suggests a plausible association between age and family-planning decisions, hinting at a greater proclivity among older women toward contraceptive practices. Social dynamics further contribute to the narrative, revealing distinctive disparities in family-planning prevalence across social groups. Notably, the prevalence is highest among GEN (81.67%) and OBC (80.20%), juxtaposed with lower figures among SC (79.82%) and ST (76.56%). Education emerges as a pivotal factor, with a discernible positive correlation between educational levels and family-planning usage. The prevalence rises from 78.14% for women who had no education to 83.30% for those who had attained higher education, underscoring the pivotal role of education in shaping family-planning choices. Economic well-being, as reflected in the wealth quintile, manifests as a driving force behind family-planning decisions. The prevalence increases with increasing wealth, reaching its zenith at 86.55% among the richest category. The influence of mass media exposure surfaces prominently in that women with mass media exposure (82.77%) exhibit a higher prevalence of the use of family-planning methods compared to those devoid of mass media exposure (75.37%). Contrary to expectations, the prevalence of family-planning methods shows relative consistency across different levels of son preference. This implies that son preference may not be a significant determinant influencing the choice of family-planning methods within this study population. Lastly, a noticeable urban–rural divide is evident, urban areas (83.80%) showcasing a higher prevalence of the use of family-planning methods compared to rural areas (79.06%).

Table 7.2 The influence of women's education, wealth quintile, mass media exposure, and other factors on their use of family-planning methods in EAG states of India, 2019-2021

Variables	UOR			AOR		
	Odds ratio	95% confidence interval		Odds ratio	95% confidence interval	
		Lower	Upper		Lower	Upper
Women's education level						
No education®	1.00			1.00		
Primary	1.22***	1.14	1.30	1.17***	1.09	1.25
Secondary	1.24***	1.15	1.22	1.20***	1.12	1.27
Higher	1.50***	1.40	1.61	1.22***	1.13	1.29
Wealth quintile						
Poorest®	1.00			1.00		
Poorer	1.27***	1.21	1.34	1.22***	1.16	1.29
Middle	1.53***	1.44	1.62	1.41***	1.33	1.51
Richer	1.75***	1.64	1.87	1.56***	1.45	1.68
Richest	2.29***	2.11	2.48	1.93***	1.75	2.12
Mass mediaedia exposure						
No®	1.00			1.00		
Yes	1.66***	1.59	1.73	1.45***	1.39	1.51
Age group (years)						
Less than 30®	1.00			1.00		
30 and above	1.56***	1.48	1.63	1.60***	1.52	1.68
Social group						
SC®	1.00			1.00		
ST	0.80***	0.75	0.85	0.89***	0.83	0.95
OBC	0.99	0.94	1.04	0.90***	0.86	0.95
GEN	1.10**	1.03	1.18	0.87***	0.81	0.93
Son preference						
0®	1.00			1.00		
1	1.09***	1.02	1.17	1.10***	1.03	1.18
>2	1.01	0.94	1.08	1.12***	1.04	1.21
Place of residence						
Rural®	1.00			1.00		
Urban	1.49	1.40	1.58	1.06	0.99	1.13

Note: *** if $p < 0.001$; ** if $p < 0.01$; CI = confidence interval; ® = reference category

7.3.3 The Influencing Factors of the Use of Family-Planning Methods Among Married Women

Table 7.2 provides pivotal insights into the factors influencing the use of family-planning methods among married women in the study. Comparing education levels with the reference group (no education) reveals noteworthy associations. For example, women with primary education exhibit an odds ratio (AOR: 1.17; 95% CI: 1.09,

1.25) indicating a 17% higher likelihood of utilizing family planning compared to those with no education. This positive correlation persists for secondary education (AOR: 1.20; 95% CI: 1.12, 1.27) and higher education (AOR: 1.22; 95% CI: 1.13, 1.29), emphasizing the link between education and family-planning usage. Similarly, wealth quintile categories, relative to the poorest, unveil a discernible trend. As wealth increases, the likelihood of family-planning usage rises, as evidenced by odds ratios of 1.22, 1.41, 1.56, and 1.93 for the poorer, middle, richer, and richest categories, respectively. Notably, women in the richest category (AOR: 1.93; 95% CI: 1.75, 2.12) have a 93% higher likelihood of utilizing family-planning methods compared to the poorest. Mass media exposure emerges as a significant influencer, with women exposed to mass media exhibiting a higher likelihood of using family-planning methods (AOR: 1.45; 95% CI: 1.39, 1.51). This suggests a 45% higher likelihood of family-planning usage among women with mass media exposure compared to those without. Furthermore, for women aged 30 years and above, the odds ratio (AOR: 1.60; 95% CI: 1.52, 1.68) signifies a 60% higher likelihood of family-planning usage compared to women aged less than 30 years. As a variable, son preference demonstrates moderate associations with family-planning usage. Women with one son (AOR: 1.10; 95% CI: 1.03, 1.18) and more than two sons (AOR: 1.12; 95% CI: 1.04, 1.21) show an increased likelihood of using family planning compared to those with no sons.

7.4 Discussion

This research delves into the multifaceted dynamics influencing the use of family-planning methods in the Empowered Action Group states of India, specifically examining the impact of women's education, wealth quintile, and mass media exposure. The findings illuminate the intricate interplay between these factors and sociodemographic elements within the context of EAG states.

The analysis unveils a substantial positive association between women with primary education and family planning, underscoring the pivotal role of basic education in enhancing women's access to information, autonomy, and decision-making power concerning their reproductive health. This aligns with established literature acknowledging the empowering effects of primary education on family-planning choices (Götmark and Andersson 2020). Similarly, the significant associations for secondary and higher education levels suggest that factors beyond formal education, such as cultural norms and regional variations, intricately shape family-planning decisions among women with advanced education. Banjo focused on women's empowerment and its correlation with the ideal family size in Nigeria (Banjo 2023). Banjo's study suggests that education empowers women, resulting in a preference for smaller family sizes and greater control over their reproductive decisions. In another study, Bongaarts' thorough review underscores the pivotal role of education in shaping outcomes related to family planning. Bongaarts argues that education not only affects contraceptive use but also plays a crucial role in influencing fertility preferences and reproductive decision-making (Bongaarts 2020).

The examination of mass media exposure's influence on family planning in the EAG states unravels a significant positive association. Women with mass media exposure demonstrate higher odds of adopting family-planning methods, aligning with the broader literature, which highlights the influential role of mass media in shaping health-related behaviors. Mass media emerges as a crucial channel for disseminating family-planning messages and information, and the positive correlation underscores the effectiveness of mass media campaigns in enhancing awareness and knowledge (Htay et al. 2023). This study emphasizes the potential of culturally sensitive messaging in mass media campaigns tailored to the unique sociocultural contexts within EAG states, amplifying the impact of mass media exposure on family-planning decisions. Ahinkorah et al. conducted a study that specifically explored the impact of mass media on family-planning attitudes and practices in sub-Saharan Africa (Ahinkorah 2020). The results contribute to understanding how mass media exposure can influence family-planning behaviors in distinct geographic contexts.

On the relationship between household wealth and family planning, the study categorizes wealth into quintiles. A noteworthy positive association is identified between the poorer wealth quintile and family planning, indicating that economic improvement within lower wealth strata enhances the likelihood of adopting family-planning methods. This positive correlation continues with the middle and richer quintiles, emphasizing the role of economic empowerment in influencing family-planning decisions. Notably, the richest quintile exhibits the highest association, signifying a nuanced distinction in higher wealth strata. This underscores that economic well-being, beyond basic improvement, significantly impacts reproductive choices. Goyal and Kumar's systematic review delved into interventions aimed at enhancing postpartum family planning (Goyal and Kumar 2021). Although not explicitly concentrating on wealth, the review underscores the socioeconomic context, offering insights into how economic factors might impact decisions related to family planning (Döring 2020).

In addition to education, wealth quintile, and mass media exposure, this chapter's analysis explores the influence of age, residence, social group, and son preference on family planning. The higher likelihood of family planning among women aged 30 years and above aligns with studies emphasizing the correlation between increased maternal age and the desire to limit family size (Bhatt et al. 2021). The negative associations observed for Scheduled Tribe (ST), Other Backward Classes (OBC), and general (GEN) categories concerning family planning compared to Scheduled Caste (SC) align with studies highlighting social disparities in reproductive health outcomes (Gaitatzi et al. 2020). The positive associations observed for women with more than one son reinforce existing literature on the influence of son preference on reproductive choices (Ngo 2020).

7.4.1 Strengths and Limitations

One notable strength of this study is its specific focus on the EAG states of India. This targeted approach provides valuable insights into family-planning dynamics within a socioeconomically less developed region. The contextual relevance of this focus enhances the applicability of the study's findings to other regions confronting similar challenges. The first limitation stems from the reliance on self-reported data, a common practice in survey-based studies. This introduces the potential for recall bias and social desirability bias, as participants might shape their responses on the basis of perceived societal norms rather than reflecting their actual behaviors. Second, a constraint of this study is the restriction of the sample to only married women. This limitation narrows the scope of the investigation, potentially overlooking the perspectives and experiences of unmarried women that could contribute to a more comprehensive understanding of family-planning dynamics. Another noteworthy limitation is the absence of a measurement of causality between outcomes and independent variables using cross-sectional data.

7.5 Conclusions

Our study delved into the complex dynamics influencing family planning in India's EAG states. Using NFHS-5 data, it uncovered key associations between women's education, wealth quintile, mass media exposure, and family-planning decisions. Contrary to expectations, a positive link was found between primary education and family planning. This challenges norms and emphasizes nuanced understanding. Additionally, according to this study, as household wealth quintile increased, a rise in family-planning utilization took place, highlighting the role of economic empowerment. Mass media exposure emerged as a significant influencer, stressing the need for targeted campaigns. Policy recommendations include tailored educational interventions emphasizing the importance of basic education. Economic empowerment programs are suggested, focusing on income opportunities and financial literacy. Targeted mass media campaigns addressing local norms are advised. Long-term sociocultural interventions and region-specific policies are recommended. The robust monitoring and evaluation of programs like Mission Parivar Vikas are vital, as is exploring technology integration for improved accessibility. The present study not only contributes academically but also offers practical implications. Translating findings into targeted policies can positively impact family-planning outcomes in the diverse sociocultural and economic landscape of the EAG states.Declaration

Availability of Data and Material The study uses secondary data, which are available on reasonable request at https://dhsprogram.com/data/dataset_admin/index.cfm.

Ethics Approval and Consent to Participate This chapter is based on secondary data, which are available in the public domain. Therefore, ethical approval is not required to conduct this study.

Competing Interests The authors declare that they have no competing interests.

Funding This chapter did not receive any specific grant from funding agencies in the public, commercial, or not-for-profit sectors.

References

Abreha SK, Zereyesus YA (2021) Women's empowerment and infant and child health status in sub-Saharan Africa: a systematic review. Matern Child Health J 25:95–106. https://doi.org/10.1136/bmjopen-2020-045952

Agrahari K, Mohanty SK, Chauhan RK (2016) Socioeconomic differentials in contraceptive discontinuation in India. SAGE Open 6(2):2158244016646612. https://doi.org/10.1177/2158244016646612

Ahinkorah BO (2020) Predictors of modern contraceptive use among adolescent girls and young women in sub-Saharan Africa: a mixed effects multilevel analysis of data from 29 demographic and health surveys. Contracept Reprod Med 5:1–12. https://doi.org/10.1186/s40834-020-00138-1

Ajzen I (2020) The theory of planned behavior: frequently asked questions. Hum Behav Emerg Technol 2(4):314–324. https://doi.org/10.1002/hbe2.195

Bairoliya N, Miller R (2021) Demographic transition, human capital and economic growth in China. J Econ Dyn Control 127:104117. https://doi.org/10.1016/j.jedc.2021.104117

Bajwa SK, Bajwa SJS, Ghai GK, Singh K, Singh N (2012) Knowledge, attitudes, beliefs, and perception of the north Indian population toward adoption of contraceptive practices. Asia Pac J Public Health 24(6):1002–1012. https://doi.org/10.1177/1010539511411473

Banjo OO (2023) Women's empowerment and completed fertility in Nigeria: what is the modulating effect of religion on the relationship? Womens Reprod Health 11:239–254. https://doi.org/10.1080/23293691.2023.2223825

Bhatt N, Bhatt B, Neupane B, Karki A, Bhatta T, Thapa J, Basnet LB, Budhathoki SS (2021) Perceptions of family planning services and its key barriers among adolescents and young people in Eastern Nepal: a qualitative study. PLoS One 16(5):e0252184. https://doi.org/10.1371/journal.pone.0252184

Bongaarts J (2020) Trends in fertility and fertility preferences in sub-Saharan Africa: the roles of education and family planning programs. Genus 76(1):1–15

Chowdhury S, Kasemi N, Singh A, Chakrabarty M, Singh S (2023) Decomposing the gap in undernutrition among under-five children between EAG and non-EAG states of India. Child Youth Serv Rev 145:106796. https://doi.org/10.1016/j.childyouth.2022.106796

Döring N (2020) How is the COVID-19 pandemic affecting our sexualities? An overview of the current media narratives and research hypotheses. Arch Sex Behav 49:1–14. https://doi.org/10.1007/s10508-020-01790-z

Ezenwaka U, Mbachu C, Ezumah N, Eze I, Agu C, Agu I, Onwujekwe O (2020) Exploring factors constraining utilization of contraceptive services among adolescents in Southeast Nigeria: an application of the socio-ecological model. BMC Public Health 20:1–11. https://doi.org/10.1186/s12889-020-09276-2

Gaitatzi F, Tsikouras P, Galazios G, Chalkidou A, Bothou A, Koutsogiannis M, Babageorgaka I, Nikolettos K, Zervoudis S, Nikolettos N (2020) Family planning laboratory review of factors affecting the choice of contraceptive methods in three teenagers' populations in Thrace, Greece. Arch Obstetr Gynaecol 1(1):13–22. https://doi.org/10.33696/Gynaecology.1.003

Götmark F, Andersson M (2020) Human fertility in relation to education, economy, religion, contraception, and family planning programs. BMC Public Health 20(1):1–17

Goyal K, Kumar S (2021) Financial literacy: a systematic review and bibliometric analysis. Int J Consum Stud 45(1):80–105. https://doi.org/10.1111/ijcs.12605

Haque R, Alam K, Rahman SM, Keramat SA, Al-Hanawi MK (2021) Women's empowerment and fertility decision-making in 53 low and middle resource countries: a pooled analysis of demographic and health surveys. BMJ Open 11(6):e045952. https://doi.org/10.1136/bmjopen-2020-045952

Htay ZW, Kiriya J, Sakamoto JL, Jimba M (2023) Association between women's empowerment and unmet family planning needs in low-and middle-income countries in Southeast Asia: a cross-sectional study. Womens Reprod Health 11:17–32. https://doi.org/10.1080/23293691.2023.2174822

Hutchinson PL, Anaba U, Abegunde D, Okoh M, Hewett PC, Johansson EW (2021) Understanding family planning outcomes in northwestern Nigeria: analysis and modeling of social and behavior change factors. BMC Public Health 21(1):1–20. https://doi.org/10.1186/s12889-021-11211-y

Kumar V, Singh P (2016) Access to healthcare among the Empowered Action Group (EAG) states of India: current status and impeding factors. Natl Med J India 29(5):267

Lesthaeghe R (2020) The second demographic transition, 1986–2020: sub-replacement fertility and rising cohabitation—a global update. Genus 76(1):1–38. https://doi.org/10.1186/s41118-020-00077-4

Maleche D, Ochanda D, Arudo MJ (2019) A comparative analysis of determinants of unmet need for current contraceptive practice among women of reproductive age living in formal and informal settlements of Eldoret town, Kenya. J Health Med Nurs 4(4):58–76

Ngo AP (2020) Effects of Vietnam's two-child policy on fertility, son preference, and female labor supply. J Popul Econ 33(3):751–794. https://doi.org/10.1007/s00148-019-00766-1

Sarkar R (2020) Association of urbanization with demographic dynamics in India. GeoJournal 85(3):779–803

Sharifi A, Khavarian-Garmsir AR (2020) The COVID-19 pandemic: impacts on cities and major lessons for urban planning, design, and management. Sci Total Environ 749:142391. https://doi.org/10.1016/j.scitotenv.2020.142391

Singh PK, Rai RK, Alagarajan M, Singh L (2012) Determinants of maternity care services utilization among married adolescents in rural India. PLoS One 7(2):e31666. https://doi.org/10.1371/journal.pone.0031666

Singh SK, Kashyap GC, Sharma H, Mondal S, Legare CH (2023) Changes in discourse on unmet need for family planning among married women in India: evidence from NFHS-5 (2019–2021). Sci Rep 13(1):20464. https://doi.org/10.1038/s41598-023-47191-9

Smith E, Sundstrom B, Delay C (2020) Listening to women: understanding and challenging systems of power to achieve reproductive justice in South Carolina. J Soc Issues 76(2):363–390. https://doi.org/10.1111/josi.12378

Thomas A, Gupta V (2021) Social capital theory, social exchange theory, social cognitive theory, financial literacy, and the role of knowledge sharing as a moderator in enhancing financial well-being: from bibliometric analysis to a conceptual framework model. Front Psychol 12:664638. https://doi.org/10.3389/fpsyg.2021.664638

Part III
Contraceptive Dynamics

Chapter 8
Understanding the Dynamics of Modern Contraception Discontinuation Among Women in India

Nanigopal Kapasia and Swagata Ghosh

Abstract Contraceptive discontinuation as a concerning issue in the domain of sexual and reproductive health simply indicates switching from one contraceptive method to another or the termination of a method. Through the dynamics of contraception discontinuation, this chapter aims to explore the levels, patterns, and determinants of the discontinuation of cause-specific modern reversible contraception in India. The chapter used data from the fifth round of the National Family Health Survey (NFHS-5), conducted in 2019–2021, and took a weighted sample of 53,213 women aged 15–49 years. The weighted frequencies and percentages for explanatory variables, bivariate results for causes behind contraceptive discontinuation, and multivariable binary logistic regression were performed to examine the association between explanatory variables and different causes for contraceptive discontinuation. Reasons for contraceptive discontinuation were desire for a child (41.7%), adverse side effects on health (14.1%), and spousal out-migration (11.7%). Older age, higher age at marriage, contraceptive methods used, women's residing in rural places, women's education, the wealth status of women, and their family size are the most significant factors in discontinuing contraceptives. The chapter's findings suggest that reproductive women be aware of newly launched modern reversible contraceptive methods and their accessibility and suggest using contraceptives under proper guidance from professional medical providers and health providers.

Keywords Contraceptive methods · Contraceptive discontinuation · Reproductive women · India

N. Kapasia (✉)
Department of Geography, Malda College, Malda, West Bengal, India

S. Ghosh
Department of Geography, University of Gour Banga, Malda, West Bengal, India

8.1 Introduction

The contraceptive discontinuation simply indicates switching from one contraceptive method to another or the termination of a method. The high contraceptive discontinuation rate is a concerning issue in the domain of reproductive health (Ali and Cleland 2010). Discontinuation is a significant determinant of contraceptive prevalence, which is emphasized in the United Nations' Sustainable Development Goal 3 (Dadzie et al. 2022), on the decline in unplanned pregnancies and on maternal and newborn deaths (Budhathoki et al. 2017). Moreover, contraceptive discontinuation is intricately linked to unwanted fertility (Rahaman et al. 2022a, b) and unsafe abortions (Rahaman et al. 2024), both of which are serious threats to maternal and child health (Ram et al. 2022). Shockingly, in regions like sub-Saharan Africa, Western Asia, Northern Africa, and Oceania (excluding Australia and New Zealand), approximately one in ten women have experienced an unwanted pregnancy each year over the past three decades (Bearak et al. 2020). Furthermore, in India, among 48.1 million pregnancies (2015), 54% and 32% were live births and induced abortions and 14% miscarriages (Singh et al. 2018).

In combating these challenges, modern reversible contraceptive methods (short-acting, long-acting, and permanent forms) have gained popularity for preventing or delaying childbirth (Rahaman et al. 2022a, b). While female sterilization remains the leading family-planning method in India (Rahaman et al. 2022a, b), long-acting reversible contraception stands out as one of the most effective options (Festin 2020). The failure rate of modern methods of contraception is much lower than that of other methods (Bradley et al. 2019).

The International Conference at Cairo underscored the right of both men and women to access safe, accessible, and effective birth control methods of their choice to address the issues of discontinuation and high unmet needs (United Nations 1994). However, a recent study revealed that contraception discontinuation rates are 38%, 55%, and 64% over the past 1, 2, and 3 years, respectively, in low- and middle-income countries (Dadzie et al. 2022). Notably, the rates of discontinuation vary among contraceptive methods, condoms, and intrauterine devices (IUDs) experiencing the highest and lowest discontinuation rates (50% vs. 12%) within 12 months. Additionally, discontinuation rates for pills, injectables, periodic abstinence, and withdrawal methods were all around 40% within the same time frame. In the context of India, contraceptive discontinuation remains a longstanding issue, prompting serious policy debates (Rana and Goli 2021; Danna et al. 2021). Recent research calculated a discontinuation rate for any method (32.6%) and modern spacing methods (43.5%) in India (Nayak et al. 2021), primarily due to pregnancy. Furthermore, method-specific causes revealed that condoms, followed by pills, injectables, IUDs, and implants, had the highest discontinuation rates in India.

Previous studies have examined predictors of reversible contraception use to limit births (Rahaman et al. 2022a, b) and to meet unmet needs for spacing births

(Rahaman et al. 2022a, b) and have examined reasons for contraceptive discontinuation (Nayak et al. 2021), highlighting health-related causes, fears of side effects, a lack of accessibility and availability, service costs, and religious beliefs as significant factors (Bellizzi et al. 2015; Diamond-Smith et al. 2012; Sedgh et al. 2016; Thobani et al. 2019). However, a detailed analysis of method-specific modern reversible contraception rates remains limited in the Indian context, hampering researchers' understanding of the dynamics of contraception discontinuation in terms of population and space. Given India's vast size and diverse population, culture, and practices, some have hypothesized that cause-specific modern spacing contraception could vary significantly across different regions. Consequently, this chapter aims to observe the levels, patterns, and determinants of people's discontinuation of cause-specific modern reversible contraception in India.

8.2 Data and Methods

8.2.1 Data

This chapter used data from the fifth round of the National Family Health Survey (NFHS-5), 2019–2021. The NFHS-5 was a representative cross-sectional survey on a national scale administered by the Ministry of Health and Family Welfare (MoHFW), government of India (International Institute for Population Sciences and ICF 2022). The MoHFW designated the IIPS, Mumbai, as a nodal surveying agency. Samples from the districts were collected to represent the national scenario; from each district, primary sampling units for rural areas and Census Enumeration Blocks (CEBs) for urban areas were selected, adopting a probability-proportional-to-sample-size approach, and finally, Households (HHs) were chosen by using systematic random sampling method. The present chapter's findings are based on a total weighted sample of 53,213 women aged 15–49 years without missing information about the reason for their most recent contraceptive discontinuation.

8.2.2 Study Variables

The outcome variable used for this chapter was the cause of contraceptive discontinuation among women of 15–49 years. This variable was considered as the percentage of reproductive-aged women who had discontinued their use of modern reversible contraceptive methods 1 year after starting to use it (International Institute for Population Sciences and ICF 2022).

8.2.2.1 Explanatory Variables

Corresponding to previous studies (Azmat et al. 2013; Nayak et al. 2021), the present chapter included a range of explanatory variables, which includes women's age (15–19, 20–24, 25–29, and above 30 years), age at marriage (below 18, 18–24, and above 24 years), caste (SC, ST, OBC, and general), religion (Hindu, Muslim, Christian, and others), educational attainment (no education, primary, secondary, or higher), residential area (urban and rural), HH size (1–4, 5–8, and above 9 members), wealth status (poorest, poorer, middle, richer, and richest), knowledge of contraception (no and yes), pregnancy loss (no and yes), contraceptive methods used (pill, IUD/injection, male condom, and others), and region (north, central, east, northeast, west, and south). The contraceptive methods used were contextual-level variables, and the remaining variables were individual-level variables.

8.2.3 Statistical Analysis

Graphical presentation (bar chart) was used to show the different causes responsible for contraception discontinuation and show method-specific contraceptive discontinuation. The different method-specific causes of contraceptive discontinuation across (Union Territories) UTs and states were presented in weighted percentage. The weighted frequencies and percentages were presented to explain the prevalence of contraceptive discontinuation among reproductive-aged women. Further, this chapter presented the bivariate results for the causes behind contraceptive discontinuation across the explanatory variables by using the chi-square test. Finally, multivariable binary logistic regression was carried out to separately study the association between explanatory variables and different causes of contraceptive discontinuation as outcome variables that were presented as adjusted odds ratios (AORs). Data analyses were performed using Stata version 16 and MS Office 2016.

8.3 Result

8.3.1 Distribution of Contraceptive Discontinuation

Among the reasons for contraceptive discontinuation, the most common is natural causes, specifically becoming pregnant due to a desire for a child (41.7%) (Fig. 8.1). This is followed by health-related causes or side effects (14.1%), reasons related to the unsuitability of the method (12.0%), and causes related to spousal out-migration (11.7%).

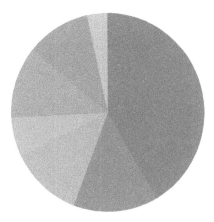

- Natural causes
- Causes for not suitable method
- Causes of Husband Migration
- Other causes
- Health related causes
- Lack of Affordability, accessibility and availability
- Causes of husband disapproval

Fig. 8.1 Causes of contraceptive discontinuation among women 15–49 years

8.3.2 Cause-Specific Discontinuation

The results reveal that 38.0% of oral pill users had discontinued its usage to become pregnant, 20.8% of users had stopped for health-related issues, and 11.7% had stopped because it was a less-effective method (Table 8.1). In addition, women who used IUD/injection had discontinued because of adverse side effects (28.1%) and because they considered it not a suitable method (15.9%). Condom users stopped using them because of spousal out-migration (13.1%) and refusal by spouses (12.3%). Eventually, other modern method users had also discontinued due to health issues and because it was a less-effective method.

8.3.3 Geographical Variation in Causes for Contraceptive Discontinuation

Figure 8.2 reveals the state-wise scenario for contraceptive discontinuation. The discontinuation rate for side effects and health concerns was especially higher in Sikkim (29.3%) and Tripura (29.3%) than in the northeastern hill states, namely Goa, Tamil Nadu, Odisha, Andhra Pradesh, Punjab, Chandigarh, Haryana, West Bengal, and Jharkhand. For the states/UTs, contraceptive discontinuation due to using an ineffective method ranges between 6.1% for Goa and 21.2% for Tamil Nadu, and it was also relatively high in Rajasthan, Chhattisgarh, Madhya Pradesh,

Table 8.1 Method-specific causes of contraceptive discontinuation among women (aged 15–49) in India, NFHS-5, 2019–2021

Contraceptive method discontinued	Natural causes	Health-related causes	Causes of an unsuitable method	Lack of affordability, accessibility, and availability	Causes of spousal out-migration	Causes of spousal disapproval	Other causes	Total
Pill	38.0	20.8	11.7	5.7	10.9	9.6	3.5	100
IUD/injection	34.9	28.1	15.9	3.8	6.8	6.1	4.4	100
Male condom	45.1	7.8	11.3	7.3	13.1	12.3	3.1	100
Other modern method	34.1	18.2	16.9	4.4	8.4	12.2	5.8	100
Total	41.7	14.1	12.1	6.4	11.7	10.7	3.4	100

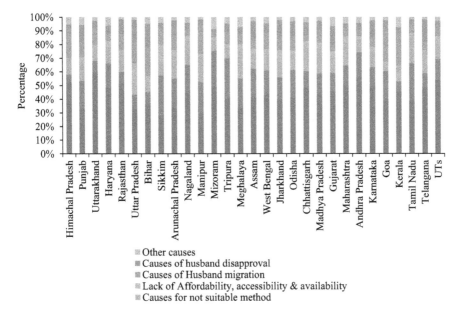

Fig. 8.2 State/UT-wise scenario of contraceptive discontinuation among women aged 15–49 years in India, NFHS-5, 2019–2021

and Maharashtra. The reason related to a lack of affordability, accessibility, and availability for discontinuation was predominantly found in Uttar Pradesh (14.6%), Sikkim (13.7%), and Jharkhand, among others. The discontinuation for spousal out-migration tends to be high in Kerala (26.3%), Goa (22.4%), Himachal Pradesh (21.4%), Bihar (21.05%), Manipur (20.9%), Punjab, Uttarakhand, Uttar Pradesh, Tripura, West Bengal, and Odisha. Discontinuation due to using a method disliked by a spouse was somewhat common in Uttar Pradesh (15.7%), Bihar (17.1%), Assam, Jharkhand, Karnataka, and Telangana.

8.3.4 Prevalence Rate for Causes of Contraceptive Discontinuation Among Women Aged 15–49 Years in India

Regarding reasons for discontinuations, the most common is wanting to become pregnant, which was predominantly observed among younger women, aged 15–19 years (51.8%), and decreases with increasing age (Table 8.2). Contrary to this natural reason, discontinuation due to adverse side effects on health was found more commonly among women aged 30 years and above than among younger women (17.6% vs. 11.3%) and more commonly among urban women than among their rural counterparts (15.1% vs. 13.6%). The incidence of no contraception use

Table 8.2 Percentage distribution of causes of contraceptive discontinuation among women 15–49 years according to background characteristics

Explanatory variables	Natural causes	Health-related causes	Causes of unsuitable method	Lack of affordability, accessibility, and availability	Causes of spousal out-migration	Causes of spousal disapproval	Other causes
Woman's age	*p*-value <0.01						
15–19	51.8	11.3	7.2	5.4	13.5	8.6	2.1
20–24	50.5	11.3	10.2	5.1	10.3	9.5	2.9
25–29	48.1	11.9	11.3	5.2	10.6	10.2	2.6
Above 30	31.0	17.6	14.0	8.2	13.2	11.8	4.2
Age at marriage or cohabitation	*p*-value <0.01						
Below 18	36.4	16.0	12.8	7.7	12.5	11.4	3.5
18–24	44.0	13.2	11.8	5.9	11.4	10.4	3.2
Above 24	46.0	14.5	10.7	5.4	10.4	10.1	3.6
Women's education	*p*-value <0.01						
No education	33.8	13.8	10.8	10.3	14.5	14.0	2.9
Primary	39.5	15.5	12.3	6.9	11.5	10.7	3.6
Secondary	42.8	14.7	12.7	5.7	10.6	10.2	3.3
Higher	47.8	11.8	11.4	4.4	12.1	9.1	3.5
Place of residence	*p*-value <0.01						
Urban	45.4	15.1	13.1	4.1	9.8	9.2	3.5
Rural	40.0	13.6	11.5	7.6	12.6	11.6	3.2
Social group	*p*-value <0.01						
SC	41.3	14.7	12.1	6.6	11.1	11.2	3.2
ST	47.2	14.6	13.9	6.0	7.1	8.1	3.2
OBC	40.2	12.8	11.5	7.5	12.8	12.1	3.1
Gen	42.7	15.3	12.4	4.9	11.7	9.2	3.8
Religion	*p*-value <0.01						
Hindu	41.3	14.1	12.4	6.6	11.5	10.9	3.2
Muslim	44.0	13.0	9.9	6.1	13.0	10.9	3.2
Christian	40.0	18.7	16.2	2.1	11.4	5.6	5.9
Others	41.0	17.3	13.9	4.9	8.6	9.1	5.3
HHs size	*p*-value <0.01						
1–4 members	39.1	16.1	12.7	5.5	12.6	10.2	3.8
5–8 members	42.6	13.5	12.0	6.6	11.1	11.1	3.2
Above 9 members	44.4	11.4	10.8	7.8	12.1	11.1	2.5

(continued)

Table 8.2 (continued)

Explanatory variables	Natural causes	Health-related causes	Causes of unsuitable method	Lack of affordability, accessibility, and availability	Causes of spousal out-migration	Causes of spousal disapproval	Other causes
Wealth index	p-value <0.01						
Poorest	37.7	13.4	11.0	9.1	13.3	11.9	3.6
Poorer	38.3	14.5	11.5	8.3	12.5	11.9	3.1
Middle	42.2	14.5	11.9	6.5	10.8	11.1	3.1
Richer	43.9	14.0	12.4	5.2	11.6	10.2	2.8
Richest	45.6	14.1	13.3	3.6	10.5	9.1	3.9
Knowledge of contraception	p-value <0.01						
No	40.1	14.9	11.7	6.9	12.3	10.4	3.9
Yes	42.3	13.8	12.2	6.3	11.4	10.8	3.1
Pregnancy loss	p-value <0.01						
No	41.4	13.4	12.1	6.7	11.8	11.2	3.3
Yes	42.8	16.5	11.9	5.2	11.3	9.1	3.3

was higher among women of a general caste (15.1%) and those who had experienced a pregnancy loss (16.5%). Unsuitable and ineffective methods played an important role in discontinuing contraceptive use among women aged 30 years above and 15–19 years, where the older age group discontinued at nearly double the rate of that of the younger group (14.0% vs. 7.2%), and this was even higher among the richest compared to poorer women (13.3% vs. 11.0%) and compared to women who had sufficient knowledge about any method of contraception (12.2%). The use of contraceptives depended mostly on individuals' affordability and physical accessibility and availability. The prevalence rate of contraceptive discontinuation among women with no education was found to be 10.3% vs. 4.4% among higher-educated women; among women residing in rural areas vs. those in urban areas, 7.6% vs. 4.1%; and among women in the poorest wealth quintile of HHs vs. the richest wealth quintile of HHs, 9.1% vs. 3.6%. Spousal out-migration is one of the prime causes of contraceptive discontinuation for users. The rate was proportionately higher for rural women than urban women (12.6% vs. 9.8%), higher for the poorest women than the richest (13.3% vs. 10.5%), and higher among Muslim women (13.0%) than among women of any other religion. Spousal dislike/disapproval for any method based on its ineffectiveness is the leading cause of contraceptive discontinuation. This was experienced by women who were uneducated (14.0%), who resided in rural areas (11.6%), and those belonging to the poorest households (11.9%).

8.3.5 Likelihood of Contraception Discontinuation

The results (Table 8.3) show that older women (above 30 years) are 1.85 times more likely to discontinue for health issues than younger women (15–29 years) are. Women who married at ages older than 24 years were less likely to discontinue contraceptives (OR: 0.75, CI: 0.68–0.82) than women who married at ages younger than 18 years. Women belonging to the Scheduled Tribe category had lower odds of discontinuation (OR: 0.83, CI: 0.76–0.92) than Scheduled Caste women. Women's wealth quintile was positively associated with the discontinuation of contraceptive use, where the richest women were 40% more likely to discontinue and switch to other methods for health problems compared to poorest women. Surprisingly, IUD/injection users had nearly 1.5 times higher odds (OR: 1.52, CI: 1.42–1.62) than oral pill users. Like health issues, women older than 30 years are 1.6-fold more likely to discontinue due to the lack of affordability, accessibility, and availability of methods that they choose. Women living in rural areas (OR: 1.28, CI: 1.15–1.43) were more likely to stop contraceptive usage due to the lack of accessibility and availability of methods than women in urban areas were. The household's wealth status had a significant association with contraceptive discontinuation. Richer women were less likely to discontinue than poorer women because richer women can afford effective contraception methods. Women who knew about contraception (OR: 1.15, CI: 1.06–1.25) were more likely to experience contraceptive cessation. The results show that the odds of discontinuation because of a method was insufficiently effective were nearly 2.5 times higher among the women aged 30 years or older (OR: 2.53, CI: 2.02–3.18) than among young women. Women with primary (OR: 1.19, CI: 1.08–1.31) and secondary (OR: 1.15, CI: 1.06–1.24) levels of education were more likely to stop contraception usage because of its effectiveness. As a method-specific cause, IUD/injection users had nearly 1.3 times higher odds (OR: 1.31, CI: 1.20–1.42) of discontinuation than pill users. On contraceptive discontinuation because of male partner refusal, women aged 30 years and above were 55% more likely to discontinue than younger women were. Higher-educated women experienced a significantly lower rate of discontinuation (OR: 0.74, CI: 0.66–0.82) due to their spouse's refusal of contraceptive use than women with no education. Women residing in the northeast region (OR: 1.72, CI: 1.54–1.92) had nearly 1.7 times higher odds of discontinuation than did women who live in the northern region of India. Contraceptive cessation due to spousal out-migration prevailed mostly among rural women (OR: 1.14, CI: 1.05–1.23), unlike their urban counterparts. Finally, women living with more than nine family members were less likely to discontinue.

Table 8.3 Likelihood of discontinuation of contraception among women 15–49 years according to background characteristics

Socioeconomic background	Health-related causes OR[95% CI]	Lack of affordability, accessibility, and availability causes OR[95% CI]	Unsuitable method–related causes OR[95% CI]	Causes of spousal disapproval OR[95% CI]	Causes of spousal out-migration OR[95% CI]
Woman's age					
15–29[a]					
20–24	1.13[0.92–1.39]	0.91[0.70–1.18]	1.56[b][1.24–1.96]	1.15[0.93–1.41]	0.74[0.62–0.89]
25–29	1.17[0.96–1.44]	1.08[0.83–1.40]	1.82[b][1.45–2.29]	1.27[1.04–1.56]	0.81[0.68–0.98]
Above 30	1.85[b][1.51–2.27]	1.60[b][1.24–2.08]	2.53[b][2.02–3.18]	1.55[b][1.26–1.91]	1.02[0.85–1.23]
Age at marriage or cohabitation					
Below 18[a]					
18–24	0.92[0.87–0.97]	0.84[b][0.77–0.91]	0.83[b][0.78–0.88]	0.91[0.85–0.96]	0.92[0.86–0.98]
Above 24	0.75[b][0.68–0.82]	0.83[0.72–0.96]	0.62[b][0.56–0.69]	0.86[b][0.77–0.96]	0.80[b][0.72–0.90]
Place of residence					
Urban[a]					
Rural	0.91[0.85–0.97]	1.28[b][1.15–1.43]	1.01[0.94–1.08]	1.17[b][1.09–1.27]	1.14[b][1.05–1.23]
Social group					
SC[a]					
ST	0.83[b][0.76–0.92]	0.95[0.83–1.09]	1.21[b][1.10–1.33]	0.77[b][0.69–0.86]	0.84[0.75–0.95]
OBC	0.91[0.85–0.98]	1.06[0.96–1.17]	0.97[0.90–1.05]	1.04[0.96–1.12]	1.11[1.03–1.21]
Gen	0.98[0.910–1.06]	0.97[0.86–1.09]	1.01[0.93–1.10]	0.91[0.83–0.99]	1.16[b][1.06–1.26]
Religion					
Hindu[a]					
Muslim	0.85[b][0.79–0.91]	1.21[b][1.10–1.35]	0.73[b][0.67–0.80]	1.07[0.99–1.16]	1.01[0.93–1.10]
Christian	0.99[0.88–1.11]	1.09[0.87–1.37]	1.12[0.99–1.27]	0.67[b][0.57–0.78]	1.29[1.08–1.54]
Others	1.25[b][1.12–1.39]	1.54[b][1.29–1.83]	1.05[0.93–1.17]	1.04[0.91–1.19]	0.98[0.83–1.15]

(continued)

Table 8.3 (continued)

Socioeconomic background	Health-related causes OR[95% CI]	Lack of affordability, accessibility, and availability causes OR[95% CI]	Unsuitable method–related causes OR[95% CI]	Causes of spousal disapproval OR[95% CI]	Causes of spousal out-migration OR[95% CI]
Women's education					
No education[a]					
Primary	1.07[0.98–1.17]	0.87[0.77–0.99]	1.19[b][1.08–1.31]	0.82[b][0.74–0.90]	0.89[0.80–0.98]
Secondary	1.02[0.95–1.10]	0.97[0.88–1.07]	1.15[b][1.06–1.24]	0.82[b][0.76–0.89]	0.97[0.89–1.05]
Higher	0.85[b][0.76–0.94]	0.91[0.79–1.05]	0.96[0.86–1.07]	0.74[b][0.66–0.82]	1.12[1.00–1.25]
HHs size					
1–4 members[a]					
5–8 members	0.85[b][0.81–0.90]	1.02[0.94–1.10]	0.99[0.93–1.05]	1.05[0.98–1.11]	0.78[b][0.73–0.83]
Above 9 members	0.79[b][0.73–0.86]	1.15[b][1.02–1.29]	0.96[0.88–1.05]	1.03[0.94–1.13]	0.78[b][0.71–0.85]
Wealth index					
Poorest[a]					
Poorer	1.13[1.05–1.22]	0.87[0.78–0.96]	1.05[0.97–1.15]	1.02[0.94–1.11]	1.01[0.92–1.10]
Middle	1.18[b][1.08–1.29]	0.74[b][0.66–0.83]	1.12[1.02–1.22]	1.10[1.00–1.21]	0.99[0.90–1.09]
Richer	1.24[b][1.13–1.36]	0.64[b][0.57–0.73]	1.08[0.98–1.20]	1.08[0.97–1.19]	1.13[1.02–1.25]
Richest	1.40[b][1.26–1.56]	0.43[b][0.37–0.51]	1.16[1.04–1.30]	0.98[0.87–1.11]	0.98[0.87–1.10]
Knowledge of contraception					
No[a]					
Yes	0.95[0.90–1.01]	1.15[b][1.06–1.25]	1.01[0.95–1.07]	1.14[b][1.07–1.22]	0.97[0.91–1.04]
Pregnancy loss					
No[a]					
Yes	1.16[b][1.09–1.23]	0.77[b][0.70–0.85]	0.92[0.86–0.99]	0.73[b][0.68–0.79]	0.92[0.86–0.99]
Reversible modern method					
Pill[a]					

8 Understanding the Dynamics of Modern Contraception Discontinuation...

IUD/Injection	1.52[b][1.42–1.62]	0.73[b][0.64–0.84]	1.31[b][1.20–1.42]	0.70[b][0.62–0.78]	
Male condom	0.34[b][0.32–0.36]	1.08[0.99–1.17]	1.09[1.02–1.16]	1.51[1.41–1.62]	
Other method	0.90[0.67–1.21]	0.68[0.39–1.21]	1.44[1.05–1.98]	1.50[1.06–2.12]	
Region					
North[a]					
Central	0.99[0.92–1.07]	2.59[b][2.33–2.88]	0.94[0.87–1.02]	1.63[b][1.50–1.77]	1.42[1.32–1.54]
East	1.17[b][1.07–1.27]	0.73[b][0.63–0.85]	0.98[0.89–1.08]	1.46[b][1.32–1.62]	1.33[1.21–1.46]
Northeast	1.41[b][1.29–1.55]	0.63[b][0.53–0.74]	1.00[0.91–1.11]	1.72[b][1.54–1.92]	0.76[0.68–0.85]
West	1.16[1.05–1.29]	1.02[0.86–1.21]	1.13[1.02–1.25]	1.27[b][1.13–1.43]	0.55[0.47–0.63]
South	1.00[0.90–1.12]	0.56[b][0.44–0.72]	1.23[b][1.10–1.38]	1.45[b][1.27–1.65]	0.80[0.70–0.91]

[a] Reference category
[b] Significant level: $p \leq 0.001$

8.3.6 Discussion

This chapter has gained insights into the levels, patterns, and determinants of cause-specific modern reversible method discontinuations in India. Along with previous relevant studies (Thobani et al. 2019; Bellizzi et al. 2020), the results show different causes of contraceptive discontinuation, such as the desire to become pregnant as a natural cause, causes related to health issues, causes from unsuitable and effective methods, a lack of affordability and accessibility, causes from spousal out-migration, and the disapproval of methods by partners. The age of women is a leading factor of contraceptive discontinuation, which is reflected in previous research (Begum et al. 2021; Bradley et al. 2009). Importantly, the probable explanation is that younger women are more inclined toward their education, careers, and personal development rather than parenthood, so they use contraception consistently. However, older women are conscious of the amount of time the have left to conceive and decide to stop contraception usage to become pregnant. Conversely, older women who have reached their desired family size opt for permanent contraceptive methods. Wanting a more effective method and wanting a new method after their current one was refused by a partner were also two other reasons for discontinuing contraceptives (Adedini and Omisakin 2023). Women also stop contraception usage for health reasons. In our chapter, nearly 14% of contraceptive users discontinued the modern reversible methods of contraception for health reasons. However, our study established that women who used IUD/Injection were 1.52 times more likely to discontinue for health issues than oral pill users were. Moreover, older women are advised against the use of hormonal contraception because it might come with higher risks of cardiovascular issues, because it is inconvenient to access and use, because it requires professional health providers to access it, or because of adverse side effects on health. These were consistent with previous studies (Nascimento Chofakian et al. 2019; Gupta et al. 2023; Felker-Kantor et al. 2023). Studies have shown the many potential health problems causing by continuing the use of certain contraceptives, problems such as irregular bleeding, depression, weight gain (Bellizzi et al. 2020), amenorrhea, the absence of menstrual periods (Weldemariam et al. 2019), headache, and vomiting, among others (Tolesa et al. 2015). Even more research has reported that some women experience earlier pregnancy loss because of health problems and stopped using contraception (Puri et al. 2015). Furthermore, women's place of residence was associated with contraception discontinuation. Women in rural areas were 28% more likely to discontinue, because of limited access to healthcare facilities (especially for contraceptive services), transportation issues, and the limited availability of certain contraceptive methods. This finding is similar to those in many previous studies (Escamilla et al. 2019; Agrahari et al. 2016; Bradley et al. 2009; Begum et al. 2021). However, other study (Kupoluyi et al. 2023) has established that low discontinuation was found among women who lived near health facilities and those who had visited one in the past 12 months when they live in rural areas. In addition, another cause of women's discontinuation was their spouse's being away from home (Samanta and Munda 2023). The wealth quintile was also linked with contraception discontinuation. Unsurprisingly, poorer women were 23% more likely to discontinue because of affordability than richer women were. Previous literature (Agrahari et al. 2016; Bearak and Jones 2017; Escamilla et al. 2019; Begum et al. 2017) has shown that wealthier women can afford effective methods, gain better access to comprehensive healthcare services (i.e., family-planning counseling and reproductive health education), and can pay transportation costs to access services that lead to the continuation of contraception. Conversely, other previous works (Nayak et al. 2021; Ghule et al. 2015) have found evidence indicating that women in the poor wealth quintile and less-educated women are more likely to discontinue, leading to unwanted births. Importantly, the educational status of women also influences contraception discontinuation. Our findings indicate that poor, educated women are much more prone to discontinue due to health issues and less-effective methods, and they are also more likely to discontinue because of their partner's preferences. This result aligns with that of other studies carried out in different settings (Mekonnen and Wubneh 2020; Nkonde et al. 2023). Contrarily, women with more education have more awareness of contraceptive options and of consistent contraception usage for limiting family size, and they are more likely to adhere to their chosen methods after consulting with their spouses. This finding collaborates other studies' findings (Compton et al. 2023; Agbana et al. 2023).

Moreover, the Ministry of Health and Family Welfare has recently taken great initiative in promoting modern contraceptive methods and providing them free of cost ("Antara" for injectable contraceptives and "Chhaya" for contraceptive pills), has launched a system for managing the supply and distribution of contraceptives (the Family-Planning Logistics Management Information System, or FP-LMIS), and has introduced family-planning strategies (Mission Parivar Vikas) to improve access to contraceptives, to increase awareness of family planning, to avoid undesirable pregnancies, to reduce maternal and infant deaths, and to reduce the total fertility rate. The government took the initiative on access to modern contraceptive methods by providing them free of cost or at a subsidized rate at health centers. People can choose from among many contraceptive methods without consulting health providers, which reflects the concern of adverse health issues. As a result, women are inclined to discontinue a contraception method or to switch to other effective methods of contraceptives.

8.3.7 Conclusion

This chapter found that a high proportion of women had discontinued modern contraception so that they could become pregnant or because of adverse side effects on their health. As a method-specific cause, women mostly discontinued oral pills, IUDs/injectables, male condoms, and less-effective methods for health reasons. Older age, women's older age at marriage, women residing in rural places, women's education, the wealth status of women, and their family size were the most significant factors to their discontinuing contraceptives. To better promote modern reversible contraceptives, healthcare providers need to tackle the discontinuation of contraception through counseling and both adequate and precise information on failure to continue and on side effects, for short-term users and for the sake of strengthening the use of contraception among women who are still at risk of becoming pregnant. The Ministry of Family and Health Welfare (MoFHW) needs to pay attention to promoting choice-based contraceptive availability, accessibility, and affordability with subsidies to reduce the discontinuation of contraception. The instructive message here for policymakers is to increase community-based family-planning outreach on contraceptive discontinuation and maternal healthcare services.

Declaration

Availability of Data and Material Data and materials for this chapter are sourced from publicly available secondary sources, accessible at https://dhsprogram.com/methodology/survey/survey-display-541.cfm. Interested individuals can register at the provided link to freely download the necessary data.

Ethics Approval and Consent to Participate This chapter is based on secondary data, which are available in the public domain. Therefore, ethical approval is not required to conduct this study.

Competing Interests The authors declare that they have no competing interests.

Funding This chapter did not receive any specific grant from funding agencies in the public, commercial, or not-for-profit sectors.

References

Adedini SA, Omisakin OA (2023) Comparing the reasons for contraceptive discontinuation between parenting adolescents and young women in sub-Saharan Africa: a multilevel analysis. Reprod Health 20(1):115

Agbana RD, Michael TO, Ojo TF (2023) Family planning method discontinuation among Nigerian women: evidence from the Nigeria demographic and health survey 2018. J Taibah Univ Med Sci 18(1):117–124

Agrahari K, Mohanty SK, Chauhan RK (2016) Socio-economic differentials in contraceptive discontinuation in India. SAGE Open 6(2):2158244016646612. https://doi.org/10.1177/2158244016646612

Ali MM, Cleland J (2010) Contraceptive switching after method-related discontinuation: levels and differentials. Stud Fam Plan 41(2):129–133. https://www.jstor.org/stable/25681353

Azmat SK, Hameed W, Mustafa G, Hussain W, Ahmed A, Bilgrami M (2013) IUD discontinuation rates, switching behavior, and user satisfaction: findings from a retrospective analysis of a mobile outreach service program in Pakistan. Int J Womens Health 5:19–27. https://doi.org/10.2147/IJWH.S36785

Bearak JM, Jones RK (2017) Did contraceptive use patterns change after the Affordable Care Act? A descriptive analysis. Womens Health Issues 27(3):316–321

Bearak J et al (2020) Unintended pregnancy and abortion by income, region, and the legal status of abortion: estimates from a comprehensive model for 1990–2019. Lancet Glob Health 8(9):e1152–e1161. https://doi.org/10.1016/S2214-109X(20)30315-6

Begum T, Rahman A, Nababan H, Hoque DME, Khan AF, Ali T, Anwar I (2017) Indications and determinants of caesarean section delivery: evidence from a population-based study in Matlab, Bangladesh. PLoS One 12(11):e0188074. https://doi.org/10.1371/journal.pone.0188074

Begum S, Chaurasia H, Moray KV, Joshi B (2021) Predictors of discontinuation of modern spacing contraceptives in India. Asia Pac J Public Health 33(1):121–125. https://doi.org/10.1177/1010539520983149

Bellizzi S, Sobel HL, Obara H, Temmerman M (2015) Underuse of modern methods of contraception: underlying causes and consequent undesired pregnancies in 35 low-and middle-income countries. Hum Reprod 30(4):973–986. https://doi.org/10.1093/humrep/deu348

Bellizzi S, Mannava P, Nagai M, Sobel HL (2020) Reasons for discontinuation of contraception among women with a current unintended pregnancy in 36 low and middle-income countries. Contraception 101(1):26–33. https://doi.org/10.1016/j.contraception.2019.09.006

Bradley SE, Schwandt H, Khan S (2009) Levels, trends, and reasons for contraceptive discontinuation. DHS analytical studies, 20. ICF Macro, Calverton. https://cedar.wwu.edu/fairhaven_facpubs/1/

Bradley SE, Polis CB, Bankole A, Croft T (2019) Global contraceptive failure rates: who is most at risk? Stud Fam Plann 50(1):3–24. https://doi.org/10.1111/sifp.12085

Budhathoki SS, Pokharel PK, Good S, Limbu S, Bhattachan M, Osborne RH (2017) The potential of health literacy to address the health related UN sustainable development goal 3 (SDG3) in Nepal: a rapid review. BMC Health Serv Res 17(1):1–13. https://doi.org/10.1186/s12913-017-2183-6

Compton SD, Manu A, Maya E, Morhe ES, Dalton VK (2023) Give women what they want: contraceptive discontinuation and method preference in urban Ghana. Contracept Reprod Med 8(1):1–7

Dadzie LK, Seidu AA, Ahinkorah BO, Tetteh JK, Salihu T, Okyere J, Yaya S (2022) Contraceptive discontinuation among women of reproductive age in Papua New Guinea. Contracept Reprod Med 7(1):8. https://doi.org/10.1186/s40834-022-00170-3

Danna K, Angel A, Kuznicki J, Lemoine L, Lerma K, Kalamar A (2021) Leveraging the client-provider interaction to address contraceptive discontinuation: a scoping review of the evidence that links them. Glob Health Sci Pract 9(4):948–963. https://doi.org/10.9745/GHSP-D-21-00235

Diamond-Smith N, Campbell M, Madan S (2012) Misinformation and fear of side-effects of family planning. Cult Health Sex 14(4):421–433. https://doi.org/10.1080/13691058.2012.664659

Escamilla V, Calhoun L, Odero N, Speizer IS (2019) Access to public transportation and health facilities offering long-acting reversible contraceptives among residents of formal and informal settlements in two cities in Kenya. Reprod Health 16(1):1–11

Felker-Kantor E, Aung YK, Wheeler J, Keller B, Paudel M, Little K, Thein ST (2023) Contraceptive method switching and discontinuation during the COVID-19 pandemic in Myanmar: findings from a longitudinal cohort study. Sex Reprod Health Matters 31(1):2215568

Festin MPR (2020) Overview of modern contraception. Best Pract Res Clin Obstet Gynaecol 66:4–14. https://doi.org/10.1016/j.bpobgyn.2020.03.004

Ghule M, Raj A, Palaye P, Dasgupta A, Nair S, Saggurti N et al (2015) Barriers to use contraceptive methods among rural young married couples in Maharashtra, India: qualitative findings. Asian J Res Soc Sci Humanit 5(6):18. https://doi.org/10.5958/2249-7315.2015.00132.X

Gupta S, Bansal R, Shergill HK, Sharma P, Garg P (2023) Correlates of post-partum intra-uterine copper-T devices (PPIUCD) acceptance and retention: an observational study from North India. Contracept Reprod Med 8(1):25

International Institute for Population Sciences (IIPS) and ICF (2022) National Family Health Survey (NFHS-5), 2019–21. IIPS, Mumbai

Kupoluyi JA, Solanke BL, Adetutu OM, Abe JO (2023) Prevalence and associated factors of modern contraceptive discontinuation among sexually active married women in Nigeria. Contracept Reprod Med 8(1):1–11. https://doi.org/10.1186/s40834-022-00205-9

Mekonnen BD, Wubneh CA (2020) Prevalence and associated factors of contraceptive discontinuation among reproductive-age women in Ethiopia: using 2016 Nationwide Survey Data. Reprod Health 17(1):1–10

Nascimento Chofakian CB, Moreau C, Borges ALV, Dos Santos OA (2019) Contraceptive discontinuation: frequency and associated factors among undergraduate women in Brazil. Reprod Health 16(1):1–12. https://doi.org/10.1186/s12978-019-0783-9

Nayak SR, Mohanty SK, Mahapatra B, Sahoo U (2021) Spatial heterogeneity in discontinuation of modern spacing method in districts of India. Reprod Health 18(1):1–12. https://doi.org/10.1186/s12978-021-01185-w

Nkonde H, Mukanga B, Daka V (2023) Male partner influence on women's choices and utilisation of family planning services in Mufulira district, Zambia. Heliyon 9(3):e14405

Puri M, Henderson JT, Harper CC, Blum M, Joshi D, Rocca CH (2015) Contraceptive discontinuation and pregnancy postabortion in Nepal: a longitudinal cohort study. Contraception 91(4):301–307. https://doi.org/10.1016/j.contraception.2014.12.011

Rahaman M, Rana MJ, Roy A, Chouhan P (2022a) Spatial heterogeneity and socio-economic correlates of unmet need for spacing contraception in India: evidences from National Family Health Survey, 2015-16. Clin Epidemiol Glob Health 15:101012

Rahaman M, Singh R, Chouhan P, Roy A, Ajmer S, Rana MJ (2022b) Levels, patterns and determinants of using reversible contraceptives for limiting family planning in India: evidence from National Family Health Survey, 2015–16. BMC Womens Health 22(1):1–13

Rahaman M, Roy A, Chouhan P, Das KC, Rana MJ (2024) Revisiting the predisposing, enabling, and need factors of unsafe abortion in India using the Heckman Probit model. J Biosoc Sci 56(3):459–479

Ram R, Kumar M, Kumari N (2022) Association between women's autonomy and unintended pregnancy in India. Clin Epidemiol Glob Health 15:101060. https://doi.org/10.1016/j.cegh.2022.101060

Rana MJ, Goli S (2021) The road from ICPD to SDGs: health returns of reducing the unmet need for family planning in India. Midwifery 103:103107. https://doi.org/10.1016/j.midw.2021.103107

Samanta R, Munda J (2023) Husband's migration status and contraceptive behaviors of women: evidence from Middle-Ganga Plain of India. BMC Womens Health 23(1):180

Sedgh G, Ashford LS, Hussain R (2016) Unmet need for contraception in developing countries: examining women's reasons for not using a method. https://www.guttmacher.org/report/unmet-need-for-contraception-in-developing-countries?utm_source=Master+List&utm_campaign=037b9b172b-NR_Intl_Unmet_Need_6_28_16&utm_medium=email&utm_term=0_9ac83dc920-037b9b172b-244275881

Singh S, Shekhar C, Acharya R, Moore AM, Stillman M, Pradhan MR et al (2018) The incidence of abortion and unintended pregnancy in India, 2015. Lancet Glob Health 6(1):e111–e120. https://doi.org/10.1016/S2214-109X(17)30453-9

Thobani R, Jessani S, Azam I, Reza S, Sami N, Rozi S et al (2019) Factors associated with the discontinuation of modern methods of contraception in the low income areas of Sukh Initiative Karachi: a community-based case control study. PLoS One 14(7):e0218952. https://doi.org/10.1371/journal.pone.0218952

Tolesa B, Alem G, Papelon T (2015) Factors associated with contraceptive discontinuation in Agarfa district, Bale Zone, south east Ethiopia. Epidemiology 5(1):179. https://www.cabdirect.org/cabdirect/abstract/20153432015

United Nations (1994) Programme of action of the international conference on population and development. A/CONF.171/13. https://www.unfpa.org/sites/default/files/event-pdf/icpd_eng_2.pdf

Weldemariam KT, Gezae KE, Abebe HT (2019) Reasons and multilevel factors associated with unscheduled contraceptive use discontinuation in Ethiopia: evidence from Ethiopian demographic and health survey 2016. BMC Public Health 19:1–15. https://doi.org/10.1186/s12889-019-8088-z

Chapter 9
Temporal, Spatial and Socioeconomic Dimensions of Hindu–Muslim Differences in Contraception Use in India

Mohai Menul Biswas

Abstract The influence of religious perspectives on contraceptive use is a well-acknowledged aspect of family-planning policy and public health research. However, literature specifically addressing Hindu–Muslim differences in contraceptive trends, patterns, and socioeconomic factors in India is limited. This chapter explores the disparities in contraceptive use, evolving patterns, and socioeconomic correlations between Hindus and Muslims in India. It utilizes data from the first four rounds of the National Family Health Survey (NFHS) conducted in 1992–1993, 1998–1999, 2005–2006, and 2015–2016. The analysis employs descriptive statistics and multivariate logistic regression to derive this chapter's findings. The results indicate that the gap in contraceptive use between Hindus and Muslims in India is gradually narrowing. However, the use of contraceptives among Muslims has been found to be significantly low compared to that of Hindus in states like Kerala, Bihar, and West Bengal. Both absolute progress and relative progress on contraceptive use among Muslims were found in most of the states. The contraceptive use among Muslims significantly varies with their socioeconomic backgrounds. The women education and wealth status are found to be strong socioeconomic correlates of contraceptive use among Muslim women. The findings of this chapter suggest that poor socioeconomic conditions are responsible for the low rate of contraceptive use in India, irrespective of religion. New policies for several vulnerable groups and state-specific interventions are needed to overcome the low rate of contraceptive use among women in India.

Keywords Hindu–Muslim · Contraception · Religion · Socioeconomic · India · NFHS

M. M. Biswas (✉)
Department of Migration and Urban Studies, International Institute for Population Sciences, IIPS, Mumbai, India

© The Author(s), under exclusive license to Springer Nature Singapore Pte Ltd. 2024
P. Chouhan et al. (eds.), *Sexual and Reproductive Health of Women*, https://doi.org/10.1007/978-981-97-8418-9_9

9.1 Introduction

Contraceptive use is a key determinant of fertility and serves as a crucial predictor of demographic transition. The level of contraceptive use in a region reflects societal attitudes toward women's roles during pregnancy and their autonomy within that society (Pleck et al. 1993; Tountas et al. 2004; Rahaman et al. 2022a, b). Additionally, the prevalence of contraception indicates the degree of gender equality and the effectiveness of public health programs (Hamid and Stephenson 2006; Dereuddre et al. 2016; James-Hawkins et al. 2018). According to Bongaarts's theoretical framework (Bongaarts 1978), variations in contraceptive use, as an intermediate fertility variable, can lead to significant changes in overall population fertility. Therefore, studying contraceptive use provides insights into its impact on demographic transitions and population development.

Globally, contraceptive use varies significantly across countries, regions, and socioeconomic groups. A notable disparity persists between developed and underdeveloped countries in the prevalence of contraceptive use. Worldwide, the contraceptive use rate stands at 64%, with developed countries at 72%, developing countries at 60%, and underdeveloped countries at 40% (UN 2015). In Africa, a particularly low rate, of 33%, is observed among underdeveloped regions. In India, contraceptive use also varies widely both between and within states and across socioeconomic groups (International Institute for Population Sciences [IIPS] 2017). States like Bihar, Uttar Pradesh, and Jharkhand exhibit lower contraceptive use rates than those of other states, indicating a need for targeted policy interventions. Additionally, contraceptive use is generally lower among Muslims and socioeconomically disadvantaged groups than among other groups (IIPS 2017).

Previous studies have identified various factors that influence the rate of contraceptive use. Existing studies have suggested that at the individual level, factors like educational level, exposure to mass media, fertility preferences, and son preference are significantly associated with the level of contraceptive use (Arokiasamy 2002; DeRose and Ezeh 2010; Karthiha 2010; Forrest et al. 2018). Factors at the household or family level, such as spousal options, communication on contraceptive use, and women's autonomy, influence the acceptance and use of contraceptives (Acharya et al. 1996; Dehlendorf et al. 2019). On the other hand, factors at the community level, such as caste, cultural norms of different groups, and religion are influencing the acceptance of family-planning methods and the percentage of contraceptive use (Bhargava et al. 2005; Ghosh and Siddiqui 2017; Sk et al. 2018; Wilonoyudho et al. 2020). Accessibility, availability, and affordability are also the major barriers to universal access to contraceptives (Sileo et al. 2015; Ghule et al. 2015; Dixit et al. 2017). The levels of, patterns among, and trends in the percentage of contraceptive use also varied across regions in India (Ghule et al. 2015). Therefore, the above information has confirmed the wide variation in the percentage of contraceptive use among regions, states, and socioeconomic groups globally and in India in particular (Jones and Dreweke 2011).

Existing studies already have found that religion as an institute plays a notable role not only in fertility levels but also in associated fertility behavior, including contraceptive use and contraceptive acceptance (Addai 1999; Jones and Dreweke 2011). Previous studies from developing countries, mainly from sub-Saharan countries, have shown that religious belief affects the acceptance of family-planning determinants, and a low percentage of contraceptive use is found among orthodox Christian communities and Muslim communities (Iyer 2002; Agadjanian et al. 2009; Omran 2012). However, studies have also suggested that people's acceptance of contraceptive use and contraceptive prevalence rates are also high in Muslim-majority countries like Indonesia, Malaysia, and Egypt (Adsera 2006; Alam et al. 2011; Wong 2012).

9.1.1 Rationale of This Study

The debate surrounding family-planning demand, choice, acceptance, and performance among Hindus and Muslims in India has been long-standing and often fueled by concerns over a potential demographic shift. Recent reports from local, unorganized media and political organizations have highlighted apprehensions that the Muslim population may surpass the Hindu population in India (Hindustan Times 2023). A scientific study on this situation is needed to comprehensively examine the patterns of contraceptive use in India from a religious perspective. Contraceptive use is a key determinant of fertility behavior and population growth (Bongaarts 1978). Therefore, examining religious differences in contraceptive practices in this chapter is crucial for gaining a nuanced understanding of the Hindu–Muslim disparity in fertility behavior, one that moves beyond common myths. Although existing studies have indicated that religion might not be a significant factor in family-planning decisions and the lack of contraceptive use in India (Bhagat 2015), distinct patterns in contraceptive choice and use based on religious backgrounds have been observed (Rahaman et al. 2022a, b). Notably, Muslim women exhibit a higher preference for spacing contraception over limiting contraception, leading to a higher demand for spacing methods among Muslims than for Hindus (Rahaman et al. 2022a, b). Additionally, evidence has shown state-level variations in contraceptive use between Hindus and Muslims, such as the higher prevalence of contraceptive use among Kerala Muslims compared to Bihar Hindus and Muslims (Bhagat 2015). Although existing research has contributed significantly to understanding the Hindu–Muslim difference in contraceptive use (Bhagat 2015; Rahaman et al. 2022a, b), an unexplored aspect remains: how the prevalence and predictors of contraception use vary across geographical units, specifically states, in India. This research gap underscores the need for a more nuanced exploration of state-specific Hindu–Muslim gaps in contraceptive use and an examination of state-level variations in predictors of contraceptive use between the two religious groups. Therefore, the present chapter aims to address the aforementioned research gap by (a) contextualizing state-level variations in the trends in contraceptive use among Hindus and

Muslims in India and (b) analyzing the associated predictors of contraceptive use at the state level. This research is pivotal because it goes beyond the existing body of literature, offering a state-level perspective on the Hindu–Muslim disparity in contraceptive use. By exploring geographical variations within India, this study aims to provide a more nuanced understanding of the factors influencing contraceptive practices among Hindus and Muslims. Such insights are crucial for designing targeted and context-specific family-planning interventions, dispelling myths, and fostering a more informed dialogue on demographic trends in India.

9.2 Data and Methods

This study utilized data from the first four rounds of the National Family Health Survey (NFHS), conducted during 1992–1993, 1998–1999, 2005–2006, and 2015–2016, respectively. The survey aims to provide reliable estimates of fertility, mortality, child nutrition, healthcare use, and women's autonomy at the national, state, and district levels. The NFHS employs a multistage sampling design, with detailed sampling methods outlined in the survey reports (IIPS 2017). This study focused on 7 Indian states where the Muslim population was approximately 15% or more, according to the 2011 Census. Table 9.1 presents the details of these states and their population sizes. Trends in contraceptive use according to religion are analyzed by using data from the first four NFHS rounds (IIPS 1995, 2000, 2007, 2017). Additionally, NFHS-4 data are used to examine the levels of, patterns among, and socioeconomic determinants of contraceptive use among Hindus and Muslims, focusing on currently married women aged 15–49 years.

Table 9.1 Selected Indian states for this study and their populations

State	Total population	Muslim population	Share of Muslim population (%)
J&K	12,541,302	8,567,485	68.31
Assam	31,205,576	10,679,345	34.2
West Bengal	91,276,115	24,654,825	27.01
Kerala	33,406,061	8,873,472	26.56
Uttar Pradesh	199,812,341	38,483,967	19.26
Bihar	104,099,452	12,971,152	16.90
Jharkhand	32,988,134	4,793,994	14.53
India	**1,210,193,422**	**172,245,178**	**14.23**

Note: J&K = Jammu and Kashmir

9.2.1 Outcome and Explanatory Variables

9.2.1.1 Outcome Variable

The dependent, or outcome, variable is contraceptive use. This variable is a binary outcome—i.e. using contraceptives, "coded as a 1," and not using them, "coded as a 0."

9.2.1.2 Explanatory Variables

Previous research has indicated significant variation in contraceptive use among women depending on socioeconomic and demographic factors (Oliveira et al. 2014). The multivariate regression models in this study include several independent variables: women's age (15–24 years, 25–34 years, 35+ years), place of residence (urban, rural), religion (Hindu, Muslim, other), education level (none, primary, secondary, higher), partner's education level (none, primary, secondary, higher), employment status (not working, working), wealth index (poor, middle, rich), exposure to mass media (none, some), and sex preference for their offspring (equal preference, daughter preference, son preference).

9.2.2 Methods

Bivariate and multivariable binary logistic regression analyses were adopted to accomplish this study objectives. Bivariate analysis is used to present the levels of contraceptive use among women belonging to the selected religions according to their background characteristics. Further, multivariable binary logistic regression models are used to assess the variations in socioeconomic correlates of contraceptive use on the basis of religious identity. The software Stata 17.0 and MS Excel are used for all the statistical analyses in this study.

9.3 Results

9.3.1 Differentials in Trends of Contraceptive Use Between Hindus and Muslims

Figure 9.1 illustrates the variations in contraceptive use trends between Hindus and Muslims across seven selected states in India. From NFHS-1 to NFHS-3, an increase in contraceptive use occurred for both religious groups in all states. Uttar Pradesh, Rajasthan, and West Bengal exhibited a consistent upward trend in contraceptive

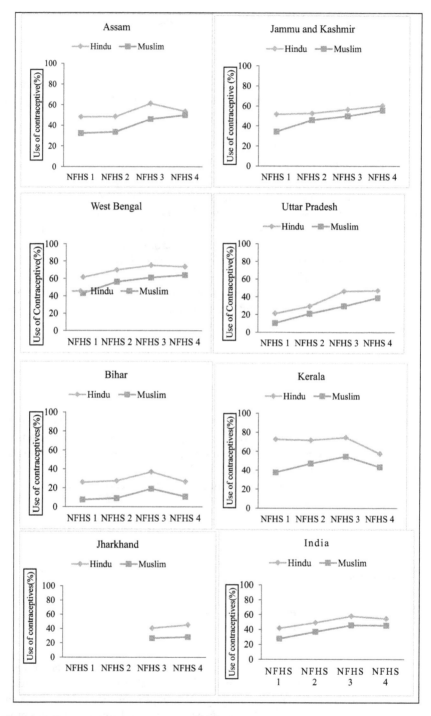

Fig. 9.1 Differentials in trends in contraceptive use between Hindus and Muslims (currently married women aged 15–49 years) in seven selected states in India, NFHS-1, -2, -3, and -4

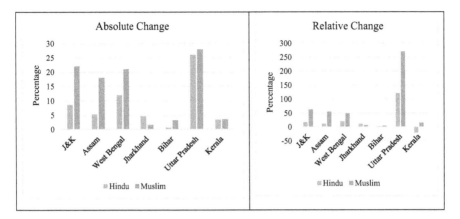

Fig. 9.2 Absolute and relative change in contraceptive use among currently married Hindu women and Muslim women in seven selected states of India. Note: J&K = Jammu and Kashmir; $^{\$}$absolute change = (NFHS-4 − NFHS-1) ÷ NFHS-1 × 100; and * relative change is shown between NFHS-3 and NFHS-4

use throughout the survey periods. However, in Kerala, contraceptive use significantly declined during NFHS-3 and NFHS-4 for women of both religions. A persistent disparity in contraceptive use between Hindus and Muslims was observed in West Bengal, Bihar, Kerala, and Jharkhand, with particularly low contraceptive use rates in Bihar and Jharkhand.

Figure 9.2 shows both the absolute and relative changes in contraceptive use among currently married Hindu and Muslim women across seven selected states. Most of the states exhibit significant increases in both absolute and relative contraceptive use, where Muslims show higher increases in most states, except Jharkhand. Conversely, Kerala saw a decrease in contraceptive use among Hindus. Uttar Pradesh experienced the highest relative increase in contraceptive use among Muslims (269.6%), followed by Jammu and Kashmir (62.6%). A notable religious gap in absolute changes in contraceptive use is evident in Jammu and Kashmir and in Assam.

9.3.2 Differences in Contraceptive Use Between Hindus and Muslims According to Background Characteristics

The percentage of contraceptive use among currently married women in seven selected states depending on their religion and according to their background characteristics is presented in Table 9.2. The analysis clearly shows that Muslims have the lowest percentage of contraceptive use, mostly because of their poor socioeconomic backgrounds. The analysis also shows that women who have a son preference reported a higher prevalence of contraceptive use among both religious groups

Table 9.2 Contraceptive prevalence rates among currently married Hindu and Muslim women in seven selected states according to their background characteristics, India, 2015–2016

Women's background characteristics	Jammu & Kashmir		Uttar Pradesh		Bihar		Jharkhand		West Bengal		Assam		Kerala	
	Hindu	Muslim	Hindu	Muslim	Hindu	Muslim	Hindu	Muslim	Hindu	Muslim	Hindu	Muslim	Hindu	Muslim
Sex preference														
Equal preference	59.3	56.3	45.9	37.2	24.0	10.1	43.7	29.1	74.3	63.5	53.3	50.8	57.7	43.6
Daughter preference	56.5	53.5	34.9	24.3	19.6	6.1	36.5	24.5	70.1	64.3	57.7	52.1	64.4	42.4
Son preference	65.1	54.9	49.6	40.6	30.0	12.0	48.7	27.1	70.0	65.7	54.1	47.1	53.1	43.8
Education														
No education	65.1	56.6	47.0	39.5	26.7	11.0	48.2	29.6	75.1	65.9	50.4	46.3	83.9	47.1
Primary education	69.1	62.2	48.5	33.5	26.1	9.0	51.3	29.2	77.2	67.2	52.0	50.0	66.2	56.3
Secondary education	57.3	54.3	46.1	38.6	26.2	12.0	40.7	25.5	72.1	60.7	55.2	52.5	61.4	45.2
Higher education	57.0	51.5	46.9	37.3	25.5	13.1	37.4	32.3	69.4	63.8	53.5	0.0	48.8	27.5
Place of residence														
Urban	72.1	61.0	59.4	46.2	39.8	15.3	50.6	33.3	70.8	62.4	56.3	48.9	59.1	59.2
Rural	57.6	58.4	43.5	32.6	24.7	10.0	43.1	25.7	74.9	64.5	53.1	50.1	56.5	51.7
Mass-media exposure														
No exposure	57.0	45.0	39.9	31.1	24.7	10.0	40.3	24.5	69.6	61.3	50.6	47.8	58.6	25.9
Exposure	61.0	58.0	50.9	42.6	28.4	13.2	48.2	30.7	74.2	65.1	54.4	52.6	58.0	43.7
Work status														
Not working	61.3	56.6	45.7	38.3	28.1	12.4	44.9	28.6	74.1	64.9	55.7	52.9	56.6	49.5
Working	68.8	57.4	57.2	46.8	33.2	19.2	51.1	34.6	82.5	76.2	63.8	61.2	60.7	60.6
Wealth index														
Poor	57.7	48.9	41.1	30.6	24.0	10.0	41.1	24.7	74.4	63.2	53.1	49.2	59.9	53.1

Middle	58.4	57.3	48.1	39.5	30.4	12.3	53.6	29.5	74.0	63.4	53.4	54.0	60.3	56.6
Rich	62.0	59.3	56.6	44.7	36.2	14.6	51.6	35.2	71.8	66.4	55.0	50.6	57.1	42.1
Partner's education														
No education	65.0	57.7	45.3	39.0	25.8	11.5	43.3	26.8	78.6	66.1	55.4	53.4	71.1	4.8
Primary education	69.9	56.9	45.5	45.3	29.7	13.0	47.9	23.3	82.3	72.8	56.9	57.7	78.9	59.1
Secondary education	62.1	56.3	49.2	37.3	30.2	14.7	46.4	30.1	72.2	63.0	56.7	52.1	58.7	40.1
Higher education	59.1	56.7	48.1	34.7	30.1	18.4	49.7	37.7	74.1	61.1	59.8	43.2	44.3	29.7

in all states except for Assam, where daughters are preferred over sons. On the other hand, the states where daughter preference is higher among Hindu women have higher contraceptive prevalence, such as in Kerala. Among both communities, the percentage of contraceptive use is higher among working women than among those who are not working. According to the analysis, the use of contraceptives increases with increasing levels of wealth in all states except for Kerala, irrespective of religion. The percentage of contraceptive use is higher in urban areas than in rural areas for both Hindus and Muslims.

The results show that women who are exposed to mass media have higher a prevalence of contraceptive use than those who are not exposed to mass media, among all states. Similarly, the working and currently married women reported higher levels of use of contraceptives among both the communities in all selected states. Among the selected states, the percentage of contraceptive use was peculiarly low in Bihar, Jharkhand, and Uttar Pradesh for both women of either religion. The gap in the percentage of contraceptive use between Hindus and Muslims was high in Bihar, Jharkhand, and Kerala across all socioeconomic groups.

9.3.3 State-Level Differences in Socioeconomic Correlates of Contraceptive Use

The adjusted odds ratios (AORs) of contraceptive use according to the socioeconomic background characteristics of women across seven states are presented in Table 9.3. The results indicate that the likelihood of using contraception generally increases with women's age in all states except for West Bengal and Assam. Bihar had the highest odds ratio (AOR: 9.28) for contraceptive use among women aged 35 years and older. Additionally, the odds of contraceptive use were consistently higher among Hindus than Muslims in all states. In Uttar Pradesh, Muslims were 83% less likely and Hindus 71% less likely to use contraception than the reference group was, namely "others." Notably, Muslims in Kerala had significantly lower odds of contraceptive use than the reference group had, with an AOR of 0.67. In Uttar Pradesh and Bihar, the likelihood of contraceptive use was 21% and 26% lower in rural areas than in urban areas, respectively. The results suggest that higher-educated women were less likely to use contraceptives than illiterate women were. In Kerala, higher-educated women (91%) were less likely to use contraceptives than illiterate women in Kerala, whereas in Uttar Pradesh, higher-educated women were 22% less likely. Wealth status was significantly associated with use of contraception, and rich women were more likely to use contraceptives than poor women were. The odds of contraceptive use were significantly higher among rich women than among poor women in states such as Uttar Pradesh (AOR: 0.50) and Jharkhand

Table 9.3 Binary logistic regression model showing adjusted odds ratios (AORs) for contraceptive use according to socioeconomic background characteristics of Hindu and Muslim women in selected states in India, 2015–2016

Women's background characteristics	J&K	Uttar Pradesh	Bihar	Jharkhand	West Bengal	Assam	Kerala
Age							
15–24®	1.00	1.00	1.00	1.00	1.00	1.00	1.00
25–34	3.46***	3.05***	6.50***	5.35***	2.75***	2.07***	4.52***
35+	5.99***	3.97***	9.28***	7.72***	1.97***	1.27**	9.11***
Religion							
Others®	1.00	1.00	1.00	1.00	1.00	1.00	1.00
Hindu	0.92	0.29**	1.13	2.64***	2.41***	1.01	1.2
Muslim	0.84	0.17***	0.41	1.23	1.45	1.01	0.67**
Place of residence							
Urban®	1.00	1.00	1.00	1.00	1.00	1.00	1.00
Rural	0.89	0.79***	0.74***	1.03	1.21	1.18	0.92
Education							
No education®	1.00	1.00	1.00	1.00	1.00	1.00	1.00
Primary education	1.24	1.01	1.19	1.2	1.18	1.21	0.11***
Secondary education	1.02	0.94	1.18*	0.78**	1.02	1.46***	0.14***
Higher education	0.72**	0.78***	0.88	0.43***	0.74	1.29	0.09***
Wealth index							
Poor®	1.00	1.00	1.00	1.00	1.00	1.00	1.00
Middle	1.07	1.31***	1.08	1.66***	1.09	0.77**	1.53
Rich	1.05	1.5***	1.22	1.65***	0.95	1.01	1.43
Mass-media exposure							
No exposure	1.00	1.00	1.00	1.00	1.00	1.00	1.00
Exposure	1.47***	1.42***	1.13	1.45***	1.20	1.19*	1.23
Work status							
No®	1.00	1.00	1.00	1.00	1.00	1.00	1.00
Yes	1.05	1.38***	1.17*	1.27***	1.54***	1.50***	1.22
Sex preference							
No preference®	1.00	1.00	1.00	1.00	1.00	1.00	1.00
Daughter preference	1.07	0.75	0.68	0.78	1.00	1.05	1.10
Son preference	1.10	1.21***	1.21***	1.01	1.13	1.07	1.08
Partner's education							
No education®	1.00	1.00	1.00	1.00	1.00	1.00	1.00
Primary education	1.42**	1.12	1.25**	1.53***	1.33*	0.95	3.5**
Secondary education	1.01	1.13**	1.29***	1.46***	0.86	0.91	2.61*
Higher education	0.99	1.01	1.15	1.63***	1.08	0.86	2.03

Note: J&K = Jammu and Kashmir; ***p <0.01, **p <0.05, and *p <0.10; and ® = reference category

(AOR: 1.65). Mass media played a positive role in increasing contraceptive use. Working women were more likely to use contraceptives than nonworking women were. The association between women's partner's education and contraceptive use was similar in relation to women's education and contraceptive use in all states except for Jharkhand. In Jharkhand, the contraceptive use rate significantly increased with increases in women's partner's education. In Jharkhand, higher-educated partners were 63% more likely to use contraceptives than illiterate partners were.

9.3.4 Differences in Socioeconomic Correlates of Contraceptive Use Prevalence Between Hindus and Muslims

The adjusted odds ratios (AOR) for contraceptive use, stratified according to religion and socioeconomic background characteristics are shown in Table 9.4, revealing notable differences across states. The data indicate that individuals aged 35 years and older, regardless of religion, are more likely to use contraception. Working women have higher contraceptive use rates than those of nonworking women. In Uttar Pradesh, factors such as place of residence, wealth quintile, and mass-media exposure significantly influence contraceptive use for both Muslims and Hindus. Contrary to expectations, higher-educated women tend to use contraception less than illiterate women do, irrespective of religion. In Kerala, higher-educated Hindu women are 92% less likely to use contraception than are illiterate women, while higher-educated Muslim women are 84% more likely to use contraception. Additionally, women engaged in work are more likely to use contraception across all selected states, regardless of religion. A preference for sons over one for daughters also shows considerable variation in its impact on contraceptive use, where Hindu women who preferred sons in Uttar Pradesh and Bihar were more likely to use contraception. In Kerala, women who preferred sons were 0.62 times less likely to use contraceptives if they were Hindu and 2.1 times more likely if they were Muslim. Women's partner's education was negatively associated with contraceptive use among both Muslims and Hindus in all states except for Jharkhand. In Jharkhand, among Hindus, higher-educated partners were 72% more likely to use contraceptives than were illiterate partners.

Table 9.4 Binary logistic regression model showing adjusted odds ratios (AORs) for contraceptive use by Hindu and Muslim women in selected states in India according to their socioeconomic background characteristics, 2015–2016

Women's background characteristics	Jammu & Kashmir		Uttar Pradesh		Bihar		Jharkhand		West Bengal		Assam		Kerala	
	Hindu	Muslim	Hindu	Muslim	Hindu	Muslim	Hindu	Muslim	Hindu	Muslim	Hindu	Muslim	Hindu	Muslim
Age														
15–24®	1.00	1.00	1.00	1.00	1.00	1.00	1.00	1.00	1.00	1.00	1.00	1.00	1.00	1.00
25–34	3.5***	3.76***	3.15***	2.49***	6.59***	6.2***	5.82***	2.47***	2.28***	4.11***	2.03***	2.22***	6.68***	3.7***
35+	5.55***	6.46***	4.39***	2.47***	9.75***	6.37***	9.11***	2.23**	1.71***	3.18***	1.33**	1.14	12.45***	7.3***
Place of residence														
Urban®	1.00	1.00	1.00	1.00	1.00	1.00	1.00	1.00	1.00	1.00	1.00	1.00	1.00	1.00
Rural	0.54***	1	0.83***	0.67***	0.71***	0.88	1.11	0.9	1.18	1.47	1.16	1.22	0.86	1.09
Education														
No education®	1.00	1.00	1.00	1.00	1.00	1.00	1.00	1.00	1.00	1.00	1.00	1.00	1.00	1.00
Primary education	1.3	1.19	1.12	0.68***	1.25*	0.98	1.19	0.77	1.17	1.55	1.12	1.38	0.18*	0
Secondary education	0.78	1.17	0.96	0.91	1.14	1.78*	0.78*	0.51*	1.06	1.33	1.53***	1.33	0.13**	1.51
Higher education	0.49**	0.86	0.81**	0.7	0.9	0.72	0.39***	0.72	0.63	1.58	1.15	2.19	0.08***	1.84*
Wealth index														
Poor®	1.00	1.00	1.00	1.00	1.00	1.00	1.00	1.00	1.00	1.00	1.00	1.00	1.00	1.00
Middle	0.87	1.17	1.32***	1.14	1.17	0.45**	1.67***	2.33**	1.12	1.05	0.74**	0.97	1.33	2.96
Rich	0.88	1.2	1.61***	1.12	1.24	0.94	1.54***	2.91***	0.93	0.97	0.93	1.28	1.68	1.86
Mass-media exposure														
No exposure	1.00	1.00	1.00	1.00	1.00	1.00	1.00	1.00	1.00	1.00	1.00	1.00	1.00	1.00
Exposure	1.16	1.59***	1.36***	1.72***	1.09	1.53*	1.52***	1.48	0.97	1.25	1.15	1.16	1.08	1.05
Work status														
No®	1.00	1.00	1.00	1.00	1.00	1.00	1.00	1.00	1.00	1.00	1.00	1.00	1.00	1.00

(continued)

Table 9.4 (continued)

Women's background characteristics	Jammu & Kashmir Hindu	Jammu & Kashmir Muslim	Uttar Pradesh Hindu	Uttar Pradesh Muslim	Bihar Hindu	Bihar Muslim	Jharkhand Hindu	Jharkhand Muslim	West Bengal Hindu	West Bengal Muslim	Assam Hindu	Assam Muslim	Kerala Hindu	Kerala Muslim
Yes	1.2	0.99	1.37***	1.45***	1.16*	1.26	1.17	1.67	1.42**	2.21**	1.48***	1.45	1.21	0.73
Sex preference														
No preference®	1.00	1.00	1.00	1.00	1.00	1.00	1.00	1.00	1.00	1.00	1.00	1.00	1.00	1.00
Daughter preference	1.3	1.06	0.7*	1.04	0.55	5.26	0.75	0.94	1.1	0.66	0.92	1.13	1.33	1.24
Son preference	1.19	1.05	1.22***	1.14	1.21***	1.11	1.05	1.15	1.14	1.05	0.97	1.11	0.62*	2.1***
Partner's education														
No education®	1.00	1.00	1.00	1.00	1.00	1.00	1.00	1.00	1.00	1.00	1.00	1.00	1.00	1.00
Primary education	1.72*	1.22	1.07	1.3*	1.26**	1.18	1.46**	1.16	1.16	1.5	0.92	0.98	3.96*	0
Secondary education	1.11	0.99	1.2***	0.9	1.3***	1.15	1.5***	1.28	0.78	0.93	0.9	0.83	2.28	1.01
Higher education	1.24	0.84	1.06	0.77	1.14	1.41	1.72***	1.17	1.1	1.06	1.01	0.47*	1.6	0.97

Note: J&K = Jammu and Kashmir; ***p <0.01, **p <0.05, and *p <0.10; and ® = reference category

9.4 Discussion

The present chapter examines how the socioeconomic correlates of contraceptive use changes with religion (Hindu and Muslim) in India. This chapter also shows the changing scenario of contraceptive use during 1992–2016. The use of contraceptives remains low in Bihar, Jharkhand, and Uttar Pradesh irrespective of religion. Over time, the gap in contraceptive use between Hindus and Muslims in India has narrowed, though the extent of religious differences varies depending on women's background characteristics across states. A decline in contraceptive use was observed in Bihar and Kerala, with a negative absolute change in Kerala among Hindus. For Muslims, the relative increase in contraceptive use was notably higher than that for Hindus. Sociodemographic factors such as women's age, place of residence, education, mass-media exposure, wealth index, and employment status similarly influenced contraceptive use for both Hindus and Muslims. These findings align with previous research (Rahaman et al. 2022a, b), which has identified these socioeconomic factors as significant determinants of contraceptive use. In all selected states, the odds of contraceptive use are higher among women aged 35 years and older, followed by those in the 25–34 age group. Contraceptive use increases with women's age because with increasing age, fertility desire wanes, and women start to use contraceptives to stop their ability to bear children (Oliveira et al. 2014). Although the disparity in contraceptive use between Hindus and Muslims remains at each educational level, both groups show an increase in contraceptive use as education levels rise (Arokiasamy 2009). Female education emerges as a crucial factor influencing contraceptive use among socioeconomic variables (Drèze and Murthi 2001; Arokiasamy 2009). This trend is evident when comparing contraceptive use within each educational level between Hindus and Muslims across the seven selected states. Additionally, the education of women's partners plays a significant role in increasing contraceptive use, particularly among Muslims in Rajasthan and Kerala. Previous research has highlighted the importance of husbands' education in enhancing contraceptive acceptance (Shakya et al. 2018). Contraceptive use also correlates with women's wealth status, where wealthier women use contraception more due to greater affordability (Mohanty and Pathak 2009). In Bihar, the gap in contraceptive use between the poor and the rich is minimal, likely because high fertility rates adversely impact contraceptive use (Mason and Smith 2000). Conversely, in Kerala, poorer women use more contraception than do wealthier women, possibly due to better public health services and higher sterilization rates among the poor (Thulaseedharan 2018). Son preference appears to increase contraceptive use among Muslim women, a finding that contrasts with earlier research (Arokiasamy 2002). Typically, urban women have higher rates of contraceptive use than those of their rural counterparts (Mohanty and Pathak 2009). However, the current study found minimal rural–urban differences in contraceptive use in Bihar, which may be due to the low awareness and acceptance of family-planning methods in urban areas in the state (Chatterjee and Sennott 2020). Recent research has suggested that India should focus on policies that promote needs-based contraception for couples (Rahaman et al. 2022a, b). This study highlights a significant demand for modern reversible contraceptives among young women with a single child, women with no sons, and those from the Muslim community in the northeast region. It calls for the government to guarantee the availability of these contraceptives to address unmet needs in India. Additionally, increasing contraceptive use is expected to improve population control and contribute to better health and well-being for women and children (Rahaman et al. 2023).

9.4.1 Limitations of This Study

The findings of this study are derived from cross-sectional survey data, limiting the establishment of causal relationships between religion and contraceptive use. This study's reliance on selected states introduces a potential limitation in that it therefore may not fully capture the variations across all Indian states. Additionally, the use of respondent-reported data raises concerns about potential biases, where the possibility of over- or underreporting affects the accuracy of the findings. Furthermore, this study did not apply multimodel tests to enhance the robustness and reliability of its findings. The absence of such rigorous testing may compromise the overall validity of the results and limit this study's ability to draw definitive conclusions on the relationship between religion and contraceptive practices. In light of these considerations, the study findings must be interpreted with caution, recognizing the inherent limitations associated with the survey data, state selection, reliance on respondent reporting, and absence of comprehensive model testing. Future research endeavors should aim to address these limitations by employing more-rigorous methods to establish causation, broadening state representation, and incorporating robust statistical analyses to increase reliability.

9.5 Conclusion

This chapter concludes that contraceptive use among Muslim women is significantly lower than that among Hindus in most states. Muslim women's lower contraceptive use compared to that of Hindu women can be attributed to factors such as religious beliefs—where conservative interpretations may prioritize childbearing and neglect family planning—along with lower levels of education and reduced exposure to mass media. The Hindu–Muslim gap in contraceptive use varies widely across states and socioeconomic groups. Notable regional variation in contraceptive use also appears within both religious communities, and even within individual states, differences appear within the same religion. The indicators used for comparison are averages for the communities within states rather than the norms for these communities. The findings of this study highlight that poor socioeconomic conditions are major barriers to contraceptive use among women in India, regardless of their religion. Therefore, targeted policy interventions, including state-specific strategies to improve contraceptive use, are needed for identified vulnerable groups (both Hindus and Muslims). Additionally, increasing the availability, accessibility, and affordability of contraceptives on the basis of women's choices could enhance contraceptive use among socioeconomically disadvantaged groups.Declaration

Availability of Data and Materials The data and materials for this chapter are sourced from publicly available secondary sources accessible at https://dhsprogram.com/methodology/survey/survey-display-541.cfm.

Interested individuals can register at the provided link to freely download the necessary data.

Ethics Approval and Consent to Participate This chapter is based on secondary data, which are available in the public domain. Therefore, ethical approval is not required to conduct this study.

Competing Interests The author declare that no competing interests.

Funding This chapter did not receive any specific grant from funding agencies in the public, commercial, or not-for-profit sectors.

References

Acharya R, Acharya R, Sureender S (1996) Inter-spouse communication, contraceptive use and family size: relationship examined in Bihar and Tamil Nadu. J Fam Welf 42(4):5–11

Addai I (1999) Does religion matter in contraceptive use among Ghanaian women? Rev Relig Res 40(3):259–277

Adsera A (2006) Religion and changes in family-size norms in developed countries. Rev Relig Res 47(3):271–286

Agadjanian V, Yabiku ST, Fawcett L (2009) History, community Milieu, and Christian-Muslim differentials in contraceptive use in sub-Saharan Africa. J Sci Study Relig 48(3):462–479

Alam SS, Mohd R, Hisham B (2011) Is religiosity an important determinant on Muslim consumer behaviour in Malaysia? J Islam Mark 2(1):83–96

Arokiasamy P (2002) Gender preference, contraceptive use and fertility in India: regional and development influences. Int J Popul Geogr 8(1):49–67

Arokiasamy P (2009) Fertility decline in India: contributions by uneducated women using contraception. Econ Polit Wkly 44:55–64

Bhagat RB (2015) Transition in Hindu and Muslim population growth rates: myth and reality. In: National seminar on 'Religious demography of India: myths and realities' organized by Centre for Culture and Development, Vadodara

Bhargava A, Chowdhury S, Singh KK (2005) Healthcare infrastructure, contraceptive use and infant mortality in Uttar Pradesh, India. Econ Hum Biol 3(3):388–404

Bongaarts J (1978) A framework for analyzing the proximate determinants of fertility. Popul Dev Rev 4:105–132

Chatterjee E, Sennott C (2020) Fertility intentions and maternal health behaviour during and after pregnancy. Popul Stud 74(1):55–74

Dehlendorf C, Fitzpatrick J, Fox E, Holt K, Vittinghoff E, Reed R et al (2019) Cluster randomized trial of a patient-centered contraceptive decision support tool, my birth control. Am J Obstet Gynecol 220(6):565.e1

Dereuddre R, Van de Velde S, Bracke P (2016) Gender inequality and the 'East–West' divide in contraception: an analysis at the individual, the couple, and the country level. Soc Sci Med 161:1–12

DeRose LF, Ezeh AC (2010) Decision-making patterns and contraceptive use: evidence from Uganda. Popul Res Policy Rev 29(3):423–439

Dixit P, Dwivedi LK, Gupta A (2017) Role of maternal and child health care services on postpartum contraceptive adoption in India. SAGE Open 7(3):2158244017733515

Drèze J, Murthi M (2001) Fertility, education, and development: evidence from India. Popul Dev Rev 27(1):33–63

Forrest W, Arunachalam D, Navaneetham K (2018) Intimate partner violence and contraceptive use in India: the moderating influence of conflicting fertility preferences and contraceptive intentions. J Biosoc Sci 50(2):212–226

Ghosh S, Siddiqui MZ (2017) Role of community and context in contraceptive behaviour in rural West Bengal, India: a multilevel multinomial approach. J Biosoc Sci 49(1):48–68

Ghule M, Raj A, Palaye P, Dasgupta A, Nair S, Saggurti N et al (2015) Barriers to use contraceptive methods among rural young married couples in Maharashtra, India: qualitative findings. Asian J Res Soc Sci Human 5(6):18

Hamid S, Stephenson R (2006) Provider and health facility influences on contraceptive adoption in urban Pakistan. Int Fam Plan Perspect 32:71–78

Hindustan Times (2023) Muslim population has grown in India, minorities decimated in Pakistan: Sitharaman. Column by Prashant Jha, New Delhi. https://www.hindustantimes.com/india-news/indian-finance-minister-debunks-perception-of-violence-against-muslims-invites-critics-to-visit-india-and-see-for-themselves-101681182577035.html

IIPS (1995) National Family Health Survey (NFHS-1), 1992–93. International Institute for Population Sciences (IIPS), Mumbai

IIPS (2000) National Family Health Survey (NFHS-2), 1998–99. International Institute for Population Sciences (IIPS), Mumbai

IIPS (2007) National Family Health Survey (NFHS-4), 2006–07. International Institute for Population Sciences (IIPS), Mumbai

IIPS (2017) National Family Health Survey (NFHS-4), 2015–16. International Institute for Population Sciences (IIPS), Mumbai, pp 791–846

Iyer S (2002) Religion and the decision to use contraception in India. J Sci Study Relig 41(4):711–722

James-Hawkins L, Peters C, VanderEnde K, Bardin L, Yount KM (2018) Women's agency and its relationship to current contraceptive use in lower-and middle-income countries: a systematic review of the literature. Glob Public Health 13(7):843–858

Jones RK, Dreweke J (2011) Countering conventional wisdom: new evidence on religion and contraceptive use. Alan Guttmacher Institute, New York

Karthiha T (2010) A study to determine the quality of life among the permanent contraceptive adopters and non-adopters at selected rural areas in Sivagangai District, Tamilnadu (Doctoral dissertation, Matha College of Nursing, Manamadurai)

Mason KO, Smith HL (2000) Husbands' versus wives' fertility goals and use of contraception: the influence of gender context in five Asian countries. Demography 37(3):299–311

Mohanty SK, Pathak PK (2009) Rich–poor gap in utilization of reproductive and child health services in India, 1992–2005. J Biosoc Sci 41(3):381–398

Oliveira ITD, Dias JG, Padmadas SS (2014) Dominance of sterilization and alternative choices of contraception in India: an appraisal of the socioeconomic impact. PLoS One 9(1):e86654

Omran AR (ed) (2012) Family planning in the legacy of Islam. Routledge, London

Pleck JH, Sonenstein FL, Ku LC (1993) Masculinity ideology: its impact on adolescent males' heterosexual relationships. J Soc Issues 49(3):11–29

Rahaman M, Rana MJ, Roy A, Chouhan P (2022a) Spatial heterogeneity and socio-economic correlates of unmet need for spacing contraception in India: evidences from National Family Health Survey, 2015-16. Clin Epidemiol Glob Health 15:101012

Rahaman M, Singh R, Chouhan P, Roy A, Ajmer S, Rana MJ (2022b) Levels, patterns and determinants of using reversible contraceptives for limiting family planning in India: evidence from National Family Health Survey, 2015–16. BMC Womens Health 22(1):1–13. https://doi.org/10.1186/s12905-022-01706-0

Rahaman M, Roy A, Chouhan P, Das KC, Rana MJ (2023) Revisiting the predisposing, enabling, and need factors of unsafe abortion in India using the Heckman Probit model. J Biosoc Sci 55(6):1–21. https://doi.org/10.1017/S002193202300024X

Shakya HB, Dasgupta A, Ghule M, Battala M, Saggurti N, Donta B et al (2018) Spousal discordance on reports of contraceptive communication, contraceptive use, and ideal family size in rural India: a cross-sectional study. BMC Womens Health 18(1):1–14

Sileo KM, Wanyenze RK, Lule H, Kiene SM (2015) Determinants of family planning service uptake and use of contraceptives among postpartum women in rural Uganda. Int J Public Health 60(8):987–997

Sk MIK, Jahangir S, Mondal NA, Biswas AB (2018) Disparities in the contraceptive use among currently married women in Muslim densely populated states of India: an evidence from the nationally representative survey. Epidemiol Biostat Public Health 15(3)

Thulaseedharan JV (2018) Contraceptive use and preferences of young married women in Kerala, India. Open Access J Contracept 9:1

Tountas Y, Dimitrakaki C, Antoniou A, Boulamatsis D, Creatsas G (2004) Attitudes and behavior towards contraception among Greek women during reproductive age: a country-wide survey. Eur J Obstet Gynecol Reprod Biol 116(2):190–195

United Nations (2015) Trends in contraceptive use worldwide 2015 (ST/ESA/SER. A/349). United Nations, Department of Economic and Social Affairs, New York

Wilonoyudho S, Salim LA, Muhtaram A (2020) The perspective of Puritan Moslem on the Family Planning Program: the case of Salafi movement in Semarang, Central Java, Indonesia. Indian J Forensic Med Toxicol 14(4):3452

Wong LP (2012) An exploration of knowledge, attitudes and behaviours of young multiethnic Muslim-majority society in Malaysia in relation to reproductive and premarital sexual practices. BMC Public Health 12(1):1–13

Chapter 10
Understanding the District-Wise Variation and Reasons of Low Fertility in West Bengal: A Cross-sectional Descriptive Study

Gita Naik, Astapati Hemram, Dinabandhu Patra, and Jagannath Behera

Abstract Fertility control behaviour is the result of reproductive decision that helps couple for rationally selecting an appropriate contraceptive method, it allow them to practise the right to have children by their own choice. This chapter tries to overview fertility behaviour among currently married women aged 15–49 years in the low fertility setting of West Bengal. This chapter emphasises spatial variation in the number of children that women have and their contraceptive use, and it aims to identify responsible factors in one of the low fertility having state (West Bengal). To achieve the above objectives, few statistical operations are carried out, like percentage distribution, bivariate analysis, chi-square test and multinomial logistic regression. The fifth round of the National Family Health Survey is the main data source. Its result shows a declining trend in the total fertility rate in West Bengal over time. Among the sample of married women, 74% are currently using modern contraceptives in Birbhum district, and 37% and 27% of the sample have two children and one child, respectively here. The percentage share for those who have more than two children is smaller, indicating that women's choice of contraceptives influences their fertility behaviour. Jalpaiguri, Kolkata, Howrah have provided significant evidence in correlation between modern contraceptive use and fewer children. Traditional contraceptives are highly used in Maldah district, where high rates of women's having more than two children have been found. Substantially more modern contraceptive use is one of the main reasons for the low fertility rate in West Bengal. Women's place of residence, wealth status and mass-media exposure are some of the other important determinants of low fertility here.

G. Naik (✉) · D. Patra · J. Behera
Department of Population Studies, Fakir Mohan University, Balasore, Odisha, India

A. Hemram
Department of Geography, Cooch Behar Panchanan Barma University,
Cooch Behar, West Bengal, India

Keywords Fertility · Contraceptive · Traditional contraceptive · Higher education · Wealth

10.1 Introduction

The greatest advancement in reproductive health over the past several decades has been a substantial increase in the use of contraceptives. Fertility control behaviour is the result of a reproductive decision that helps couples in rationally selecting an appropriate contraceptive method, allowing them to practise the right to have children by their own choice (Speizer and Calhoun 2021; Dasgupta et al. 2022). Most notably, the increased usage of contraception has made a substantial contribution to contemporary declines in fertility (Canning and Schultz 2012; Lindberg et al. 2018). Globally, the contraceptive prevalence rate (CPR) of any method was estimated to be 65%, modern methods accounting for 58.7% of women in a marriage or civil union in 2022 (WHO 2023). However, the total fertility rate (TFR) of developing countries has fallen from 6.1 in 1955 to 2.6 in 2020 (Bongaarts and Hodgson 2022).

In India, a fertility transition began in late 1960s and has recently gained momentum. During the past decade in particular, fertility levels have declined throughout the country to varying degrees. Nationally, contraceptive use increased from 1992–1993 to 2019–2021, where the proportion of married women of reproductive age using any method of contraception has increasing from 40.7% to 66.7% over the same period (IIPS and ICF 2021; Kumar et al. 2022). Notably, declines in fertility occur due to active engagement in family-planning programmes. Studies have pointed out that acceptance of family-planning methods depends on demographic, socioeconomic and cultural factors, including women's age of marriage, education level, economic status and mass-media exposure (Adhikari 2010; Ahinkorah et al. 2021; Kassim and Ndumbaro 2022; Rahaman et al. 2022). For instance, in the state of Tamil Nadu, age of marriage and education level were directly linked with acceptance of family planning (FP), whereas in other Indian states, exemplified by Karnataka, Meghalaya and Bihar, economic status and mass-media exposure were responsible for the same (Potdar et al. 2015; Pal et al. 2018; Passah 2020; Osborn et al. 2021). Fertility decline in any region or country is not solely determined by the use of contraceptive methods; other behavioural, sociodemographic and economic factors also contribute to the acceleration of fertility decline (Bongaarts 2015; Majumder and Ram 2015). However, a recent study has found that contraceptive prevalence and women's education level both had significant effects on fertility, with contraceptive prevalence having a significantly higher effect on the acceleration of fertility reduction (Liu and Raftery 2020).

Among the eastern states of India, West Bengal in particular has been experiencing fertility decline over the past four decades. Women of childbearing age in West

Bengal are having fewer children than the national average and using more family planning, leading to an increase in the use of effective contraceptive methods. Earlier studies on contraceptive use and fertility dynamics have shown that women in West Bengal often practise traditional contraception and that their acceptance of family-planning programmes is low, although couples have a wide selection of contraceptive methods to limit their family size (Paul and Kulkarni 2006). A study conducted by Das and Ghosh (2020) showed how the dynamics of contraceptive use affect fertility behaviour in West Bengal. Das and Ghosh's study found that choice and time in the adoption of contraceptive methods has strong positive impacts on fertility, where after having a boy, couples often choose modern methods over traditional methods. Another study, conducted by Haque and Patel (2015), has revealed that contraceptive methods, age at marriage and female education level have had heavy influences on fertility decline in West Bengal. That study also found that although the use of traditional methods of contraception remains high in the state, the use of modern family-planning methods has increased significantly over time.

The use of family-planning programmes and fertility behaviour vary across the region, depending on the socioeconomic group. Studying which factors play significant roles in the low fertility behaviour in West Bengal is crucial. Although numerous studies have been carried out to identify fertility behaviour and its related factors, the situation in West Bengal remains unclear and warrants district-specific exploration to better inform district-specific family-planning advice. Therefore, this chapter examines the influence of contraception and other socioeconomic factors on the declining fertility in West Bengal. Further, this chapter also seeks to shed light on the district-wise prevalence of contraception in West Bengal.

10.2 Data and Methods

10.2.1 Study Setting

Recently, India became the most populous country in the world after overtaking China. Currently, 28 states and 8 union territories (UTs) make up the Indian federal union. West Bengal is one of the densest and most populous states in India. Indian states can be further divided into districts and these districts into census enumeration areas (EAs) for rural areas and into wards for urban areas. The narrowest divisions are villages and municipalities for rural and urban areas, respectively. This chapter focuses on how fertility is determined by different factors in West Bengal because its total fertility rate is below the replacement level (according to NFHS-5). West Bengal is divided into 20 districts, and all these districts are considered to show the spatial variation in contraceptive use and the number of children that women have.

10.2.2 Study Design and Study Population

The present research is based on the data from the fifth round of the National Family Health Survey (NFHS). This survey was conducted by International Institute for Population Sciences (IIPS) under the Ministry of Health and Family Welfare. Its data on women are utilised to gain insights into the linkages between the fertility rate and fertility-determining factors in West Bengal. This chapter is based on data on currently married women aged 15–49 years, and its total sample size is 16,522.

10.2.3 Dependent Variable

The dependent variable in this study is the "number of children" that women have, and we classified it in the following way: "no children," "one child," "two children" and "more than two children." We carried out multinomial logistic regression, and "two children" was the base outcome.

10.2.4 Predictor Variables

Current contraceptive use and other socioeconomic background characteristics of the respondents are the major predictor variables in our multinomial logistic regression model. In this study, women's place of residence, highest education level of the respondent and of their spouse, wealth index score, mass-media exposure to family planning, caste, religion, age group, contraceptive decision-making and desire for children are the major socioeconomic predictor variables that can influence fertility.

10.2.5 Statistical Analysis

Simple percentage distribution, bivariate cross-tabulation, chi-square test and relative risk ratio in multinominal logistic regression are employed in this chapter's data analysis. The STATA 17 and QGIS statistical tools are used for data analysis and for the bivariate graphical representation.

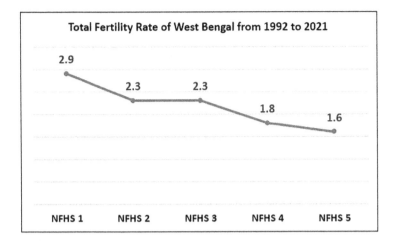

Fig. 10.1 Declining trend of TFR in West Bengal

10.3 Results

10.3.1 Change in Total Fertility Rate

The total fertility rate in West Bengal underwent a sharp decline from 1992 to 2021 (Fig. 10.1). In 1992–1993 (NFHS-1), the TFR of West Bengal was 2.9, but more recently, in 2019–2021 (NFHS-5), it was 1.6. This large gap represents a progressive sign towards a fertility transition in West Bengal. A previous study has underscored fact that it is one of the states with high traditional contraceptive use and low fertility. But in reality, it should be high due to the high failure rate of traditional contraception. Therefore, this study examines the linkages between fertility on one hand and other socioeconomic factors and contraceptive use on another in West Bengal.

10.3.2 District-Wise Spatial Variation in Fertility

Table 10.1 presents the district-wise variation in fertility, classifying women into those with no child, one child, two children and more than two children. Among the districts, Kolkata (43.9%), Paschim Medinipur (45.6%) and Uttar Dinajpur (35.9%) had the highest percentage of women with one child, two children and more than two children, respectively. On the other hand, the districts with the lowest percentage of women with one child, two children and more than two children were Malda (21.4%), Uttar Dinajpur (31.4%) and Hugli (10.7%), respectively.

Table 10.1 District-wise fertility variation among currently married women aged 15–49 years in West Bengal

District	No child	One child	Two children	>2 children
Darjeeling	11.27	33.77	35.18	19.78
Jalpaiguri	10.13	28.81	36.57	24.5
Koch Bihar	9.2	26.73	38.69	25.38
Uttar Dinajpur	11.09	21.47	31.48	35.96
Dakshin Dinajpur	9.99	31.53	39.19	19.29
Maldah	9.43	21.43	34.98	34.17
Murshidabad	9.85	24.25	34.88	31.02
Birbhum	8.87	27.46	39.4	24.26
Nadia	8.98	32.84	39.49	18.69
North 24 Pargana	9.37	39.7	36.07	14.85
Hugli	10.97	37.82	40.49	10.72
Bankura	8.83	27.33	43.83	20.01
Puruliya	8.31	22.27	38.97	30.44
Haora	9.66	35.58	37.53	17.23
Kolkata	9.04	43.96	34.41	12.6
South 24 Pargana	11.04	30.47	37.75	20.74
Paschim Medinipur	9.11	25.32	45.65	19.92
Purba Medinipur	7.81	35.59	42.74	13.85
Paschim Bardhhaman	10.48	34.26	35.82	19.44
Purba Bardhhaman	7.86	30.37	45.11	16.65
Total (*n*)	1577	5136	6379	3430

10.3.3 District-Wise Contraceptive Use

Table 10.2 displays the district-wise diversity in contraceptive use among women. The types of family-planning methods are categorised into two groups: modern contraceptives and traditional contraceptives. In West Bengal, 61% of women use modern contraceptives, and 14% use traditional contraceptives. Birbhum (74%) has the highest percentage of modern contraceptive use, followed by Kolkata (72%) and Jalpaiguri (70%). Conversely, modern contraceptives are used less often in Puruliya (41%), Purba Medinipur (48%) and Nadia (49%). On the other hand, traditional contraceptives, which are less effective, are used more often in Maldah (21%), Murshidabad (21%), Uttar Dinajpur (20%) and Dakshin Dinajpur (20%).

Figure 10.2 displays four bivariate maps (Fig. 10.2a–d) showing the variation in the number of children and contraceptive use in geographical units (districts) across West Bengal. Generally, most of the districts in West Bengal, where modern contraceptive use is high (63.0–73.8%), the rate of women with more than 2 children moderate (19.1–27.5%). Howrah and Murshidabad are exceptions in that Howrah has a low and Murshidabad a high percentage of women with more than two children (Fig. 10.1b). The Hugli and North 24 Parganas districts have high percentages of women with one child (36.5–44.0%), and the percentages of modern

Table 10.2 District-wise contraceptive type used by currently married women aged 15–49 years in West Bengal

District	Modern contraceptives	Traditional contraceptives
Darjeeling	67.01	15.16
Jalpaiguri	70.11	12.6
Koch Bihar	67.67	14.01
Uttar Dinajpur	60.93	20.26
Dakshin Dinajpur	58.98	19.62
Maldah	54.65	20.61
Murshidabad	64.89	20.52
Birbhum	73.85	8.3
Nadia	49.32	10.56
North 24 Parganas	60.99	17.83
Hugli	61.27	13.63
Bankura	51.85	4.8
Puruliya	41.31	9.71
Haora	68.41	16.11
Kolkata	71.72	12.96
South 24 Parganas	67.89	14.97
Paschim Medinipur	55.58	5.16
Purba Medinipur	48.08	11.19
Paschim Bardhhaman	54.02	11.28
Purba Bardhhaman	58.51	9.38
Total (*n*)	10,035	2253
Total (%)	60.74	13.64

contraceptive use among women in these districts are moderate (52.2–63.0%) (Fig. 10.1a). The low use of both traditional and modern contraceptives in Puruliya might be reflected in its high percentage of women with more than two children (Fig. 10.1b,d). This chapter also discovered that districts such as Uttar Dinajpur, Maldah and Murshidabad are high in both women with more than two children and traditional contraceptive use.

10.3.4 Contraceptive Use According to Background Characteristics

Table 10.3 shows how fertility differs according to women's socioeconomic background characteristics. Urban women have lower rates of having two children and more than two children than rural women do (Table 10.3). Also, with an increase in women's education level, the percentage of women with more than two children decreases; besides that, better-educated women are more likely to have no children or only one child. Their spouse's education level has the same impact on the number

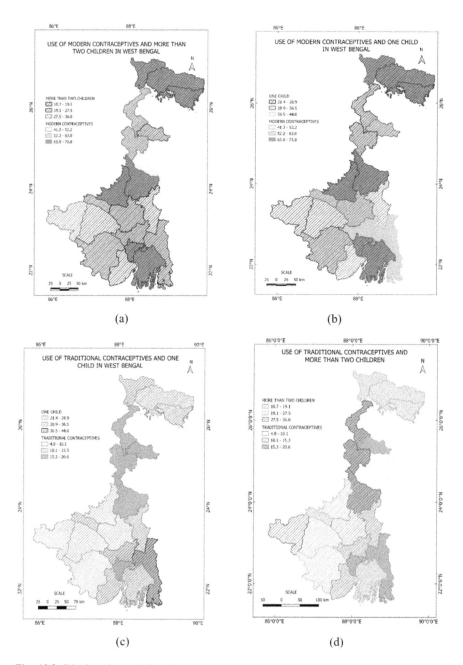

Fig. 10.2 District-wise variation in contraceptive use and the number of children of married women aged 15–49 years in West Bengal: (**a**) the use of modern contraceptives and one child; (**b**) the use of modern contraceptives and more than two children; (**c**) the use of traditional contraceptives and one child; and (**d**) the use of traditional contraceptives and more than two children

Table 10.3 Fertility in relation to contraceptive use and other socioeconomic factors (%)

Socioeconomic factors	No child	One child	Two children	>2 children	Chi-square (p-value)
Current contraceptive use					<0.001
Modern method	3.22	27.08	45.83	23.87	
Traditional method	7.68	46.81	29.02	16.48	
Place of residence					<0.001
Urban	10.34	39.75	34.84	15.07	
Rural	9.19	27.28	40.26	23.27	
Women's education level					<0.001
No education	3.97	11.69	37.45	46.89	
Primary	4.32	17.82	47.24	30.62	
Secondary	11.69	39.56	38.87	9.88	
Higher	22.65	58.11	18.55	0.69	
Spouses' education level					<0.001
No education	4.66	13.82	39.06	42.46	
Primary	7.18	23.19	42.25	27.39	
Secondary	12.00	36.39	40.10	11.51	
Higher	15.03	52.66	27.62	4.70	
Wealth index					<0.001
Poorest	8.31	21.43	41.32	28.94	
Poorer	9.06	29.38	38.16	23.40	
Middle	10.22	32.79	38.88	18.10	
Richer	11.19	43.89	35.28	9.65	
Richest	11.81	50.98	34.00	3.21	
Mass-media exposure to FP					<0.001
Not exposed	7.91	23.91	39.83	28.34	
Exposed	10.58	35.67	37.83	15.92	
Caste					<0.001
SC	9.53	28.68	41.81	19.98	
ST	13.37	25.05	37.34	24.24	
OBC	9.19	28.82	39.53	22.46	
General	9.00	35.49	36.86	18.64	
Religion					<0.001
Hindu	9.55	33.56	40.67	16.22	
Muslim	9.37	24.69	33.57	32.37	
Christian	13.62	31.15	35.74	19.48	
Others	13.26	40.62	31.51	14.61	

(continued)

Table 10.3 (continued)

Socioeconomic factors	No child	One child	Two children	>2 children	Chi-square (p-value)
Age group					<0.001
15–19	54.91	42.62	2.25	0.22	
20–24	19.19	55.19	22.85	2.77	
25–29	8.66	36.77	44.82	9.74	
30–34	3.91	25.81	49.17	21.11	
35–39	2.77	22.09	47.77	27.38	
40–44	2.45	18.98	44.27	34.31	
45+	2.75	19.82	35.19	42.24	
Contraceptive decision-making					<0.001
Mainly by respondent	3.37	31.24	40.44	24.95	
Mainly by spouse/partner	4.54	28.58	38.67	28.21	
Joint	4.08	30.72	43.30	21.89	
Desire for more children					<0.001
Wants within 2 years	54.54	39.35	4.79	1.32	
Wants after 2+ years	19.26	73.74	5.91	1.08	
Undecided	16.19	53.03	21.39	9.39	
Does not want	1.98	31.09	44.09	22.85	
Sterilised	0.20	6.97	59.10	33.73	
Total (n)	16,522				

of children that they have; thus, in addition to women's education level, their spouse's education level is also important in how many children they have.

An increase in family wealth also decreases fertility; in Table 10.3, fertility decreases more with every step upward in their wealth index score, leading women to more often have only one child. Mass-media exposure as a background characteristic has shown a connection to the number of children that women have. Among all women exposed to mass media, nearly 36% had only one child, whereas among all women not thus exposed, nearly 24% had one child. Similarly, women exposed to mass media were less likely to have more than two children (16%) than those not thus exposed (28%).

Caste-wise data highlight that the General caste (19%) has the lowest percentage of women with more than two children, followed by SC (20%), OBC (22%) and ST (24%). We also found here that among religious women, Muslims had the lowest percentage of women with one child (25%) and the highest percentage of women with more than two children (32%). The percentage of women with two children was highest for Hindu women (41%), followed by Christian women (36%), Muslim women (34%) and women espousing other religions (32%).

The percentage of women with more than two children was lower when couples engaged in joint decision-making for contraceptive used than when couples engaged in women-only or spouse-only decision-making. Among women who wanted children within 2 years or after 2 years, most of them had no children or only one child. Nearly 59% of women had two children, and 34% had more than two children, whereas among those who were sterilised, 7% had only one child. On the other hand, 31% of women with only one child and 44% with two children desired no more children. The chi-square result shows a strong correlation between all the identified independent variables and the dependent variable.

10.3.5 Results from Multinominal Logistic Regression

Table 10.4 shows the adjusted relative risk ratios (aRRRs) of the number of children that women have to their contraceptive use and socioeconomic background characteristics in West Bengal. The multinominal logistic regression analysis indicates that the relative risk ratio (RRR) of no children to two children was 1.75 (CI: 1.34–2.27) and that the RRR of one child to two children was 1.25 (CI: 1.08–1.44) among currently married traditional contraceptive users. Thus, these results show that traditional contraceptive users are more likely to have no children. The RRR of no children to two children was 0.59 (CI: 0.47–0.74) in the rural areas of West Bengal, and that of one child to two children was 0.75 (CI: 0.66–0.85) in these areas. The relative risk ratio decreased with increasing levels of education and higher wealth index scores among women with more than two children. Women who were exposed to mass media had a 48% higher chance of not having children than women not thus exposed. ST women were 1.15 (CI: 0.94–1.39) times more likely to have more than two children than only two children. The RRR of no children was 0.39 (CI: 0.31–0.49) times higher than that of two children; on the other hand, it was 3.00 (CI: 2.65–3.39) times higher among Muslim women with more than two children than among Muslim women with only two children. On contraceptive decision-making made by women's spouse/partner, the RRR was 0.87 (CI: 0.45–1.68) times higher among women with no children than among those with two children, but it was 1.15 (CI: 0.88–1.49) times higher among women with more than two children than those with only two children. These results show that women's contraceptive use, their place of residence, the education level of the respondent and that of their spouse/partner, their wealth status, their mass-media exposure, their religion and their contraceptive decision-making affected the fertility of currently married women in West Bengal

Table 10.4 Multinomial logistic regression for the number of children that women have in West Bengal

Socioeconomic factors	No child vs. two children			One child vs. two children			>2 children vs. two children		
	RRR	CI	p-Value	RRR	CI	p-Value	RRR	CI	p-Value
Current contraceptive use									
Modern method®									
Traditional method	1.75	1.34, 2.27	0.000	1.25	1.08, 1.44	0.002	1.07	0.90, 1.27	0.422
Place of residence									
Urban®									
Rural	0.59	0.47, 0.74	0.000	0.75	0.66, 0.85	0.000	0.81	0.71, 0.92	0.002
Women's education level									
No educated®									
Primary	0.52	0.37, 0.74	0.000	0.80	0.67, 0.95	0.014	0.70	0.62, 0.79	0.000
Secondary	0.66	0.48, 0.89	0.007	1.29	1.09, 1.51	0.002	0.38	0.34, 0.43	0.000
Higher	5.58	3.75, 8.29	0.000	3.20	2.50, 4.09	0.000	0.10	0.05, 0.19	0.000
Spouses' education level									
No educated®									
Primary	0.88	0.42, 1.89	0.746	0.95	0.61, 1.45	0.797	0.91	0.67, 1.23	0.533
Secondary	0.94	0.48, 1.81	0.850	1.05	0.71, 1.53	0.813	0.71	0.52, 0.96	0.027
Higher	1.78	0.78, 4.04	0.171	1.52	0.92, 2.52	0.103	0.93	0.47, 1.86	0.846
Wealth index									
Poorest®									
Poorer	1.60	1.27, 2.03	0.000	1.40	1.22, 1.60	0.000	0.91	0.82, 1.02	0.117
Middle	1.91	1.46, 2.49	0.000	1.38	1.17, 1.61	0.000	0.72	0.62, 0.83	0.000
Richer	3.09	2.22, 4.28	0.000	1.99	1.65, 2.40	0.000	0.51	0.41, 0.62	0.000
Richest	2.60	1.68, 4.00	0.000	1.86	1.45, 2.37	0.000	0.26	0.18, 0.37	0.000
Mass-media exposure to FP									
Not exposed®									

(continued)

Table 10.4 (continued)

Socioeconomic factors	No child vs. two children			One child vs. two children			>2 children vs. two children		
	RRR	CI	p-Value	RRR	CI	p-Value	RRR	CI	p-Value
Exposed	1.48	1.23, 1.79	0.000	1.07	0.96, 1.18	0.240	0.82	0.75, 0.91	0.000
Caste									
SC®									
ST	1.55	1.09, 2.19	0.014	1.04	0.83, 1.31	0.728	1.15	0.94, 1.39	0.165
OBC	0.87	0.64, 1.18	0.374	1.04	0.87, 1.23	0.663	0.89	0.75, 1.05	0.171
General	1.08	0.85, 1.37	0.520	1.28	1.11, 1.45	0.000	0.77	0.67, 0.89	0.000
Religion									
Hindu®									
Muslim	0.39	0.31, 0.49	0.000	0.38	0.33, 0.43	0.000	3.00	2.65, 3.39	0.000
Christian	1.72	0.71, 4.15	0.226	1.01	0.60, 1.68	0.982	1.04	0.62, 1.75	0.881
Others	1.98	0.76, 5.13	0.162	1.55	0.85, 2.81	0.152	0.82	0.41, 1.67	0.590
Age group									
15–19®									
20–24	0.03	0.02, 0.05	0.000	0.19	0.11, 0.30	0.000	1.44	0.33, 6.31	0.628
25–29	0.01	0.004, 0.01	0.000	0.08	0.04, 0.12	0.000	2.50	0.59, 10.80	0.220
30–34	0.00	0.00, 0.00	0.000	0.07	0.45, 0.11	0.000	5.19	1.20, 22.39	0.027
35–39	0.00	0.00, 0.00	0.000	0.08	0.05, 0.13	0.000	6.98	1.61, 30.14	0.009
40–44	0.01	0.004, 0.02	0.000	0.09	0.05, 0.14	0.000	9.54	2.20, 41.25	0.003
45+	0.01	0.005, 0.02	0.000	0.13	0.08, 0.22	0.000	15.05	3.48, 65.10	0.000
Contraceptive decision-making									
Mainly by respondent®									
Mainly by spouse/partner	0.87	0.45, 1.68	0.684	0.74	0.54, 1.00	0.057	1.15	0.88, 1.49	0.303
Joint	0.91	0.59, 1.40	0.655	0.80	0.66, 0.97	0.022	0.89	0.75, 1.05	0.184
Desire for more children									

(continued)

Table 10.4 (continued)

Socioeconomic factors	No child vs. two children			One child vs. two children			>2 children vs. two children		
	RRR	CI	p-Value	RRR	CI	p-Value	RRR	CI	p-Value
Wants within 2 years®									
Wants after 2+ years	0.15	0.10, 0.21	0.000	1.13	0.81, 1.56	0.473	1.18	0.58, 2.39	0.644
Undecided	0.03	0.02, 0.04	0.000	0.23	1.17, 0.32	0.000	1.64	0.89, 3.01	0.109
Does not want	0.00	0.00, 0.00	0.000	0.07	0.05, 0.09	0.000	1.64	0.96, 2.79	0.069
Sterilised	0.00	0.00, 0.00	0.000	0.01	0.009, 0.017	0.000	1.58	0.92, 2.72	0.097

® = Reference category

10.4 Discussion

The effective and consistent use of contraceptive by a couple can limit the number of children that they have. Findings from this study show that the rate of using any modern contraceptive method among currently married women is 60.7%. This finding differs from that of previous studies conducted in India, which have shown that in West Bengal, about 57% of currently married women are using modern contraception (New et al. 2017).

Another study has found that the prevalence of modern contraception methods is higher among women who have more than two children. This finding is similar to that of a previous study conducted in West Bengal (Haque and Patel 2015). Notably, a significant relationship exists between women using contraception and the number of children they have, as revealed by an adjusted RRR. Nevertheless, a significant difference appeared on the subject of the number of children a woman has, that between women who reported using modern methods and those who reported using traditional methods. However, this study indicates that traditional contraceptive users are more likely to have no children. This result is similar to that of a study conducted in Uttar Pradesh (Halli et al. 2022). Traditional contraceptive users mostly are mostly women in the wealthy, urban section of society (Ram et al. 2014; Gebreselassie et al. 2017). Several studies conducted in different parts of the world have found that affluent, urban women have a lower chance of having children than their poorer, rural counterparts (Rahman et al. 2022; Cherie et al. 2023). Given our results, this theme seems to repeat in the case of West Bengal.

Our study findings revealed that rural women were more likely to have more children in all categories than women from urban areas in West Bengal. Similar results were also found in previous studies (Matsumoto and Yamabe 2013; Rahman et al. 2022). The higher number in rural areas could be attributed to the lower use of contraceptive methods; notably, women from rural areas tend to marry at an early age, and rural women are comparatively less concerned about family-planning methods (Boateng et al. 2023).

This study has shown that the relative risk ratio of having more than two children decreased with increasing levels of education and wealth status. The educated and richest women were less likely to have more children than their less-educated, poorer counterparts. These findings are consistent with those of other studies (Matsumoto and Yamabe 2013; Liu and Raftery 2020; Chouhan et al. 2020; Das and Ghosh 2020; Rahman et al. 2022). A plausible reason could be that access to education improves women's understanding of effective contraceptive use, raises pregnancy awareness and helps to avoid early marriage. Moreover, higher-educated women devote more time to training or knowledge acquisition. Having access to education enables individuals to set other priorities first and put off having children until they have established a secure career (Boahen and Yamauchi 2017). Also, this study found that wealth status was inversely related to the number of children that a woman has. The number of children that a woman has was lower among women in the richest wealth index households compared with those from households with a poorest wealth index. The richest people tend to be able to afford the cost of childcare and provide the basic needs of the child, including food and medical care; this could explain why the number of children that women have was kept small by those in the richest wealth index households (Boateng et al. 2023). In contrast, the poorest households perceive their children as sources of income, which encourages them to have more children. Additionally, the poorest people lack family-planning knowledge and pregnancy-related awareness (Chauhan and Nagarajan 2021).

This study found that women who were exposed to mass media had a higher likelihood of not having a child than women who were not exposed to mass media. This finding is similar to that found in previous research conducted in India and other developing countries (Chouhan et al. 2020; Ahinkorah et al. 2020; Chauhan and Nagarajan 2021; Boateng et al. 2023). Perhaps the impact of mass media increases information and alters perceptions of women's ideal number of children, thus together shaping contraceptive use patterns (Das et al. 2021).

Also, a significant correlation was shown between women's social group position and their having more children in West Bengal. ST women have higher a relative risk ratio of having more than two children than having only two children. This finding corroborates previous studies conducted in India (Chouhan et al. 2020; Nagadeve and Dongardive 2021). The probable explanation is that ST women lack knowledge on family-planning methods. Additionally, fear and unconcern about family-planning methods and limited pregnancy-related awareness led them to have higher fertility (Palo et al. 2020). We noted that Muslim women were more likely to have more children than their counterparts were. Our study's finding here aligns with that of previous research conducted in India and in South Asia (Adhikari 2010; Saikia et al. 2019; Chouhan et al. 2020; Rahman et al. 2022). Attitudes, beliefs and practices greatly differ between Muslim and non-Muslim women on marriage, reproductive behaviour and fertility control behaviour. These differences are supposed to have distinct impacts on the intermediate factors of fertility behaviour between Muslim women and women espousing other religions.

10.5 Conclusion

The findings of our study showed the key role of modern contraceptive in low fertility in West Bengal. Previous studies have shown that women in West Bengal and those in Kerala exhibit different fertility behaviour even though both states are low fertility settings with high traditional contraceptive use. The multinomial model of this chapter showed a similar result for traditional contraceptive use in West Bengal. Women's education level, wealth, mass-media exposure and place of residence were other important factors in bringing low fertility here. Family-planning programmes worked well but required more awareness for modern contraceptive use because traditional contraceptive use is still high in West Bengal.

Declaration

Availability of Data and Materials The data and materials for this chapter are sourced from publicly available secondary sources accessible at https://dhsprogram.com/methodology/survey/survey-display-541.cfm. Interested individuals can register at the provided link to freely download the necessary data.

Ethics Approval and Consent to Participate This chapter is based on secondary data, which are available in the public domain. Therefore, ethical approval is not required to conduct this study.

Competing Interests The authors declare that they have no competing interests.

Funding This chapter did not receive any specific grant from funding agencies in the public, commercial or not-for-profit sectors.

References

Adhikari R (2010) Demographic, socio-economic, and cultural factors affecting fertility differentials in Nepal. BMC Pregnancy Childbirth 10(1):19. https://doi.org/10.1186/1471-2393-10-19

Ahinkorah BO, Seidu A, Armah-Ansah EK, Budu E, Ameyaw EK, Agbaglo E, Yaya S (2020) Drivers of desire for more children among childbearing women in sub-Saharan Africa: implications for fertility control. BMC Pregnancy Childbirth 20(1):778. https://doi.org/10.1186/s12884-020-03470-1

Ahinkorah BO, Seidu A, Armah-Ansah EK, Ameyaw EK, Budu E, Yaya S (2021) Socio-economic and demographic factors associated with fertility preferences among women of reproductive age in Ghana: evidence from the 2014 demographic and health survey. Reprod Health 18(1):2. https://doi.org/10.1186/s12978-020-01057-9

Boahen EA, Yamauchi C (2017) The effect of female education on adolescent fertility and early marriage: evidence from free compulsory universal basic education in Ghana. J Afr Econ 27(2):227–248. https://doi.org/10.1093/jae/ejx025

Boateng D, Oppong FB, Senkyire EK, Logo DD (2023) Socioeconomic factors associated with the number of children ever born by married Ghanaian females: a cross-sectional analysis. BMJ Open 13(2):e067348. https://doi.org/10.1136/bmjopen-2022-067348

Bongaarts J (2015) Modeling the fertility impact of the proximate determinants: time for a tune-up. Demogr Res 33:535–560. https://doi.org/10.4054/demres.2015.33.19

Bongaarts J, Hodgson D (2022) Fertility transition in the developing world. Springer, Berlin

Canning D, Schultz T (2012) The economic consequences of reproductive health and family planning. Lancet 380(9837):165–171. https://doi.org/10.1016/s0140-6736(12)60827-7

Chauhan BG, Nagarajan R (2021) Trend and determinants of fertility in a declining fertility regime: a study of rural Uttar Pradesh. Commun Health Equity Res Policy 43(2):143–152. https://doi.org/10.1177/0272684x211004947

Cherie N, Getacher L, Belay AS, Gultie T, Mekuria A, Sileshi S, Degu G (2023) Modeling on number of children ever born and its determinants among married women of reproductive age in Ethiopia: a Poisson regression analysis. Heliyon 9(3):e13948. https://doi.org/10.1016/j.heliyon.2023.e13948

Chouhan P, Saha J, Zaveri A (2020) Covariates of fertility behavior among ever-married women in West Bengal, India: analysis of the National Family Health Survey-4. Child Youth Serv Rev 113:104956. https://doi.org/10.1016/j.childyouth.2020.104956

Das K, Ghosh S (2020) Rural–urban fertility convergence, differential stopping behavior, and contraceptive method mix in West Bengal, India: a spatiotemporal analysis. J Fam History. https://doi.org/10.1177/0363199020959785

Das P, Samad N, Banna HA, Sodunke TE, Hagan JE, Ahinkorah BO, Seidu A (2021) Association between media exposure and family planning in Myanmar and Philippines: evidence from nationally representative survey data. Contracept Reprod Med 6(1):11. https://doi.org/10.1186/s40834-021-00154-9

Dasgupta A, Wheldon MC, Kantorová V, Ueffing P (2022) Contraceptive use and fertility transitions: the distinctive experience of sub-Saharan Africa. Demogr Res 46:97–130. https://doi.org/10.4054/demres.2022.46.4

Gebreselassie T, Bietsch K, Staveteig S, Pullum TW (2017) Trends, determinants, and dynamics of traditional contraceptive method use. ICF, Lexington

Halli SS, Alam MT, Joseph A, Prakash R, Isac S, Becker M, Anand P, Vasanthakumar N, Ramesh BM, Blanchard J (2022) Declining fertility and increasing use of traditional methods of family planning: a paradox in Uttar Pradesh, India? J Biosoc Sci 55(2):224–237. https://doi.org/10.1017/s0021932022000086

Haque I, Patel PP (2015) Socioeconomic and cultural differentials of contraceptive usage in West Bengal. J Fam Hist 40(2):230–249. https://doi.org/10.1177/0363199015572753

IIPS, ICF (2021) National Family Health Survey (NFHS–5), 2019-21. International Institute for Population Sciences, Mumbai. https://rchiips.org/nfhs/NFHS-5_FCTS/India.pdf

Kassim M, Ndumbaro F (2022) Factors affecting family planning literacy among women of childbearing age in the rural Lake zone, Tanzania. BMC Public Health 22(1):646. https://doi.org/10.1186/s12889-022-13103-1

Kumar K, Singh A, Tsui AO (2022) Measuring contraceptive use in India: implications of recent fieldwork design and implementation of the National Family Health Survey. Demogr Res 47:73–110. https://doi.org/10.4054/demres.2022.47.4

Lindberg LD, Santelli J, Desai S (2018) Changing patterns of contraceptive use and the decline in rates of pregnancy and birth among U.S. adolescents, 2007–2014. J Adolesc Health 63(2):253–256. https://doi.org/10.1016/j.jadohealth.2018.05.017

Liu DH, Raftery AE (2020) How do education and family planning accelerate fertility decline? Popul Dev Rev 46(3):409–441. https://doi.org/10.1111/padr.12347

Majumder N, Ram F (2015) Explaining the role of proximate determinants on fertility decline among poor and non-poor in Asian countries. PLoS One 10(2):e0115441. https://doi.org/10.1371/journal.pone.0115441

Matsumoto Y, Yamabe S (2013) Family size preference and factors affecting the fertility rate in Hyogo, Japan. Reprod Health 10(1):6. https://doi.org/10.1186/1742-4755-10-6

Nagadeve DA, Dongardive PB (2021) Fertility and family planning differentials among social groups in India. Demography India 50(1):1–16

New JR, Cahill N, Stover J, Gupta YP, Alkema L (2017) Levels and trends in contraceptive prevalence, unmet need, and demand for family planning for 29 states and union territories in India:

a modelling study using the family planning estimation tool. Lancet Glob Health 5(3):e350–e358. https://doi.org/10.1016/s2214-109x(17)30033-5

Osborn J, Sriram R, Shanmugam K, Ravishankar S (2021) A study on contraceptive prevalence rate and factors influencing it in a rural area of Coimbatore, South India. J Family Med Prim Care 10(6):2246. https://doi.org/10.4103/jfmpc.jfmpc_2345_20

Pal A, Yadav J, Sunita S, Singh KJ (2018) Factors associated with unmet need of family planning in Bihar, India: a spatial and multilevel analysis. Int J Reprod Contracep Obstet Gynecol 7(9):3638. https://doi.org/10.18203/2320-1770.ijrcog20183768

Palo SK, Samal M, Behera J, Pati S (2020) Tribal eligible couple and care providers' perspective on family planning: a qualitative study in Keonjhar district, Odisha, India. Clin Epidemiol Glob Health 8(1):60–65. https://doi.org/10.1016/j.cegh.2019.04.008

Passah MC (2020) Influence of sociodemographic factors on the utilization of contraceptive methods among the married women of Jowai town, West Jaintia Hills district, Meghalaya. Oriental Anthropol 20(1):181–193. https://doi.org/10.1177/0972558x20913726

Paul P, Kulkarni PM (2006).The dynamics of fertility transition in West Bengal, India. In: European population conference, Liverpool, UK, 21st–24th June

Potdar PA, Raikar VR, Potdar AB (2015) Socio-demographic determinants of contraceptive use among married women from urban area of North Karnataka. Indian J Public Health Res Dev 6(4):104. https://doi.org/10.5958/0976-5506.2015.00208.9

Rahaman M, Singh R, Chouhan P, Roy A, Ajmer S, Rana MJ (2022) Levels, patterns and determinants of using reversible contraceptives for limiting family planning in India: evidence from National Family Health Survey, 2015–16. BMC Womens Health 22(1):1–13

Rahman AS, Hossain Z, Rahman ML, Kabir E (2022) Determinants of children ever born among ever-married women in Bangladesh: evidence from the demographic and health survey 2017–2018. BMJ Open 12(6):e055223. https://doi.org/10.1136/bmjopen-2021-055223

Ram F, Shekhar C, Chowdhury B (2014) Use of traditional contraceptive methods in India & its socio-demographic determinants. PubMed 140(Suppl):S17–S28. https://pubmed.ncbi.nlm.nih.gov/25673538

Saikia N, Moradhvaj, Saha A, Chutia U (2019) Actual and ideal fertility differential among natives, immigrants, and descendants of immigrants in a northeastern state of India. Popul Space Place 25(4):e2238. https://doi.org/10.1002/psp.2238

Speizer IS, Calhoun LM (2021) Her, his, and their fertility desires and contraceptive behaviours: a focus on young couples in six countries. Glob Public Health 17(7):1282–1298. https://doi.org/10.1080/17441692.2021.1922732

World Health Organization (2023) Family planning/contraception methods. www.who.int. Accessed 18 Sep 2023 https://www.who.int/news-room/fact-sheets/detail/family-planning-contraception

Part IV
Sexually Transmitted Infections

Chapter 11
Knowledge of Sexual and Reproductive Health Matters Among Girls in India: Does Parent–Adolescent Communication Play a Role?

Pintu Paul and Ria Saha

Abstract Adequate knowledge of sexual and reproductive health (SRH) is critical in making informed decisions on safe sexual practices. However, knowledge of SRH among girls is limited in India, leading to adverse SRH outcomes. Parent–adolescent communication may play a crucial role in gaining accurate knowledge of SRH matters among girls. In this chapter, we use data from the UDAYA survey to examine the level of sufficient/adequate knowledge of SRH matters and its sociodemographic correlates among adolescents and young girls in Uttar Pradesh and Bihar. We further assess the relationship between parent–adolescent communication and girls' knowledge of SRH matters. Overall, adequate knowledge of SRH among adolescents and young girls is critically low in the study setting. Over two-thirds of girls (69%) discuss the physical changes of puberty/menstruation, and only 3% of girls discuss pregnancy-related issues with their parents, where most of these discussions occur with mothers only. Our findings indicate that parent–adolescent communication is positively associated with knowledge of SRH matters. This study underscores the importance of parent–adolescent communication in girls' gaining accurate information on SRH. The findings suggest that well-designed, culturally appropriate interventions tailored to specific contexts should be aimed at developing equitable attitudes towards gender-differential parental control or monitoring ado-

---

This chapter is an extended study of our original research, namely "Association between exposure to social media and knowledge of sexual and reproductive health among adolescent girls: Evidence from the UDAYA survey in Bihar and Uttar Pradesh, India," which was published in *Reproductive Health* in 2022.

P. Paul (✉)
Ashoka University, Sonipat, India
e-mail: pintupaul383@gmail.com

R. Saha
Business Development & Research Intelligence, Somerset Council, Somerset, UK
e-mail: ria.saha@somerset.gov.uk

© The Author(s), under exclusive license to Springer Nature Singapore Pte Ltd. 2024
P. Chouhan et al. (eds.), *Sexual and Reproductive Health of Women*,
https://doi.org/10.1007/978-981-97-8418-9_11

lescents and suggest raising awareness and encouraging parents to enhance their positive involvement in advocating for the SRH issues of their children.

Keywords Sexual and reproductive health (SRH) · Parent–adolescent communication · Adolescents and young girls · India

11.1 Background

According to Census 2011, India has the largest number of adolescents aged 10–19 years globally (253 million), of which 47.3% are female (UNFPA 2014). Adolescence is a crucial developmental phase between childhood and adulthood that shapes an individual's long-term health and well-being. In this phase, adolescents undergo rapid physical and emotional changes and reach sexual maturity. This stage often brings many questions and uncertainties about sexuality, leading to anxiety and confusion. However, discussing sexual and reproductive health (SRH) remains a social taboo in India (Paul et al. 2017; Khanna et al. 2022). The government of India has formulated several policies and programmes, including the SABLA scheme (2011) and the Rashtriya Kishor Swasthya Karyakram (RKSK) of 2014, to safeguard the SRH of adolescents and young adults (Barua et al. 2020; Bhat and Shankar 2021; Population Council 2017). Despite these government initiatives, adolescents and other young girls continue to face substantial hindrances to accessing adequate and accurate information on SRH matters (Janighorban et al. 2022; Deshmukh and Chaniana 2020).

Previous studies have documented that girls' knowledge of SRH matters is limited in India, especially among those in rural areas and those living in socially and economically disadvantaged communities (Santhya and Jejeebhoy 2012; Saha et al. 2022; Meena et al. 2015; Banerjee et al. 2015; Khanna et al. 2022; Deshmukh and Chaniana 2020; Rose-Clarke et al. 2019). For instance, awareness of contraceptive methods is critically low among adolescent girls in diverse Indian contexts, ranging from 19% to 48% (Patel et al. 2018; Shankar et al. 2017; Gupta et al. 2015). A previous study conducted in Uttar Pradesh and Bihar using the UDAYA dataset found substantial gender differences in HIV/AIDS awareness, where girls were significantly less informed than boys. They found that only 30% of adolescent girls had heard of HIV/AIDS in 2015–2016, which has increased to 39% after 3 years (Srivastava et al. 2021). Our recent study found that a small proportion of girls (<10%) have sufficient knowledge of SRH in the states of Uttar Pradesh and Bihar (Saha et al. 2022).

Poor knowledge of SRH not only adversely affects the physical health of girls but also has significant detrimental effects on their mental health. Adolescents ang young girls with insufficient SRH knowledge are vulnerable to unhealthy and unsafe menstrual hygiene practices, high-risk sexual behaviours, sexual abuse, limited access to modern contraceptives, and sexually transmitted infections (STIs) (Parida et al. 2021; Hamdanieh et al. 2021). A lack of adequate SRH information can negatively influence fertility decisions, resulting in teenage pregnancies, unwanted pregnancies, and unsafe abortions (Liu et al. 2023; Murro et al. 2021). This lack of information can result in severe health outcomes, including premature births, low birth weight, and maternal and neonatal mortality. Additionally, it increases the risk of preventable gynaecological issues, such as irregular menstrual cycles, urethral discharge, and burning during urination (Kumar et al. 2021; Banke-Thomas et al. 2017; Hardon et al. 2019).

Studies have indicated that the social stigma around SRH, low levels of education, and a lack of efficacy and agency prevent girls specifically from socioeconomically disadvantaged communities from accessing adequate SRH information (Barua et al. 2020; Santhya and Jejeebhoy 2012; Saha et al. 2022; Hardon et al. 2019; Sanneving et al. 2013; Singh and Srinivasan 2000). In India, conservative sociocultural norms and poor parent–adolescent communication often restrict girls from gaining SRH knowledge from parents, household members, and peers. Adolescents and young girls also encounter misinformation on sexual health topics, contributing to the worsening of their SRH issues (Munakampe et al. 2018; Janighorban et al. 2022).

Evidence indicates that parents can serve as key sources of information for SRH-related matters (Bobhate and Shrivastava 2011; Yadav and Kumar 2023). Parents who are actively involved in their children's lives and maintain positive relationships are more likely to prioritize their children's education, health, and well-being (Raj et al. 2019, 2021). For instance, parental engagement significantly delays marriage time for adolescent girls in India (Paul et al. 2023; Bhan et al. 2019). It helps keep girls in school until they become adults, which can also positively impact their gaining SRH information from their parents, schools, and peer groups. Studies have also demonstrated that parent–adolescent communication and connectedness can significantly influence sexual behaviour and SRH outcomes. This includes reduced levels of unprotected sex, delayed sexual initiation, the prevention of teenage pregnancy, and a decreased risk of STIs (Markham et al. 2010; Santa Maria et al. 2014; Deptula et al. 2010; Okigbo et al. 2015). Positive dialogue with parents can empower adolescents and young girls to make informed decisions on their SRH issues (Usonwu et al. 2021; Wamoyi et al. 2010). Hence, parental communication about SRH matters may play a vital role in girls' obtaining accurate SRH knowledge (Jejeebhoy and Santhya 2011; Sandra Byers et al. 2021). In this context, this study aims to examine the extent of knowledge about SRH and its variations across sociodemographic factors. The study further explores how parental communication about SRH matters is linked to the SRH knowledge of girls in Uttar Pradesh and Bihar.

11.2 Data and Methods

11.2.1 Data Source

We used data from the Understanding the Lives of Adolescents and Young Adults (UDAYA) survey, conducted by the Population Council. This longitudinal survey collected data on adolescent boys and girls (aged 10–19 years) in Bihar and Uttar Pradesh in 2015–2016 (wave 1) and again followed up in 2018–2019 (wave 2). The UDAYA survey adopted a multistage sampling design, selecting 150 primary sampling units from rural and urban areas by using the Census 2011 list. We analysed data from 10,425 participants in wave 2 by including the cohorts of unmarried and married girls (aged 15–19 in wave 1). For the analysis of the association between parent–adolescent communication and girls' SRH knowledge, we used a subsample featuring 6168 unmarried girls interviewed in both waves.

11.2.2 Measures

We assessed girls' SRH knowledge by using three variables: (1) sexual intercourse and pregnancy, (2) contraceptive methods, and (3) HIV/AIDS. Each variable was categorized into two groups: girls with sufficient knowledge and girls with insufficient knowledge. Knowledge about sexual intercourse and pregnancy was assessed by using two questions: whether a woman can get pregnant the first time she has sexual intercourse and whether pregnancy is more likely on certain days between menstrual periods. If respondents answered yes to the second question, they were asked when this occurs. Those who answered "halfway between two periods" were considered knowledgeable. A dichotomous variable was created, categorizing participants with correct answers to both questions as having sufficient knowledge. Contraceptive knowledge was evaluated with three questions on family planning: how often to take oral pills, when to take contraceptive pills after sexual intercourse, and how many times one condom can be used. Participants who gave correct answers to any two questions were deemed knowledgeable. HIV/AIDS knowledge was measured through five questions addressing misconceptions about HIV transmission and two major prevention methods. Participants who rejected all the misconceptions and knew about prevention methods were considered knowledgeable. Those who answered all five questions correctly were categorized as having sufficient knowledge. A detailed description of the measures for sufficient SRH knowledge is provided elsewhere (Saha et al. 2022).

Parental interaction or communication with girls may play a crucial role in girls' gaining accurate knowledge of SRH and in providing the necessary support for their successful transitions to adulthood. We assessed parent–adolescent communication about SRH issues via two items: whether girls and their parents had had any discussion about (a) physical changes during puberty/menstruation and (b) how pregnancy occurs. In addition, sociodemographic variables were included in this analysis: girls' current age, place of residence (urban or rural), caste, religion, education, wealth quintile, and state.

11.2.3 Analytical Strategies

First, we analysed the level of SRH knowledge in both study states. Next, we examined the relationship between sufficient SRH knowledge and various sociodemographic characteristics through bivariate analysis. Third, we assessed parent–adolescent communication about SRH issues across both states. Finally, we assessed whether parent–adolescent communication at wave 1 was significantly associated with SRH knowledge at wave 2 among adolescents and young girls. To determine this association, we initially calculated the bivariate percentage distribution between the two factors. We used sample weights for percentage estimation and tested differences by using Pearson's chi-square statistic. Additionally, a binary logistic regression model was employed to examine both the unadjusted and adjusted associations between parent–adolescent communication and SRH knowledge. All the analyses were conducted by using Stata software (StataCorp, College Station, TX, USA).

11.3 Results and Discussion

11.3.1 Knowledge of SRH Matters

Overall, adolescents and young girls in the study setting have significantly low levels of adequate knowledge about sexual and reproductive health (SRH) issues. More than half of the girls (52%) lack an understanding of sexual intercourse and pregnancy, and only 9% possess the correct knowledge on both questions related to sexual intercourse and pregnancy. Concerning contraceptive methods, 58% of girls have no knowledge, 31% of girls use any method of contraception, and only 12% have the correct knowledge on at least two contraceptive methods (referred to as sufficient knowledge about contraceptive use). Nearly two-thirds of girls (65%) do not have the correct knowledge about HIV/AIDS. Only 7% of girls reported correct answers for all five questions about HIV/AIDS (referred to as sufficient knowledge of HIV/AIDS) (Fig. 11.1).

The level of sufficient SRH knowledge differs considerably across the studied states. Girls living in Bihar have a higher understanding of sexual intercourse and pregnancy (11% vs. 7%) and contraceptive methods (12% vs. 11%) compared to those living in Uttar Pradesh. Conversely, knowledge about HIV/AIDS is somewhat greater among girls in Uttar Pradesh than among those in Bihar (7% vs. 6%)

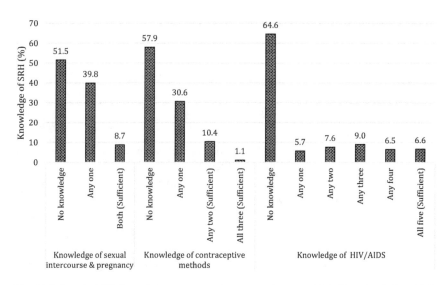

Fig. 11.1 Level of SRH knowledge among adolescents and young girls in Uttar Pradesh and Bihar

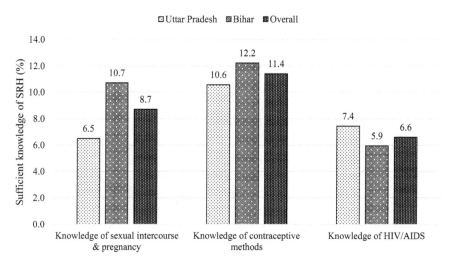

Fig. 11.2 Sufficient knowledge of SRH matters among adolescents and young girls in Uttar Pradesh and Bihar

(Fig. 11.2). The lack of SRH knowledge in this area is attributed mainly to cultural barriers, taboos, restricted female agency, low education, and low access to digital technology (Saha et al. 2022). Additionally, disrupted and diminished services and limited local health facilities can contribute to adolescents' lack of SRH knowledge and awareness. Adolescent girls in these states have a limited understanding of government initiatives on SRH (e.g. the RKSK), which inhibits them from accessing the benefits of the programme. For instance, only 2–3% of girls in Bihar and 1–5% of girls in Uttar Pradesh were aware of a peer education programme, one of the key components of the RKSK programme (Santhya et al. 2017a, b). Girls' lack of knowledge on SRH matters may lead to critical reproductive health issues among women, including the high burden of unwanted pregnancies and maternal mortality in the study region (Dehingia et al. 2020; Sharma and Singh 2023).

Table 11.1 Knowledge of SRH matters according to socioeconomic characteristics of adolescents and young girls

Variables	Sufficient knowledge of SRH					
	Sexual intercourse and pregnancy		Contraceptive methods		HIV/AIDS	
	%	p-Value	%	p-Value	%	p-Value
Current age of girls		<0.001		<0.001		<0.001
18	6.4		7.4		4.6	
19	6.9		7.1		5.4	
20	8.9		11.5		6.5	
21	10.6		14.3		8.6	
22	12.0		19.4		8.8	
Place of residence		0.430		<0.001		<0.001
Urban	8.8		13.7		13.5	
Rural	8.7		11.0		5.4	
Caste		0.003		<0.001		<0.001
SC/ST	7.8		9.0		3.9	
OBC	8.9		11.5		6.5	
General	9.3		13.7		10.4	
Religion		0.213		0.088		<0.001
Hindu	8.9		11.7		6.6	
Non-Hindu	8.0		10.4		7.0	
Education		0.001		<0.001		<0.001
Illiterate	6.3		9.1		0.7	
Primary	7.3		7.2		1.8	
Secondary	9.2		10.8		5.2	
Higher	9.3		17.0		17.7	
Marital status		<0.001		<0.001		<0.001
Unmarried	4.9		7.6		7.6	
Married	13.2		16.0		5.5	
Wealth quintile		<0.001		<0.001		<0.001
Poorest	6.0		8.2		1.9	
Poorer	8.4		10.1		3.8	
Middle	7.8		11.3		5.4	
Richer	10.2		12.7		9.2	
Richest	12.3		16.1		15.1	

Note: p-values were derived from Pearson's chi-square test of association

11.3.2 Knowledge of SRH Matters According to Socioeconomic Characteristics

Table 11.1 displays the level of sufficient knowledge on SRH matters according to selected sociodemographic characteristics. The data show that the proportion of girls with sufficient knowledge increases with age across all three measures of SRH knowledge, indicating that younger girls (under 18 years) are more susceptible to lacking adequate SRH information than older girls. Girls residing in urban areas possess greater knowledge of contraceptive methods (14% vs. 11%) and HIV/AIDS (14% vs. 5%) than their rural counterparts. The lack of SRH knowledge among girls in rural areas is often attributed to regressive social norms, social stigma, disrupted and reduced services, and limited local health facilities (Meena et al. 2015; Saha et al. 2022; Anand 2014).

Girls from socially disadvantaged backgrounds—such as those belonging to a Scheduled Caste (SC), Scheduled Tribe (ST), or Other Backward Class (OBC)—encounter substantial barriers to accessing SRH information. For example, only 9% of girls from SC/ST groups have adequate knowledge of contraceptive methods, compared to 14% of girls from the General caste. Girls from the SC/ST groups are the least informed about HIV/AIDS, with only 4% having adequate knowledge, followed by OBC girls, at 7%. In contrast, 10% of girls from the General caste are sufficiently informed about HIV/AIDS. Hindu girls have slightly more knowledge about contraceptive methods than non-Hindu girls (12% vs. 10%; p<0.088). However, non-Hindu girls possess a slightly higher level of knowledge about HIV/AIDS than Hindu girls (p<0.001).

A clear positive relationship exists between girls' educational attainment and their knowledge of SRH, with SRH knowledge increasing as educational levels rise. Girls with secondary and higher education are more informed about sexual intercourse and pregnancy, contraceptive methods, and HIV/AIDS than those with no education. Girls with little or no education often have reduced self-efficacy and lack agency or autonomy, which can limit their access to SRH information. Even when exposed to SRH information, their lack of education can hamper their ability to contextualize and respond appropriately. Education enables young girls to access diverse health awareness programmes and online resources, stay updated on health recommendations, and develop the confidence and motivation required to engage in health and knowledge-seeking behaviours (Saha et al. 2022).

Married girls reported significantly higher levels of sufficient knowledge about sexual intercourse and pregnancy (13% vs. 5%) and contraceptive methods (16% vs. 8%) than unmarried girls. This difference may be attributed to married girls' increased exposure to and support from mainstream maternal health outreach programmes, which may enhance their awareness of healthy sexual practices. These findings underscore a critical area of concern and emphasize the need to strengthen efforts towards more-inclusive, age- and context-specific adolescent health programmes. However, married girls are less informed about HIV/AIDS than their unmarried counterparts are (8% vs. 6%). This could be due to a lack of or weak advocacy for programmes related to HIV/AIDS, which receive little attention in maternal healthcare policies, as well as social stigma and a lack of awareness campaigns, leading to insufficient knowledge about HIV/AIDS among married adolescents and young girls (Plesons et al. 2020).

The economic status of a household is positively correlated with girls' knowledge of SRH. Girls from the wealthiest quintile exhibit significantly higher levels of sufficient knowledge about sexual intercourse and pregnancy (12% vs. 6%), contraceptive methods (16% vs. 8%), and HIV/AIDS (15% vs. 2%) than those from the poorest quintile. Poor families often face multiple barriers to accessing healthcare information and services, grappling with social marginalization, low levels of education, and limited exposure to health awareness programmes. Furthermore, the pervasiveness of early marriage and child labour hinders girls belonging to poor families from obtaining critical healthcare information, including that on SRH matters (Srivastava et al. 2021; Oginni et al. 2017).

11.3.3 Parent–Adolescent Communication on SRH Issues

In the study setting, discussing SRH issues with children is often considered a matter of disgrace to the community/society. Parents often feel discomfort when discussing SRH-related topics with their children. Moreover, social stigma around SRH matters and a lack of both education and SRH knowledge among parents stand out as major barriers to parent–adolescent communication (Maina et al. 2020). Other obstacles to parent–adolescent dialogue on SRH topics are the prevailing cultural beliefs of parents that adolescents are too immature for conversations on sexual topics and an unfavourable conversational atmosphere (Toru et al. 2022).

In this study, we found that over two-thirds of girls (69%) discuss physical changes during puberty/menstruation and that only 3% of girls discuss

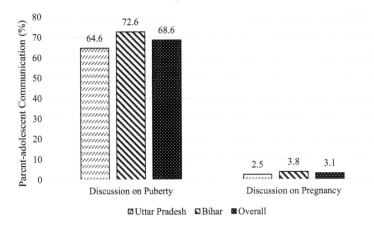

Fig. 11.3 Parent–adolescent communication on SRH issues in Uttar Pradesh and Bihar

Table 11.2 Parent–adolescent communication on SRH issues in Uttar Pradesh and Bihar (combined)

Parent–adolescent communication	Discussing puberty/menstruation		Discussing pregnancy	
	N	%	N	%
Mother	4241	68.2	154	2.5
Father	11	0.2	18	0.4
Both	21	0.3	12	0.3
Neither	1694	28.8	5783	94.3
NA	201	2.6	201	2.6
Total	6168	100.0	6168	100.0

Note: NA refers to not applicable

pregnancy-related issues with their parents. Girls from Bihar have a relatively higher proportion of parent–adolescent communication on menstruation (73% vs. 65%) and pregnancy (4% vs. 3%) than those from Uttar Pradesh (Fig. 11.3). Although discussion related to menstruation with parents occurs at the time of physical changes or puberty, pregnancy is likely to occur after marriage, leading to low parent–adolescent communication on pregnancy during adolescence (Paul et al. 2023). In the Tanzanian context, parents have limited communication with their daughters on pregnancy issues, which tends to be always delivered as general warnings (Wamoyi et al. 2010). Similarly, in Ghana, condoms (5%) and other contraceptive methods (9%) are hardly discussed between parents and adolescents (Manu et al. 2015).

Interestingly, the majority of girls indicated that they discussed these SRH issues only with their mothers. According to Table 11.2, over one-third of girls (68%) communicate about menstruation issues, and 3% of girls discuss issues related to pregnancy with their mothers only. Only a few proportions of girls (0.2% for menstruation and 0.4% for pregnancy) discuss SRH issues solely with their fathers (Table 11.2). Our findings resonate with those of other studies on similar socioeconomic settings like Nepal and Ethiopia, where the majority of adolescents interacted with their mothers only (Singh et al. 2023; Toru et al. 2022). Ironically, fathers mostly decide their daughters' social mobility, education, marriage, and other aspects of life in such patriarchal settings. In this context, daughters are submissive to their fathers—an asymmetrical power relationship—which is historically, socially, and economically produced and reproduced through the process of social interaction (Basu et al. 2017).

Table 11.3 Sufficient knowledge of SRH matters depending on parent–adolescent communication on SRH issues

Parent–adolescent communication	Knowledge of sexual intercourse and pregnancy		Knowledge of contraceptive methods		Knowledge of HIV/AIDS	
	%	p-Value	%	p-Value	%	p-Value
Discussion on menstruation		0.003		0.005		<0.001
No	5.8		8.0		5.1	
Yes	8.2		9.5		7.7	
Discussion on pregnancy		0.195		<0.001		<0.001
No	7.4		8.8		6.6	
Yes	9.0		17.0		15.8	
Overall	7.5		9.1		6.9	

11.3.4 Relationship Between Parent–Adolescent Communication and Girls' Knowledge of SRH Matters

A positive correlation exists between parent–adolescent communication and girls' knowledge of SRH matters. Girls who communicated with parents around puberty/menstruation have a significantly higher percentage of adequate knowledge of sexual intercourse and pregnancy (8% vs. 6%), contraceptive methods (10% vs. 8%), and HIV/AIDS (8% vs. 5%) relative to those without such communication. Similarly, girls who had discussions with their parents about pregnancy issues have a notably higher percentage of sufficient knowledge about contraceptive methods (17% vs. 9%) and HIV/AIDS (16% vs. 7%) than those who do not engage in these conversations (Table 11.3).

We conducted both crude and multivariable binary logistic regression analyses to examine the link between parent–adolescent communication and adolescents and young girls' knowledge of sexual and reproductive health (SRH) issues. The unadjusted regression results reveal that girls who talked with their parents about puberty or menstruation are more likely to have sufficient knowledge about sexual intercourse and pregnancy (OR: 1.38; 95% CI: 1.11, 1.73), contraceptive methods (OR: 1.27; 95% CI: 1.05, 1.54), and HIV/AIDS (OR: 1.53; 95% CI: 1.25, 1.87). Similarly, discussions about pregnancy are strongly associated with increased knowledge about contraceptive methods (OR: 2.22; 95% CI: 1.53, 3.23) and HIV/AIDS (OR: 1.91; 95% CI: 1.29, 2.81). Even after adjusting for key sociodemographic factors, the association between parent–adolescent communication about menstruation and knowledge of sexual intercourse and pregnancy (AOR: 1.33; 95% CI: 1.06, 1.68) and HIV/AIDS (AOR: 1.31; 95% CI: 1.06, 1.61) remains statistically significant. However, an adjusted analysis shows that parental discussions about pregnancy are significantly associated only with girls' knowledge of contraceptive methods (AOR: 1.91; 95% CI: 1.30, 2.81). While the odds of knowledge about sexual intercourse

Table 11.4 Binary logistic regression results showing the relationship between parent–adolescent communication and knowledge of SRH matters among adolescents and young girls

Parent–adolescent communication	Knowledge of sexual intercourse and pregnancy	95% CI		Knowledge of contraceptive methods	95% CI		Knowledge of HIV/AIDS	95% CI	
	OR	LB	UB	OR	LB	UB	OR	LB	UB
Unadjusted model									
Discussing puberty	1.38**	1.11	1.73	1.27*	1.05	1.54	1.53**	1.25	1.87
Discussing pregnancy	1.29	0.79	2.13	2.22**	1.53	3.23	1.91**	1.29	2.81
Adjusted model									
Discussing puberty	1.33*	1.06	1.68	1.15	0.95	1.40	1.31*	1.06	1.61
Discussing pregnancy	1.14	0.69	1.91	1.91**	1.30	2.81	1.49	0.99	2.26

and pregnancy are higher among girls who discuss pregnancy with their parents than among those who do not, this association is statistically insignificant in both unadjusted and adjusted analyses, possibly due to smaller sample sizes (Table 11.4).

A Global Early Adolescent Study conducted in four countries found that parental communication with adolescents is positively associated with pregnancy knowledge and contraceptive awareness (Sievwright et al. 2023). Parental support during adolescence can enhance girls' self-efficacy and empower them, aiding them in operationalizing their agency and raising their voices against conservative societal norms. Conversely, parental restriction and control, especially when fathers are overly strict, psychologically controlling, and less likely to recognize their children's positive behaviour, is linked to lower self-esteem in girls (Kernis et al. 2000). Parental support coupled with the agency and decision-making power of girls can help them to stay in school longer and gain adequate knowledge of SRH, resulting in their better management of menstrual hygiene and safer sexual practices (Singh et al. 2023; Malango et al. 2022). In addition, mother–daughter communication about sexual practices has been observed to be associated with daughters' enhanced communication with their immediate partners, leading to the establishment of inner confidence in contraception selection and use (Hutchinson and Cooney 1998).

However, unidirectional, fear-based, or admonishing conversations are found to be less effective in making a positive measurable impact (Wamoyi et al. 2010; Sievwright et al. 2023). A strict and authoritative parental style may lead to anxiety and depression among adolescent girls, and they thus become vulnerable to poor SRH outcomes (Yap et al. 2014; Janighorban et al. 2022). More so, initiating such discussions when parents suspect their adolescents are engaging in sexual activity can be counterproductive (Magnani et al. 2002). In contrast, positive parental engagement with adolescent girls can help reduce risky sexual behaviours, such as early sexual initiation and unprotected sex, and can help decrease the risk of STIs, including HIV/AIDS (Coakley et al. 2017; Widman et al. 2016). Thus, having a timely and quality dialogue between parents and their children regarding SRH issues is pertinent to ensuring the good health and well-being of adolescents and young girls.

Importantly, our measure of parent–adolescent communication on SRH issues lacks comprehensiveness in that it encompasses only two dimensions of SRH matters: puberty/menstruation and pregnancy. Moreover, the quality of communication is inadequately elucidated by these two questions on parent–adolescent communication, thereby impeding the development of tailored policies to address the poor SRH outcomes of girls. Future studies can explore more dimensions of parent–adolescent communication about SRH issues (e.g. contraceptive methods and the risk of STIs) in designing their studies to provide much-more-informed and better-targeted policy recommendations.

11.4 Conclusion

The sociocultural mosaic of Uttar Pradesh and Bihar is largely patriarchal, characterized by conservative social norms, low female education, son preference, lower female age at marriage, widespread dowries, and the submissive status of women. The sufficient knowledge of SRH among girls is critically low in the study region. Adolescents and young girls face significant obstacles to accessing adequate SRH information. For example, girls from rural areas, those with lower education levels, those socially marginalized, and those from economically disadvantaged families often have limited SRH knowledge. In the study area, inadequate SRH knowledge is frequently a result of conservative social norms, social stigma, disrupted and poor-quality services, and limited local health facilities.

We further found that communication between parents and adolescents about sexual and reproductive health (SRH) is positively linked to increased knowledge about sexual intercourse and pregnancy, contraceptive methods, and HIV/AIDS. The study highlighted the crucial role of parent–adolescent dialogue in gaining accurate information on SRH for adolescents and young girls. Although parental engagement was found to be a positive catalyst in facilitating SRH information among adolescents and young girls, excessive parental control or restrictive behaviour may risk this protective association of SRH on girls (Markham et al. 2010). In the patriarchal setting of Bihar and Uttar Pradesh, parents (fathers in particular) often exert their gender-differentiated attitudes towards the behaviours of adolescents, where girls (daughters) are overmonitored compared to their male counterparts when they reach puberty and try to settle their marriage at an early age. This potentially results in girls' being poorly informed about SRH issues, which may further negatively impact their future fertility behaviours. The findings of this study highlight the necessity for targeted interventions designed for specific contexts, focusing on fostering equitable beliefs about and attitudes towards gender differences in the parental control or monitoring of adolescents. These interventions should raise awareness of SRH issues and encourage parents to become more actively involved in supporting their children's SRH issues. Additionally, the findings underscore the need for culturally appropriate policies and programmes to guide community stakeholders and support a comprehensive approach to enhancing the SRH of adolescents and young girls in India.

Declaration

Availability of Data and Materials The data and materials for this study are accessible through the Harvard Dataverse repository (https://www.1015237projectudaya.in/).

Ethics Approval and Consent to Participate The UDAYA survey was approved by the Population Council's ethical review board. The privacy and confidentiality of respondents were rigorously upheld during the interviews. Consent was obtained from all participants, with additional consent from parents or guardians for unmarried minors.

Competing Interests The authors declare that they have no known financial or personal conflicts of interest that could have influenced the reported work.

Funding This study did not receive any specific funding from external grant agencies.

References

Anand M (2014) Health status and health care services in Uttar Pradesh and Bihar: a comparative study. Indian J Public Health 58(3):174–179

Banerjee SK, Andersen KL, Warvadekar J, Aich P, Rawat A, Upadhyay B (2015) How prepared are young, rural women in India to address their sexual and reproductive health needs? A cross-sectional assessment of youth in Jharkhand. Reprod Health 12:1–10

Banke-Thomas OE, Banke-Thomas AO, Ameh CA (2017) Factors influencing utilisation of maternal health services by adolescent mothers in low- and middle-income countries: a systematic review. BMC Pregnancy Childbirth 17(1):1–14

Barua A, Watson K, Plesons M, Chandra-Mouli V, Sharma K (2020) Adolescent health programming in India: a rapid review. Reprod Health 17(1):1–10

Basu S, Zuo X, Lou C, Acharya R, Lundgren R (2017) Learning to be gendered: gender socialization in early adolescence among urban poor in Delhi, India, and Shanghai, China. J Adolesc Health 61(4):S24–S29

Bhan N, Gautsch L, McDougal L, Lapsansky C, Obregon R, Raj A (2019) Effects of parent–child relationships on child marriage of girls in Ethiopia, India, Peru, and Vietnam: evidence from a prospective cohort. J Adolesc Health 65(4):498–506

Bhat N, Shankar P (2021) India's adolescents: taking charge of the future. Lancet Child Adolesc Health 5(12):847–849

Bobhate PS, Shrivastava SR (2011) A cross sectional study of knowledge and practices about reproductive health among female adolescents in an urban slum of Mumbai. J Fam Reprod Health 5(4):117–124

Coakley TM, Randolph S, Shears J, Beamon ER, Collins P, Sides T (2017) Parent–youth communication to reduce at-risk sexual behavior: a systematic literature review. J Hum Behav Soc Environ 27(6):609–624

Dehingia N, Dixit A, Atmavilas Y, Chandurkar D, Singh K, Silverman J, Raj A (2020) Unintended pregnancy and maternal health complications: cross-sectional analysis of data from rural Uttar Pradesh, India. BMC Pregnancy Childbirth 20:1–11

Deptula DP, Henry DB, Schoeny ME (2010) How can parents make a difference? Longitudinal associations with adolescent sexual behavior. J Fam Psychol 24(6):731

Deshmukh DD, Chaniana SS (2020) Knowledge about sexual and reproductive health in adolescent school-going children of 8th, 9th, and 10th standards. J Psychosexual Health 2(1):56–62

Gupta M, Bhatnagar N, Bahugana P (2015) Inequity in awareness and utilization of adolescent reproductive and sexual health services in union territory, Chandigarh, North India. Indian J Public Health 59(1):9–17

Hamdanieh M, Ftouni L, Al Jardali BA, Ftouni R, Rawas C, Ghotmi M et al (2021) Assessment of sexual and reproductive health knowledge and awareness among single unmarried women living in Lebanon: a cross-sectional study. Reprod Health 18:1–12

Hardon A, Pell C, Taqueban E, Narasimhan M (2019) Sexual and reproductive self care among women and girls: insights from ethnographic studies. BMJ 365:l1333

Hutchinson KM, Cooney TM (1998) Patterns of parent-teen sexual risk communication: implications for intervention. Fam Relat 47:185–194

Janighorban M, Boroumandfar Z, Pourkazemi R, Mostafavi F (2022) Barriers to vulnerable adolescent girls' access to sexual and reproductive health. BMC Public Health 22(1):1–16

Jejeebhoy SJ, Santhya KG (2011) Parent-child communication on sexual and reproductive health matters: perspectives of mothers and fathers of youth in India. Population Council, New Delhi

Kernis MH, Brown AC, Brody GH (2000) Fragile self-esteem in children and its associations with perceived patterns of parent-child communication. J Pers 68(2):225–252

Khanna R, Sheth M, Talati P, Damor K, Chauhan B (2022) Social and economic marginalisation and sexual and reproductive health and rights of urban poor young women: a qualitative study from Vadodara, Gujarat, India. Sex Reprod Health Matters 29(2):2059898

Kumar P, Srivastava S, Chauhan S, Patel R, Marbaniang SP, Dhillon P (2021) Factors associated with gynaecological morbidities and treatment-seeking behaviour among adolescent girls residing in Bihar and Uttar Pradesh, India. PLoS One 16(6):e0252521

Liu R, Dong X, Ji X, Chen S, Yuan Q, Tao Y et al (2023) Associations between sexual and reproductive health knowledge, attitude and practice of partners and the occurrence of unintended pregnancy. Front Public Health 10:1042879

Magnani RJ, Karim AM, Weiss LA, Bond KC, Lemba M, Morgan GT (2002) Reproductive health risk and protective factors among youth in Lusaka, Zambia. J Adolesc Health 30(1):76–86

Maina BW, Ushie BA, Kabiru CW (2020) Parent-child sexual and reproductive health communication among very young adolescents in Korogocho informal settlement in Nairobi, Kenya. Reprod Health 17(1):1–14

Malango NT, Hegena TY, Assefa NA (2022) Parent–adolescent discussion on sexual and reproductive health issues and its associated factors among parents in Sawla town, Gofa zone, Ethiopia. Reprod Health 19(1):108

Manu AA, Mba CJ, Asare GQ, Odoi-Agyarko K, Asante RKO (2015) Parent–child communication about sexual and reproductive health: evidence from the Brong Ahafo region, Ghana. Reprod Health 12:1–13

Markham CM, Lormand D, Gloppen KM, Peskin MF, Flores B, Low B, House LD (2010) Connectedness as a predictor of sexual and reproductive health outcomes for youth. J Adolesc Health 46(3):S23–S41

Meena JK, Verma A, Kishore J, Ingle GK (2015) Sexual and reproductive health: knowledge, attitude, and perceptions among young unmarried male residents of Delhi. Int J Reprod Med 2015(1):431460

Munkampe MN, Zulu JM, Michelo C (2018) Contraception and abortion knowledge, attitudes and practices among adolescents from low and middle-income countries: a systematic review. BMC Health Serv Res 18(1):1–13

Murro R, Chawla R, Pyne S, Venkatesh S, Sully EA (2021) Adding it up: investing in the sexual and reproductive health of adolescents in India. Guttmacher Institute, New York. https://www.guttmacher.org/sites/default/files/report_pdf/investing-in-sexual-reproductive-health-adolescents-india.pdf. Accessed 19 Jul 2022

Oginni AB, Adebajo SB, Ahonsi BA (2017) Trends and determinants of comprehensive knowledge of HIV among adolescents and young adults in Nigeria: 2003-2013. Afr J Reprod Health 21(1):26–34

Okigbo CC, Kabiru CW, Mumah JN, Mojola SA, Beguy D (2015) Influence of parental factors on adolescents' transition to first sexual intercourse in Nairobi, Kenya: a longitudinal study. Reprod Health 12:1–12

Parida SP, Gajjala A, Giri PP (2021) Empowering adolescent girls, is sexual and reproductive health education a solution? J Family Med Prim Care 10(1):66

Patel P, Puwar T, Shah N, Saxena D, Trivedi P, Patel K et al (2018) Improving adolescent health: learnings from an interventional study in Gujarat, India. Indian J Commun Med 43(Suppl 1):S12

Paul M, Essén B, Sariola S, Iyengar S, Soni S, Klingberg Allvin M (2017) Negotiating collective and individual agency: a qualitative study of young women's reproductive health in rural India. Qual Health Res 27(3):311–324

Paul P, Closson K, Raj A (2023) Is parental engagement associated with subsequent delayed marriage and marital choices of adolescent girls? Evidence from the understanding the lives of adolescents and young adults (UDAYA) survey in Uttar Pradesh and Bihar, India. SSM Popul Health 24:101523

Plesons M, Khanna A, Ziauddin M, Gogoi A, Chandra-Mouli V (2020) Building an enabling environment and responding to resistance to sexuality education programmes: experience from Jharkhand, India. Reprod Health 17:1–9

Population Council (2017) Adolescent health priorities and opportunities for Rashtriya Kishor SwasthyaKaryakram (RKSK) in Uttar Pradesh. https://www.popcouncil.org/uploads/pdfs/2017PGY_UDAYA-RKSKPolicyBriefUP.pdf. Accessed 19 Jul 2022

Raj A, Salazar M, Jackson EC, Wyss N, McClendon KA, Khanna A et al (2019) Students and brides: a qualitative analysis of the relationship between girls' education and early marriage in Ethiopia and India. BMC Public Health 19(1):1–20

Raj A, Johns NE, Bhan N, Silverman JG, Lundgren R (2021) Effects of gender role beliefs on social connectivity and marital safety: findings from a cross-sectional study among married adolescent girls in India. J Adolesc Health 69(6):S65–S73

Rose-Clarke K, Pradhan H, Rath S, Rath S, Samal S, Gagrai S et al (2019) Adolescent girls' health, nutrition and wellbeing in rural eastern India: a descriptive, cross-sectional community-based study. BMC Public Health 19(1):1–11

Saha R, Paul P, Yaya S, Banke-Thomas A (2022) Association between exposure to social media and knowledge of sexual and reproductive health among adolescent girls: evidence from the UDAYA survey in Bihar and Uttar Pradesh, India. Reprod Health 19(1):1–15

Sandra Byers E, O'Sullivan LF, Mitra K, Sears HA (2021) Parent–adolescent sexual communication in India: responses of middle class parents. J Fam Issues 42(4):762–784

Sanneving L, Trygg N, Saxena D, Mavalankar D, Thomsen S (2013) Inequity in India: the case of maternal and reproductive health. Glob Health Action 6(1):19145

Santa Maria D, Markham C, Swank P, Baumler E, McCurdy S, Tortolero S (2014) Does parental monitoring moderate the relation between parent–child communication and pre-coital sexual behaviours among urban, minority early adolescents? Sex Educ 14(3):286–298

Santhya KG, Jejeebhoy SJ (2012) The sexual and reproductive health and rights of young people in India: a review of the situation. Population Council, New Delhi

Santhya KG, Acharya R, Pandey N et al (2017a) Understanding the lives of adolescents and young adults (UDAYA) in Uttar Pradesh, India. Population Council, New Delhi

Santhya KG, Acharya R, Pandey N et al (2017b) Understanding the lives of adolescents and young adults (UDAYA) in Bihar, India. Population Council, New Delhi

Shankar P, Dudeja P, Gadekar T, Mukherji S (2017) Reproductive health awareness among adolescent girls of a government school in an urban slum of Pune City. Med J Dr DY Patil Univ 10(2):133

Sharma H, Singh SK (2023) The burden of unintended pregnancies among Indian adolescent girls in Bihar and Uttar Pradesh: findings from the UDAYA survey (2015–16 & 2018–19). Arch Public Health 81(1):1–16

Sievwright KM, Moreau C, Li M, Ramaiya A, Gayles J, Blum RW (2023) Adolescent–parent relationships and communication: consequences for pregnancy knowledge and family planning service awareness. J Adolesc Health 73(1):S43–S54

Singh LP, Srinivasan K (2000) Family planning and the scheduled tribes of Rajasthan: taking stock and moving forward. J Health Manag 2(1):55–80

Singh DR, Shrestha S, Karki K, Sunuwar DR, Khadka DB, Maharjan D et al (2023) Parental knowledge and communication with their adolescent on sexual and reproductive health issues in Nepal. PLoS One 18(7):e0289116

Srivastava S, Chauhan S, Patel R, Kumar P (2021) A study of awareness on HIV/AIDS among adolescents: a longitudinal study on UDAYA data. Sci Rep 11(1):22841

Toru T, Sahlu D, Worku Y, Beya M (2022) Parent–adolescent communication on sexual and reproductive health issues and associated factors among students in high school and preparatory in Arekit, southwest, Ethiopia, 2020. Int J Afr Nurs Sci 17:100509

United Nations Population Fund (UNFPA) (2014) A profile of adolescents and youth in India. Office of the Registrar General & Census Commissioner, India. 2014 [cited/accessed 2022 19 Jan]. https://india.unfpa.org/sites/default/files/pub-pdf/AProfileofAdolescentsandYouthinIndia_0.pdf

Usonwu I, Ahmad R, Curtis-Tyler K (2021) Parent–adolescent communication on adolescent sexual and reproductive health in sub-Saharan Africa: a qualitative review and thematic synthesis. Reprod Health 18(1):1–15

Wamoyi J, Fenwick A, Urassa M, Zaba B, Stones W (2010) Parent-child communication about sexual and reproductive health in rural Tanzania: implications for young people's sexual health interventions. Reprod Health 7(1):1–18

Widman L, Choukas-Bradley S, Noar SM, Nesi J, Garrett K (2016) Parent–adolescent sexual communication and adolescent safer sex behavior: a meta-analysis. JAMA Pediatr 170(1):52–61

Yadav N, Kumar D (2023) The impact of reproductive and sexual health education among school going adolescents in Andaman and Nicobar Islands. Clin Epidemiol Global Health 24:101416

Yap MBH, Pilkington PD, Ryan SM, Jorm AF (2014) Parental factors associated with depression and anxiety in young people: a systematic review and meta-analysis. J Affect Disord 156:8–23

Chapter 12
Do Menstrual Hygiene Practices Reduce Sexual Diseases? A Cross-sectional Study

Swagata Karjee and Prites Chandra Biswas

Abstract Menstrual unhygienic practices have negative impacts on the reproductive and maternal health of women. This chapter aims to investigate menstrual hygiene practices and their associations with sexual diseases among women. Primary household survey data were included in the analysis to fulfil the chapter objectives. Multivariable logistic regression analyses examined the association between menstrual hygienic practices and sexual diseases. Overall, 81% of women in Koch Bihar district use hygienic products during menstruation. Only 53.6% of women who have unimproved toilets use hygienic methods. More than half of the women (60%) have experienced at least one sexual disease. Rural women (AOR: 1.28; 95% CI: 1.24–1.30) are more vulnerable to sexual diseases than urban women are. This chapter finds that menstrual hygienic practices (AOR: 0.64; 95% CI: 0.58–0.72) are significantly associated with various sexual diseases. Interventions that ensure women have access to private facilities with water for menstrual hygiene management (MHM) and that educate women about safer, low-cost MHM materials could reduce sexual disease among women. Further studies on the effects of specific practices for managing hygienically reusable pads are needed.

Keywords Menstrual hygiene · Sexual disease · Women · India

S. Karjee
Department of Geography, Cooch Behar Panchanan Barma University, Cooch Behar, West Bengal, India

P. C. Biswas (✉)
Department of Geography, Acharya Brojendra Nath Seal College, Cooch Behar, West Bengal, India

© The Author(s), under exclusive license to Springer Nature Singapore Pte Ltd. 2024
P. Chouhan et al. (eds.), *Sexual and Reproductive Health of Women*, https://doi.org/10.1007/978-981-97-8418-9_12

12.1 Introduction

The World Health Organization (WHO) has recognized sexual diseases as major global public health concerns. Sexual diseases are more common in the form of sexually transmitted infections and reproductive tract infections (RTIs). These infections are caused by various pathogens, including bacteria, fungi, viruses, and (other) parasites (Chakrabarty and Singh 2023; Galvin and Cohen 2004; Patel et al. 2006; Bradford and Ravel 2017). The burden is significantly higher on this population because of the distinct anatomical and physiological traits that make women more prone to infections (Klouman et al. 1997; Anbesu et al. 2023). Worldwide, about one million new sexually transmitted infections (STIs) are acquired every day, and 90% of them occur in low- and middle-income countries (LMICs) (WHO 2021). Sexual diseases may result in women's reproductive organ injury, infertility, scarring, obstructions, and deficiencies in fallopian tube function and pregnancy-related problems like postpartum haemorrhage and sepsis (Johnson et al. 2011; Racicot and Mor 2017; Zeng et al. 2022). Moreover, women who have sexually transmitted diseases (STDs) are at a higher risk of contracting HIV because these infections can lead to vaginal inflammation and ulceration, which gives the virus a place to enter the body (Galvin and Cohen 2004; Passmore et al. 2016; Mwatelah et al. 2019). Similarly, RTI symptoms, which include itching, abnormal discharge, and soreness, can cause women a great deal of psychological suffering and can lead to stigmatization, social isolation, humiliation, and shame (Bilardi et al. 2013; Galvin and Cohen 2004). In light of this, minimizing sexual diseases is essential to enhancing the general health and well-being of women. Such initiatives may also advance gender parity and allow women to fully engage in socioeconomic and political life.

Proper menstrual hygiene management (MHM) during menstruation is crucial for women's reproductive health because it decreases the risk of sexual disease (Karjee et al. 2023; Roy et al. 2021). According to previous research from Nepal, Bangladesh, and African countries, using sanitary products like tampons, menstrual cups, or sanitary pads might help reduce the replication of potentially harmful bacteria and minimize the incidence of sexual diseases (Bhusal 2020; Austrian et al. 2021; Feng et al. 2021). Most earlier studies in India that looked at the connection between women's RTIs and their usage of sanitary products were based on secondary data (Anand et al. 2015; Chakrabarty and Singh 2023). Thus, the purpose of this chapter is to examine the impact of menstrual hygienic practices on the prevalence of sexual diseases among women in a particular geographic region through a primary field survey.

12.2 Database and Methodology

12.2.1 Sample

In this chapter, women aged 15–24 years were selected for the sample. In total, 237 samples were included in this chapter by using a simple random sampling method in different community development blocks of Koch Bihar district of West Bengal. The sample size was calculated by using a single population proportion formula (Yamane 1967). The respondents were asked several questions related to socioeconomic conditions, menstrual practices, and sexual diseases through a structured survey schedule.

12.2.2 Variables

Women were asked about which protection methods they use to avoid bloodstains throughout their menstrual cycle (survey question: what do you use for protection?). Hygienic practices include sanitary napkins, locally prepared napkins, tampons, and menstrual cups. Any of these four products that a woman uses throughout her menstrual cycle is considered a hygienic practice (coded as 1), and anything else is considered an unhygienic practice (coded as 0). To investigate factors linked to menstrual hygienic practices, women's age, religion, social group, education, monthly household income, mass-media exposure, toilet type, availability of soap for handwashing, water source, and place of residence were included in the analysis.

To examine the prevalence of sexual diseases, women were asked, have you experienced genital sore/ulcer, genital discharge, or genital pain in the past 12 months? If a woman experienced any of these symptoms in the past 12 months, it was considered a sexual disease, coded as 1; otherwise, it was coded as 0. Women's age, religion, social group, education, monthly household income, mass-media exposure, toilet type, availability of soap for handwashing, water source, and place of residence were included in the analysis.

12.2.3 Statistical Analysis

We employed both a bivariate analysis and a multivariate analysis to accomplish the chapter's objectives. The chi-square test was applied to investigate the relationship between the independent and dependent variables in the bivariate analysis. To investigate the factors linked to menstrual hygienic practices and the association between menstrual hygienic practices and the prevalence of sexual diseases, we employed a multivariable logistic regression model. STATA 12.1 software was used to conduct the analysis.

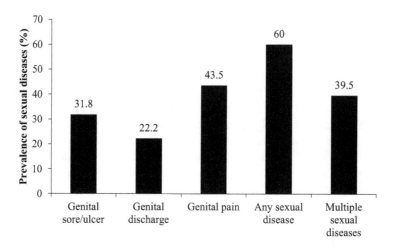

Fig. 12.1 Prevalence of different sexual diseases among young women in Koch Bihar district

12.3 Results

Figure 12.1 shows the prevalence of sexual diseases among women. About 60% of women had experienced at least one sexual disease in Koch Bihar district, whereas nearly 40% of women reported that they had experienced multiple sexual diseases in Koch Bihar district. Moreover, about 43.5% of women had experienced genital pain, followed by genital sore/ulcer (31.8%) and abnormal genital discharge (2.2%).

Table 12.1 shows the prevalence and likelihood of menstrual hygienic practices among young women in Koch Bihar district. The prevalence of hygienic practices is partially higher among women aged 15–19 years than those aged 20–24. Hindu and Muslim women used more hygienic products than women espousing the other religions. However, the probability of hygienic practices was higher among Muslim women than among Hindu women. Among all the social groups, hygienic practices are significantly low among Scheduled Tribe (ST) women (62.4%). Women belonging to other social groups used 2.15 times more hygienic methods than Scheduled Caste (SC) women. Women's education also played a pivotal role in using hygienic methods. Higher-educated women had a 7.22 times higher probability of using hygienic methods than illiterate women had. The results also indicate that women with a monthly household income below INR 20,000 used considerably low hygienic products (63.6%) than women with more than INR 40,000 (97.1%). Similarly, women with higher exposure to mass media have a higher prevalence of hygienic practices (88.2%). Hygienic practices are significantly higher (83.2%) among women who use improved toilets than those who use unimproved toilets (53.6%). Likewise, the availability of soap for handwashing and water sources in household premises positively impacts menstrual hygiene methods. Women in urban areas used more hygienic methods (98.1%) during menstruation than rural women (67.3%).

Table 12.1 Prevalence and likelihood of menstrual hygienic practice among young women in Koch Bihar district

Women's socioeconomic correlates	%	aOR	95% CI
Age			
15–19 years	87.6	[Ref.]	
20–24 years	85.1	0.71*	0.67–0.92
Religion			
Hindu	82.3	[Ref.]	
Muslim	78.4	1.25	0.87–1.72
Others	76.4	1.18	0.69–2.02
Social group			
SC	74.1	[Ref.]	
ST	62.4	0.54***	0.52–0.67
Others	87.8	2.15***	2.14–2.18
Education			
Illiterate	37.3	[Ref.]	
Primary	43.3	1.02	0.81–1.53
Secondary	84.9	3.59***	3.50–3.62
Higher	98.6	7.22***	7.18–7.37
Monthly household income (INR)			
Below 20,000	63.6	[Ref.]	
20,000–40,000	83.4	2.86***	2.79–2.90
Above 40,000	97.1	6.54***	6.36–7.06
Mass-media exposure			
No	44.1	[Ref.]	
Partial	68.4	1.06	0.92–1.83
High	88.2	1.33**	1.25–1.76
Toilet type			
Improved	83.2	[Ref.]	
Unimproved	53.6	0.52***	0.50–0.63
Availability of soap for handwashing			
Available	72.9	[Ref.]	
Unavailable	59.1	0.49***	0.46–0.56
Water source			
Available	66.8	[Ref.]	
Unavailable	43	0.37**	0.32–0.42
Place of residence			
Urban	98.1	[Ref.]	
Rural	67.3	0.64*	0.61–0.87

Note: aOR = adjusted odds ratio; CI = confidence interval; Ref. = reference category; and significance level at *** ≤0.001, ** ≤0.01, and * ≤0.05

Table 12.2 shows the prevalence and likelihood of young women's having had any sexual disease according to various characteristics. Women's having any sexual disease is considerably higher among those who opted for unhygienic methods

Table 12.2 Prevalence and likelihood of women's having a sexual disease, in Koch Bihar district

Women's socioeconomic correlates	%	Model I	Model II
Menstrual practice			
Unhygienic	12.4	[Ref.]	[Ref.]
Hygienic	8.2	0.26*** [0.21–0.33]	0.64* [0.58–0.72]
Toilet type			
Improved	7.7	[Ref.]	[Ref.]
Unimproved	8.9	1.15* [1.12–1.24]	1.07 [1.02–1.30]
Availability of soap for handwashing			
Available	6.6	[Ref.]	[Ref.]
Unavailable	12	1.77** [1.72–1.80]	1.28* [1.22–1.36]
Water source			
Available	11.5	[Ref.]	[Ref.]
Unavailable	10.2	1.10 [0.87–1.35]	1.05 [0.77–1.24]
Age			
15–19 years	10.6		[Ref.]
20–24 years	9.1		0.99 [0.57–1.50]
Religion			
Hindu	6.3		[Ref.]
Muslim	8.9		1.12* [1.08–1.22]
Others	6.4		0.66 [0.53–1.81]
Social group			
SC	11.1		[Ref.]
ST	10.4		0.98 [0.84–1.56]
Others	9.8		0.62 [0.34–1.21]
Education			
Illiterate	10.9		[Ref.]
Primary	9.5		1.17 [1.02–1.89]
Secondary	9.2		0.56* [0.47–0.62]
Higher	2.3		0.38*** [0.36–0.41]
Monthly household income (INR)			
Below 20,000	13.6		[Ref.]
20,000–40,000	12.4		0.91 [0.77–1.10]
Above 40,000	7.1		0.52* [0.49–0.74]
Mass-media exposure			
No	8.1		[Ref.]
Partial	10.4		1.24* [1.19–1.30]
High	9.6		1.11* [1.07–1.23]
Place of residence			
Urban	6.8		[Ref.]
Rural	17.3		1.28*** [1.24–1.30]

Note: aOR = adjusted odds ratio; CI = confidence interval; Ref. = reference category; and significance level at *** ≤0.001, ** ≤0.01, and * ≤0.05

(12.4%) during their menstrual cycle than those who used hygienic methods. Women who used unimproved toilets (8.9%) have a higher risk of sexual diseases than women who used improved toilets (7.7%). The unavailability of soap (12%) for handwashing also increased the risk of women's having any sexual disease. Moreover, women aged 15–19 years who are Muslim or belong to an SC have a higher risk of sexual diseases than their counterparts do. Similarly, women with low education and those belonging to poor households (income less than INR 20,000) have a higher risk of having a sexual disease. Rural women were 17.8% more vulnerable to having a sexual disease than urban women were.

With all the factors in model II adjusted for, the results indicate that women who used menstrual hygiene practices were less likely to be at risk of having a sexual disease (aOR: 0.64; 95% CI: 0.58–0.72) than those who used unhygienic methods. The unavailability of soap for handwashing also accelerated the risk of any sexual diseases. For instance, women who did not have soap available for washing their hands had a higher likelihood of having a sexual disease (aOR: 1.28; 95% CI: 1.22–1.36). Moreover, Muslim women experienced a 1.12 times higher likelihood of having a sexual disease than Hindu women did. Similarly, women with higher education, who belong to a rich family, and who have higher exposure to mass media have a lower likelihood of having a sexual disease. The probability of women's having a sexual disease was significantly higher among women who lived in rural areas (aOR: 1.28; 95% CI: 1.24–1.30) than among urban women.

12.4 Discussion

The prime objective of the present chapter is to assess the prevalence of sexual diseases among women and those diseases' associations with menstrual hygienic practices in Koch Bihar district. Overall, almost 81% of the respondents reported that they had used hygienic methods during menstruation. Being aged 20–24 years, belonging to the Muslim religion, belonging to a Scheduled Tribe, being illiterate, having a monthly household income below INR 20,000, having no exposure to mass media, having access to unimproved toilet facilities, and being a rural resident were the factors associated with unhygienic menstrual practices. Previous cross-sectional studies in India have also suggested a strong correlation between education and income on one hand and hygienic practices on the other (Roy et al. 2021; Karjee et al. 2023). Similar results were also reported by a small geographical study conducted in Indian villages (Bhagwat and Jijina 2020). Our results also align with those of previous research in Bangladesh, Nepal, and Ethiopia (Ha and Alam 2022; Bhusal 2020; Habtegiorgis et al. 2021).

Our study confirms the association between menstrual hygiene practices and women's having a sexual disease. Women who used unhygienic menstrual products like cloths and rags were more likely to be vulnerable to sexual diseases than women who used hygienic products during menstruation to prevent blood stains. A few studies conducted in India have confirmed that menstrual hygienic products reduce symptoms of urinary tract infections and reduce menstrual morbidities, which supports our study findings (Chakrabarty and Singh 2023; Yaliwal et al. 2020). Previous studies in Kenya and Tanzania have also suggested that hygienic practices were significantly associated with a lower prevalence of sexually transmitted diseases (Phillips-Howard et al. 2016; Baisley et al. 2009). Furthermore, several studies have revealed that fabric and reusable materials take longer to dry, encouraging many women to use and even store them wet (Das et al. 2015). This maintains damp surroundings, raising women's risk of vaginitis or vulvovaginal candidiasis (VVC) even more (Das et al. 2023). These elements could be involved in the increased risk of RTIs in women who use unclean materials such as cloths and rags during their periods. The other variables that were associated with women's having a sexual disease in a multivariable binary logistic regression analysis are women's availability of soap for handwashing, education, exposure to mass media, and place of residence. The availability of soap and water in a toilet facilitates maintaining hygiene during menstruation. Most girls clean their external genital area with soap and water; therefore, having soap and water in a toilet is significant to retaining personal hygiene. One of the key findings of our chapter is that menstrual unhygienic practice is expected to decrease with increased access to improved toilets and water availability.

12.4.1 Limitations

This chapter contains several limitations. First, reporting bias might have existed due to the study's use of self-reported data. Furthermore, this chapter did not look into which specific sexual disease categories are most common among women or whether using sanitary materials lowers the incidence of sexual diseases of all kinds as well. Because experimental data are required to prove a causal link between predictors and outcome variables, this study could not prove this.

12.5 Conclusion

Neglecting personal hygiene increases the chances of women's having sexual diseases. The current chapter indicates that women who maintain hygienic practices during menstruation have a lower risk of sexual diseases. Therefore, hygienic practices are essential to reduce sexual diseases like STIs and RTIs. Health education, awareness, menstrual hygiene management, successful diagnosis and treatment for these people, and the proper diagnosis of at-risk people are all important components of effective preventative programmes.

Declaration

Availability of Data and Material The data analysed in this study are available from the corresponding author upon reasonable request. The corresponding author takes responsibility for the integrity and accuracy of the data analysis in this chapter.

Ethics Approval and Consent to Participate Verbal consent was to be obtained from all adult study participants, and we obtained verbal consent from adult participants (parents and key informants) and women ages below 18 years who were considered emancipated minors in this context.

Competing Interests The authors declare that they have no competing interests.

Funding This research received no specific grant from public, commercial, or not-for-profit funding agencies.

References

Anand E, Singh J, Unisa S (2015) Menstrual hygiene practices and its association with reproductive tract infections and abnormal vaginal discharge among women in India. Sex Reprod Healthc 6(4):249–254

Anbesu EW, Aychiluhm SB, Alemayehu M, Asgedom DK, Kifle ME (2023) A systematic review and meta-analysis of sexually transmitted infection prevention practices among Ethiopian young people. SAGE Open Med 11:20503121221145640

Austrian K, Kangwana B, Muthengi E, Soler-Hampejsek E (2021) Effects of sanitary pad distribution and reproductive health education on upper primary school attendance and reproductive health knowledge and attitudes in Kenya: a cluster randomized controlled trial. Reprod Health 18(1):1–13

Baisley K, Changalucha J, Weiss H, Mugeye K, Everett D, Hambleton I et al (2009) Bacterial vaginosis in female facility workers in north-western Tanzania: prevalence and risk factors. Sex Transm Infect 85:370

Bhagwat A, Jijina P (2020) A psychosocial lens on an indigenous initiative to address menstrual health and hygiene in Indian villages. Soc Work Public Health 35(3):73–89

Bhusal CK (2020) Practice of menstrual hygiene and associated factors among adolescent school girls in Dang district, Nepal. Adv Prev Med 2020:1292070

Bilardi JE, Walker S, Temple-Smith M, McNair R, Mooney-Somers J, Bellhouse C et al (2013) The burden of bacterial vaginosis: women's experience and the psychosocial impact of living with recurrent bacterial vaginosis. PLoS One 8(9):e74378

Bradford LL, Ravel J (2017) The vaginal mycobiome: a contemporary perspective on fungi in women's health and diseases. Virulence 8(3):342–351

Chakrabarty M, Singh A (2023) Assessing the link between hygienic material use during menstruation and self-reported reproductive tract infections among women in India: a propensity score matching approach. PeerJ 11:e16430

Das P, Baker KK, Dutta A, Swain T, Sahoo S, Das BS et al (2015) Menstrual hygiene practices, WASH access and the risk of urogenital infection in women from Odisha, India. PLoS One 10(6):e0130777

Das S, Bhattacharjee MJ, Mukherjee AK, Khan MR (2023) Recent advances in understanding of multifaceted changes in the vaginal microenvironment: implications in vaginal health and therapeutics. Crit Rev Microbiol 49(2):256–282

Feng C, Li R, Shamim AA, Ullah MB, Li M, Dev R et al (2021) High-resolution mapping of reproductive tract infections among women of childbearing age in Bangladesh: a spatial-temporal analysis of the demographic and health survey. BMC Public Health 21:1–16

Galvin SR, Cohen MS (2004) The role of sexually transmitted diseases in HIV transmission. Nat Rev Microbiol 2(1):33–42

Ha MAT, Alam MZ (2022) Menstrual hygiene management practice among adolescent girls: an urban–rural comparative study in Rajshahi division, Bangladesh. BMC Womens Health 22(1):86

Habtegiorgis Y, Sisay T, Kloos H, Malede A, Yalew M, Arefaynie M et al (2021) Menstrual hygiene practices among high school girls in urban areas in Northeastern Ethiopia: a neglected issue in water, sanitation, and hygiene research. PLoS One 16(6):e0248825

Johnson HL, Ghanem KG, Zenilman JM, Erbelding EJ (2011) Sexually transmitted infections and adverse pregnancy outcomes among women attending inner city public sexually transmitted diseases clinics. Sex Transm Dis 38:167–171

Karjee S, Rahaman M, Biswas PC (2023) Contextualizing the socio-economic and spatial patterns of using menstrual hygienic methods among young women (15–24 years) in India: a cross-sectional study using the nationally representative survey. Clin Epidemiol Glob Health 20:101253

Klouman E, Masenga EJ, Klepp KI, Sam NE, Nkya W, Nkya C (1997) HIV and reproductive tract infections in a total village population in rural Kilimanjaro, Tanzania: women at increased risk. JAIDS J Acquir Immune Defic Syndr 14(2):163–168

Mwatelah R, McKinnon LR, Baxter C, Abdool Karim Q, Abdool Karim SS (2019) Mechanisms of sexually transmitted infection-induced inflammation in women: implications for HIV risk. J Int AIDS Soc 22:e25346

Passmore JAS, Jaspan HB, Masson L (2016) Genital inflammation, immune activation and risk of sexual HIV acquisition. Curr Opin HIV AIDS 11(2):156

Patel V, Weiss HA, Mabey D, West B, D'Souza S, Patil V et al (2006) The burden and determinants of reproductive tract infections in India: a population based study of women in Goa, India. Sex Transm Infect 82(3):243

Phillips-Howard PA, Nyothach E, Ter Kuile FO, Omoto J, Wang D, Zeh C et al (2016) Menstrual cups and sanitary pads to reduce school attrition, and sexually transmitted and reproductive tract infections: a cluster randomized controlled feasibility study in rural Western Kenya. BMJ Open 6(11):e013229

Racicot K, Mor G (2017) Risks associated with viral infections during pregnancy. J Clin Invest 127(5):1591–1599

Roy A, Paul P, Saha J, Barman B, Kapasia N, Chouhan P (2021) Prevalence and correlates of menstrual hygiene practices among young currently married women aged 15–24 years: an analysis from a nationally representative survey of India. Eur J Contracept Reprod Health Care 26(1):1–10

World Health Organization (2021) Accelerating the global sexually transmitted infections response: report on the first informal think-tank meeting. World Health Organization, Geneva

Yaliwal RG, Biradar AM, Kori SS, Mudanur SR, Pujeri SU, Shannanwaz M (2020, 2020) Menstrual morbidities, menstrual hygiene, cultural practices during menstruation, and WASH practices at schools in adolescent girls of North Karnataka, India: a cross-sectional prospective study. Obstet Gynecol Int:6238193

Yamane T (1967) Taro Yamane method for sample size calculation. The survey causes of mathematics anxiety among secondary school students in Minna Metropolis. Math Assoc Niger (MAN) 46(1):188

Zeng M, Yang L, Mao Y, He Y, Li M, Liu J et al (2022) Preconception reproductive tract infections status and adverse pregnancy outcomes: a population-based retrospective cohort study. BMC Pregnancy Childbirth 22(1):501

Part V
Maternal Health: Key Issues

Chapter 13
Maternal Healthcare Scenario in India: Evaluating Implications of the National Health Policy

Ankita Zaveri and **Salim Mandal**

Abstract The significance of maternal health in India is undeniable in that it profoundly affects the well-being of both mothers and children. This chapter seeks to examine the present state of maternal healthcare in India and analyse the effects of the National Health Policy on maternal well-being. The research in this chapter combines a comprehensive review of existing literature, National Family and Health Survey (NFHS) data for analysis, and a policy evaluation to provide a holistic understanding of the challenges and opportunities within the maternal health landscape. This chapter includes indicators such as antenatal care (ANC) coverage, institutional delivery rates, skilled providers, and postnatal health checkups to gauge the overall status of maternal health in India and track maternal mortality rates (MMRs) to meet the target of the National Health Policy on maternal health. The study reveals that ANC coverage increased by 30.6% from NFHS-1 (1992–1993) to NFHS-5 (2019–2021). Institutional delivery and delivery by skilled providers have contributed to this increase (62.6% and 55.4%, respectively) over the study period (NFHS-1 to NFHS-5). The postnatal care taken within 2 days of delivery rose by 44.4% from NFHS-3 (2005–2006) to NFHS-5 (2019–2021). The chapter results shows that India has engaged in significant development in maternal healthcare services over time and achieved an MMR below 100 per 100,000 live births—one of the goals of the National Health Policy (2017). Furthermore, the research explores the socioeconomic and cultural factors influencing maternal health in India, acknowledging the diverse and complex nature of the country.

Keywords Maternal healthcare · Antenatal care · Institutional delivery · Maternal mortality · India

---

A. Zaveri
Department of Geography, University of Gour Banga, Malda, India

S. Mandal (✉)
Department of Geography, Darjeeling Govt. College, Darjeeling, India

13.1 Introduction

Maternal well-being is paramount in advancing the prosperity and equality of any nation. Maternal health, a linchpin in societal progress, extends beyond the individual sphere, influencing broader issues such as economic development and social equity. The significance lies not only in safeguarding the health and survival of mothers but also in addressing multifaceted challenges that resonate across various facets of society. To achieve safe outcomes, pregnant women and infants must be provided with specialized care and attention throughout the phases of pregnancy and childbirth (UNICEF 2008). This commitment to maternal health not only nurtures the individuals involved but also contributes to the overall resilience and advancement of the community at large.

According to WHO estimates, India accounts for about 22% of the total maternal deaths that occur worldwide each year (Hill et al. 2007; Zureick-Brown et al. 2013; Hogan et al. 2010). Millions more have pregnancy-related morbidity on top of this. India's health indicators have improved significantly over the past 2–3 decades thanks to public health initiatives. During the 1990s, certain vital metrics, notably the maternal mortality ratio (MMR) and infant mortality rate (IMR), plateaued at approximately 400 per 100,000 live births and 60 per 1000 live births, respectively (MoHFW 2004). A decrease of about 43% in the global maternal mortality was documented during 1990–2015. Remarkably, India showed a better decline, of about 70% in maternal mortality during the same period (Kamal et al. 2015; Shahabuddin et al. 2017). Unfortunately, even with this notable decrease, India still contributes 15% of the world's maternal deaths and is ranked second, only to Nigeria, in terms of the total maternal deaths (WHO 2015).

One of the goals of National Health Policy of 2002 was to reduce the MMR to 100 per lakh live births by 2010, which failed given that the MMR was 178 per lakh live births during 2010–2012. The National Health Policy of 2017 states that by 2020, the target MMR is 100 per lakh live births. And this target was achieved during the period 2018–2020, when the MMR decreased to 97 per lakh live births. India pledged to meet the most recent Sustainable Development Goals (SDGs) set by the UN, which is to achieve a maternal mortality rate of 70 per lakh live births by 2030. In underdeveloped nations, about half of the maternal deaths occurred within the first 48 hours after giving birth or during labour. Key variables influencing the reduction in these fatalities encompass the type of personnel aiding pregnant women during childbirth and the delivery location (Koblinsky 2003). A minimum of four antenatal care (ANC) visits are needed to comprehensively assess the health of both the mother and the child, allowing for systematic monitoring. The primary objectives of ANC include monitoring foetal growth and pre-emptively addressing and preventing potential issues for the mother. Another pivotal factor impacting the well-being of both mothers and children is the quality of delivery care. Opting for institutional childbirth is associated with advantages linked to the availability of life-saving equipment and hygienic conditions, thereby diminishing the risks of maternal and/or paediatric illnesses and fatalities (Shariff and Singh 2002; Singh et al. 2012; Arokiasamy and Pradhan 2013; Hamal et al. 2020; Yadav et al. 2021). The provision of maternal healthcare coverage is contingent on the accessibility and use of health services; it needs a minimum of four antenatal care visits, postnatal care, and care during delivery (Gopalakrishnan and Immanuel 2018; Ghosh and Ghosh 2020; Gandhi et al. 2022). The rationale for this research is rooted in the significance of maternal health as a crucial indicator of a nation's overall well-being and development. Understanding the current scenario in India will shed light on existing challenges, successes, and areas requiring intervention. The research will identify disparities in maternal healthcare utilization across various demographic factors, including socioeconomic status, education, and geographic location. Overall, the study on the maternal healthcare scenario in India and the evaluation of the implications of the National Health Policy is a vital undertaking that holds the potential to inform policy decisions, improve healthcare practices, and contribute to the overall well-being of women in the country.

The objective of this chapter is to underscore the advancements in maternal healthcare in India. This will be achieved through a comparative analysis of factors such as the utilization of antenatal care (ANC), the rates of institutional delivery, and the use of postnatal care (PNC). Additionally, this chapter will assess the implications of the National Health Policy on these aspects.

13.2 Data Sources and Methods

To overview the maternal well-being in India, nationally represented data from NFHS-1 (1991–1992) to NFHS-5 (2019–2021) have been incorporated. The government of India's Ministry of Health and Family Welfare launched the country's first National Family Health Survey (NFHS-1), conducted 1992–1993, to gather data at the federal, state, and local levels on family planning, ANC use, child health and nutrition, immunization, and mother and child well-being. Aiding researchers, administrators, and policymakers in the evaluation of population and family welfare programmes was the aim. This chapter incorporated the population of 24 states, along with the National Capital Territory of Delhi. The household survey sample contained a total of 89,777 women aged 13 to 49 who had ever been married. In 1998–1999, a subsequent study (NFHS-2) was conducted, which covered all 26 states and featuring a sample size exceeding 90,000 women aged 15–49 who had ever been married. The third National Family Health Survey (NFHS-3), conducted in 2005–2006, provides comprehensive data on HIV-related knowledge, family planning, fertility, mortality, and various aspects of healthcare, nutrition, and health. NFHS-3 collected information from 109,041 households, 124,385 women, and 74,369 men across all 29 states, constituting a nationally representative sample. The fourth National Family Health Survey (NFHS-4), conducted in 2015–2016, provided population, health, and nutrition data for all states, union territories (UTs), and the entire country. For NFHS-4's district-level estimates, a two-stage sampling methodology was employed in both the rural and urban areas of each Indian district.

The survey included 601,509 families, 699,686 women, and 112,122 men aged 15 to 54, sampled from 28,586 primary sampling units (PSUs) that were distributed across 640 districts in India. The fifth edition of the National Family Health Survey (NFHS-5: 2019–2021) collected data from 636,699 households, featuring 724,115 women and 101,839 men. NFHS-5 offers comprehensive data on population, health, and nutrition for India—every state and union territory and 707 districts.

Bivariate analysis has been integrated to visualize the maternal healthcare scenario in India by using data from consecutive NFHSs. To show the trend in the maternal mortality rate, information from a sample registration survey (SRS) was used..

13.2.1 Variables

Four maternal healthcare coverage domains that were taken from the NFHSs were used in this investigation. First, the number of antenatal care (ANC) visits during an individual's most recent pregnancy was recorded, and only those who received four or more ANC visits were included. ANC visits serve as a gauge for women's access to professional prenatal care. Second, whether the delivery was carried out in a medical facility where professional delivery care is available was factored in. Third, whether the delivery was administered by proficient healthcare providers and whether postnatal health checkups were conducted within the initial 2 days following childbirth were also factored in.

The use of facility-based delivery and ANC visits are affected by sociodemographic and socioeconomic determinants, among various other factors. The maternal background characteristics examined in this study draw on existing empirical literature that has explored factors pertinent to maternal healthcare services. The mother's age at birth (categorized as below 20, 20–34, and 35–49 years), birth order (one, two to three, four to five, and six or higher), type of residence (rural or urban), number of schooling years (no schooling, < 5 years, 5–7 years, 8–9 years, 10–11 years, and 12 or more years), religion (Hindu, Muslim, Christian, Buddhist, Jain and others), caste (Schedule Caste, Schedule Tribe, Other Backward Class, and others), and household's wealth index category (poorest, poor, middle, richer, and richest) are among these variables.

13.3 Results

The fundamental components of maternal healthcare (MHC) services encompass the completion of four or more ANC visits, receiving institutional delivery care, receiving assistance from a skilled provider, and undergoing a postnatal health checkup within the initial 2 days following childbirth. Data from five consecutive NFHSs, featuring nationally representative data, show an increasing trend in maternal healthcare services. During NFHS-1 (1992–1993), only 27.9% of women had four and more ANC visits, which increased to 29.99% during NFHS-2 (1998–1999) and 37.26% during NFHS-3 (2005–2006). Afterwards, the proportion of four or more ANC visits rapidly reached 51.2% during NFHS-4 (2015–2016) and during the latest NFHS-5 (2019–2021) reached 58.5% (Fig. 13.1).

Regarding institutional delivery (child delivered in a health facility), the proportion increased from 26% during NFHS-1 to 88.6% during NFHS-5 (IIPS & ICF 2021). A remarkable, steep change of 40.2% can be found from NFHS-3 (38.7%) to NFHS-4 (78.9%). A similar trend to that of institutional delivery can be observed for delivery by a skilled provider, in that it was initially 34% (NFHS-1) but rose to 89.4% (NFHS-5), with a sharp increase (from 46.6% to 81.4%) during NFHS-4. But information on another MHC service, i.e. postnatal care within the first 2 days after childbirth, was not available for NFHS-1 or − 2, but starting from 37.3% during NFHS-3, it increased to 65.1% during NFHS-4 and 81.7% during NFHS-5 (Fig. 13.1).

Table 13.1 shows the distribution of maternal background characteristics: at least four ANC visits, institutional delivery, assistance by a skilled birth attendant, and PNC within 2 days of delivery over the study period 2005–2006 to 2019–2021. The proportions of mothers who received all maternal healthcare services significantly increased for all age groups from NFHS-3 to NFHS-5. All maternal healthcare services (NFHS-3 to NFHS-5) increased over time, but the rate of increase for delivery in a health facility and for assistance by a skilled birth attendant was comparatively higher in that delivery in a health facility increased from 67.5 to 93.8 in urban areas and from 28.9 to 86.7 in rural areas. The rural–urban gap in all maternal healthcare services was reduced over time. On the other hand, the rate of increase in assistance by a skilled birth provider was very high among all quintiles of the wealth index. For example, from 2005–2006 to 2019–2021, for those in the second wealth quintile, it increased from 31.8 to 88.2, and for those in the middle wealth quintile, it increased by 43%.

Table 13.2 illustrates the current status of several maternal background characteristics across Indian states: four or more ANC visits, institutional delivery, assistance by skilled birth attendants, and postnatal health checkups within 2 days of

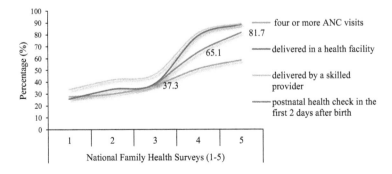

Fig. 13.1 Trends of different MHC services

Table 13.1 Description of maternal background characteristics: four or more ANC visits, delivered in health facility (i.e. institutional delivery), delivered by a skilled provider, and postnatal care within the 2 days after childbirth (2005–2021)

Maternal Background Characteristics	4 or More ANC Visits			Delivered in Health Facility			Delivered by Skilled Provider			PNC Within 2 d		
	NFHS-3	NFHS-4	NFHS-5	NFHS-3	NFHS-4	NFHS-5	NFHS-3	NFHS-4	NFHS-5	NFHS-3	NFHS-4	NFHS-5
Age at birth (years)												
<20	30.3	54.53	61.0	38.0	81.4	88.9	47.2	83.7	89.7	34.9	65.5	59.1
20–34	39.6	52.84	59.6	39.8	79.3	88.9	47.5	81.7	89.6	38.8	65.6	61.7
35–49	22.9	39.49	55.8	21.7	61.8	81.2	28	65.6	84.1	23.1	54.3	58.0
Birth order												
1	53.3	62.27	66.3	57.0	88.2	94.1	65.2	89.3	93.7	51.2	72.1	61.1
2–3	42.3	52.5	59.3	39.4	77.7	88.0	47.7	80.6	89	40.9	65.2	61.9
4–5	17.6	28.9	42.9	19.6	60.3	75.0	27.3	65	79	21.5	51.3	60.2
6 or higher	7.30	16.03	31.8	10.9	48	63.5	16.5	52.5	68.3	11.8	42.9	55.3
Residence type												
Urban	63.0	67.08	69.6	67.5	88.7	93.8	73.5	90	94	61.0	73.1	62.4
Rural	27.9	45.14	55.2	28.9	75.1	86.7	37.5	78	87.8	28.6	61.7	60.8
Schooling												
No schooling	16.1	28.18	40.2	18.4	61.6	74.8	26.1	66	78.4	19.1	51.0	59.0
<5 years completed	35.3	47.99	55.6	36.3	69.9	82.7	45.0	74.1	84.5	33.6	59.4	61.0
5–7 years completed	45.1	52.81	57.5	47.9	80.2	87.4	56.9	82.8	88.6	43.8	65.1	62.4
8–9 years completed	53.5	56.58	60.5	57.7	85.3	90.6	67.1	87.3	91.3	50.3	68.4	61.7
10–11 years complete	68.2	65.55	65.9	72.2	91.5	94.5	80.3	92.3	94.2	65.1	73.5	62.2
12 or more years completed	81.7	70.53	69.5	86.4	94.7	96.9	91.0	94.9	95.8	77.5	77.6	61.6
Religion												
Hindu	37.5	51.25	59.2	39.1	80.8	89.5	47.5	82.8	90	37.6	65.8	61.6
Muslim	31.6	49.32	58.0	33.0	69.2	84.3	38.8	73.6	86.8	32.0	58.9	59.5

Christian	55.9	63.02	67.6	53.4	78.5	83.3	60.2	80.8	85.4	54.1	68.9	54.9
Sikh	64.3	67.64	61.5	58.3	92.5	96.1	75.4	95.4	96.9	64.4	86.6	66.3
Buddhist	49.7	75.14	67.4	58.8	92.2	93.8	64.9	93.4	94.6	47.3	79.1	68.9
Jain	86.4	71.0	87.4	93.1	98.1	99.7	94.3	97.8	98.5	70.2	82.6	62.2
Other	16.6	54.7	50.1	10.4	51.0	73.4	14.6	61	78	12.4	55.6	63.3
Caste												
Scheduled Caste	30.0	49.0	55.9	32.9	78.3	87.3	40.6	80.7	88.5	32.4	64.4	61.4
Scheduled Tribe	22.3	46.21	58.4	17.7	68.0	82.3	25.4	71.5	84.5	23.0	59.0	61.7
Other Backward Class	35.5	48.62	57.7	37.7	79.8	89.5	46.7	82	89.9	35.6	64.9	61.6
Other	50.4	61.77	65.7	51	82.9	91.2	57.8	85.3	91.8	47.6	69.1	60.4
Don't know	38.9	47.74	59.8	43.4	73.6	85.7	54.2	78.2	86.8	37.1	53.2	56.3
Wealth quintile												
Lowest	12.2	25.15	42.3	12.7	59.6	76.2	19.4	64.1	79.3	14.4	47.9	57.5
Second	21.3	44.67	54.2	23.5	75.1	87.2	31.8	78.3	88.2	22.8	59.9	61.2
Middle	36.8	57.65	63.3	39.2	85.0	92.3	49	86.8	92.4	36.8	69.4	62.4
Fourth	53.4	66.45	68.5	57.9	90.5	95.4	67.2	91.8	95.0	52.1	75.0	63.1
Highest	78.3	73.9	72.9	83.7	95.3	97.4	88.8	95.5	96.8	74.6	79.5	62.9

Source: NFHS-3 to –5 (IIPS and Macro International (2007), IIPS & ICF (2017), IIPS & ICF (2021)

Table 13.2 Four or more ANC visits, deliveries in a health facility, deliveries assisted by a skilled provider, and postnatal health checkup for the mother within 2 days of childbirth in Indian states according to percentages (NFHS-5)

	State/UTs	Percentage who had four or more ANC visits (%)	Percentage of births delivered in a health facility (%)	Percentage of deliveries assisted by a skilled provider (%)	Percentage of deliveries with a postnatal health checkup for the mother within 2 days of childbirth (%)
North	Chandigarh	79.4	96.9	97	91.3
	Delhi	77.8	91.8	93.4	88.3
	Haryana	60.9	94.9	94.4	93.3
	Himachal Pradesh	70.6	88.2	87.1	90.5
	Jammu & Kashmir	81.1	92.4	95.1	85.7
	Ladakh	78.9	95.1	97	82.5
	Punjab	59.7	94.3	95.6	88.5
	Rajasthan	55.4	94.9	95.6	86.3
	Uttarakhand	61.8	83.2	83.7	84.6
Central	Chhattisgarh	60.4	85.7	88.8	89.3
	Madhya Pradesh	57.5	90.7	89.3	86.8
	Uttar Pradesh	42.4	83.4	84.8	79.3
East	Bihar	25.2	76.2	78.9	64.4
	Jharkhand	38.7	75.8	82.5	75.9
	Odisha	78.1	92.2	91.8	92.5
	West Bengal	76.7	91.7	94.1	70.1
Northeast	Arunachal Pradesh	36.6	79.2	82.1	59.2
	Assam	50.7	84.1	86.1	69.6
	Manipur	79.4	79.9	85.6	75.3
	Meghalaya	52.2	58.1	64	56.4
	Mizoram	58.1	85.8	87.7	70.2
	Nagaland	20.7	45.7	55.3	47.7
	Sikkim	58.4	94.7	96.5	71.2
	Tripura	55.2	89.2	89.2	73.2
West	Dadra & Nagar Haveli and Daman & Diu	86.2	96.5	97.8	92.2
	Goa	93	99.7	99.1	95.4
	Gujarat	77.2	94.3	93.2	91.5
	Maharashtra	71.4	94.7	93.8	86.3

(continued)

Table 13.2 (continued)

	State/UTs	Percentage who had four or more ANC visits (%)	Percentage of births delivered in a health facility (%)	Percentage of deliveries assisted by a skilled provider (%)	Percentage of deliveries with a postnatal health checkup for the mother within 2 days of childbirth (%)
South	Andaman & Nicobar Islands	83.6	98.9	97.3	89.1
	Andhra Pradesh	67.5	96.5	96.1	91.3
	Karnataka	70.9	97	93.8	88.5
	Kerala	81.3	99.8	100	93.2
	Lakshadweep	92.1	99.6	100	92.6
	Puducherry	87.4	99.6	99.9	93.1
	Tamil Nadu	90.6	99.6	99.8	93.2
	Telangana	70.5	97	93.6	88.5

Source: NFHS-5 (2019–2021)

childbirth. Despite notable increases in the utilization of maternal healthcare services by women, considerable disparities persist among states. The prevalence of pregnant women undergoing at least four ANC visits is notably high in Goa (93%), followed by Lakshadweep (92.1%) and Tamil Nadu (90.6%), whereas it is as low as 20.7% in Nagaland, followed by a lower prevalence in Bihar (25.2%), Arunachal Pradesh (36.6%), and Jharkhand (38.7%). The interstate variation in the percentage of pregnant women with at least four ANC visits (ranging from 20.7% to 93%) is more pronounced than the variation in institutional delivery, the percentage of deliveries assisted by skilled providers, and the percentage of deliveries with a postnatal health checkup for the mother within two days of childbirth. The highest percentage of births delivered in a health facility is observed in the southern region, whereas the lowest is in the central and eastern regions of India. Interestingly, the scenario differs for the percentage of deliveries assisted by skilled providers and for the percentage of deliveries with a postnatal health check within two days of birth, with the highest in the central region and the lowest in the northern region..

Figure 13.2 describes the trend in the maternal mortality rate (MMR) from 1997–1998 to 2018–2020. The trend shows that the maternal mortality rate gradually declined from 398 per lakh live births during 1997–1998 to 301 per lakh live births during 2001–2003, when the National Health Policy of 2002 was introduced.

Afterwards, the MMR again sharply declined from 301 to 113 per lakh live births during 2016–2018, when the latest National Health Policy of 2017 was launched, and a target was set for a reduction in MMR to 100 per lakh births by 2020, which was achieved when MMR decreased to 97 per lakh live births during 2018–2020 (Fig. 13.2).

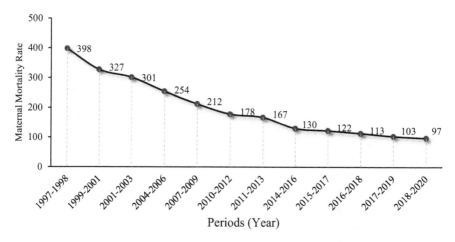

Fig. 13.2 Trends in the maternal mortality rate (MMR) (SRSs: 1997–1998 to 2018–2020)

13.4 Discussion

The research reveals that women's use of maternal healthcare services is influenced by diverse maternal factors such as their birth order, place of residence, education, religion, social group, and wealth quintile (Singh et al. 2012; Kumar et al. 2019; Tarekegn et al. 2014). Our results indicate that Muslim women are less likely to opt for four or more antenatal care (ANC) visits and skilled birth attendance (SBA) than their Hindu counterparts are. The lower coverage among Muslims and Scheduled Caste/Scheduled Tribe (SC/ST) women may be linked to their reduced autonomy and lower socioeconomic status (Basant 2007; Nayar 2007; Mistry et al. 2009). Educational status emerges as a significant determinant of maternal healthcare services, with educated women exhibiting the capability to access health information, make informed decisions, and effectively utilize healthcare resources (Zaveri et al. 2023). The study also highlights substantial disparities in maternal healthcare service utilization across economic groups (Pathak et al. 2010). Women from wealthier households are more likely to avail themselves of maternal healthcare services than those from poorer backgrounds are. Moreover, a noticeable decline took place in the percentage of all maternal healthcare services after an increase in birth order, which is consistent with the findings from other studies (Singh et al. 2012; Kumar et al. 2019; Tarekegn et al. 2014).

The data reveal a positive trend in the percentage of women receiving four or more antenatal care (ANC) visits over the years. Starting at 27.9% during NFHS-1 (1992–1993), this proportion has steadily increased to 58.5% during the latest NFHS-5 (2019–2021). This upward trajectory indicates an improvement in women's awareness and in the accessibility of antenatal care services, highlighting efforts to promote maternal health (Carroli et al. 2001; Bhutta et al. 2005). This chapter demonstrates that pregnant women who had four or more antenatal care

(ANC) visits were more likely to deliver in a health facility than those who did not attend four or more ANC visits. Similar observations have been reported in several other studies (Rockers et al. 2009; Tann et al. 2007; Oguntunde et al. 2010). Institutional delivery is crucial for ensuring a safe and controlled environment for childbirth. It plays a vital role in reducing maternal mortality. Some studies have found that increased access to skilled care at hospitals is proving to be a lifesaver for mothers, resulting in a significant decline in the maternal mortality rate (Ranvive et al. 2013; Ng et al. 2014). Policies and interventions promoting institutional deliveries may have contributed to improved maternal and child health outcomes. This upward trajectory underscores the success of interventions and policies aimed at promoting deliveries in health facilities, emphasizing the importance of professional care during childbirth. Ensuring that deliveries are attended by skilled healthcare providers is essential for reducing maternal and neonatal mortality (WHO 2018). This positive trend reflects an increasing reliance on skilled healthcare professionals during childbirth, ensuring a safer and more controlled environment for both mothers and newborns. Determining whether a corresponding increase in postnatal health checkups has taken place would be valuable to ensuring comprehensive care for mothers and newborns. This underscores a growing recognition of the significance of postnatal health checkups in ensuring the well-being of both mothers and infants in the critical days following childbirth. The positive trends in maternal healthcare services may be attributed to various government initiatives, policies, and awareness campaigns. Understanding the factors that contributed to this improvement can help policymakers identify successful strategies and further strengthen maternal health programmes. While progress is evident, challenges in reaching the entire population might persist, particularly in remote or underserved areas. Understanding the disparities in maternal healthcare utilization across different regions and socioeconomic groups is crucial for designing targeted interventions. The findings suggest progress, but continued efforts are needed to ensure equitable access to quality maternal healthcare services for all women across the country.

The observed trends suggest a positive correlation between increased institutional deliveries, skilled assistance during childbirth, and a focus on postnatal care. Government initiatives, awareness campaigns, and improvements in healthcare infrastructure may have contributed to these positive changes. However, ongoing efforts are required to ensure that these positive trends continue so that they reach all segments of the population and address any remaining disparities in maternal healthcare access and utilization.

The introduction of the National Health Policy of 2017 appears to have played a pivotal role in driving the decline in the MMR. Policies that focus on improving maternal healthcare services, enhancing healthcare infrastructure, and increasing access to prenatal and postnatal care can contribute significantly to reducing maternal mortality. Setting specific targets, such as reducing the MMR to 100 per lakh births by 2020, provides a clear roadmap for healthcare providers and policymakers. Achieving and even surpassing these targets would indicate the successful implementation of strategies outlined in the policy.

Improvements in healthcare infrastructure and accessibility are often critical factors in reducing maternal mortality. These could include ensuring that pregnant women have access to skilled healthcare professionals, well-equipped facilities, and essential maternal health services. Community engagement and awareness campaigns may have also played roles in the success of the policy. Educating communities about the importance of maternal healthcare, family planning, and detecting complications early can lead to better health-seeking behaviours. The success in reducing the MMR underscores the importance of the ongoing monitoring and evaluation of healthcare policies (SRS 2019, 2022). Regular assessments help identify areas of improvement, refine strategies, and ensure that the positive trends are sustained over time. Effective maternal health policies often take a multisectoral approach, addressing not only healthcare services but also social, economic, and cultural factors that impact maternal health. Collaboration between different sectors and stakeholders is crucial for comprehensive and sustainable outcomes. Although this achievement should be celebrated, remaining vigilant and continuing efforts to further improve maternal health outcomes are essential. Sustainable progress will depend on maintaining the momentum of effective policies, addressing emerging challenges, and adapting strategies to evolving healthcare needs. Additionally, sharing success stories and lessons learned can contribute to global efforts to reduce maternal mortality and improve overall maternal health worldwide.

13.5 Conclusion

Maternal healthcare in India has been a major public health concern, and the implications of the National Health Policy play crucial roles in shaping the landscape. The National Health Policy in India aims to address various aspects of healthcare, including maternal health, with a focus on improving accessibility, affordability, and the quality of services. Several positive strides have been made in recent years. Initiatives such as the Pradhan Mantri Surakshit Matritva Abhiyan (PMSMA) and Janani Suraksha Yojana (JSY) have aimed to increase institutional deliveries and provide financial assistance to pregnant women. However, challenges persist, including regional disparities, inadequate infrastructure, and sociocultural factors affecting healthcare utilization. The implications of the National Health Policy need continuous evaluation to ensure its effectiveness in achieving maternal health goals. Key areas of concern include the need for improved infrastructure, skilled healthcare providers, and increased community awareness. Monitoring and assessment mechanisms should be strengthened to track progress and address emerging challenges.

Policymakers must consider not only quantitative indicators such as maternal mortality rates but also qualitative aspects such as the overall experience of pregnant women in accessing healthcare. The inclusion of community engagement, education, and empowerment is crucial to achieving sustainable improvements in maternal health. In conclusion, although progress has been made in addressing maternal health in India through the National Health Policy, ongoing efforts are needed to overcome persistent challenges. A comprehensive approach that combines infrastructure development, capacity building, community engagement, and continuous evaluation is essential to ensure positive and lasting impacts on maternal health outcomes.

Declaration

Availability of Data and Material The data and materials for this chapter are sourced from publicly available secondary sources accessible at https://dhsprogram.com/methodology/survey/survey-display-541.cfm. Interested individuals can register at the provided link to freely download the necessary data.

Ethics Approval and Consent to Participate This chapter is based on secondary data, which are available in the public domain. Therefore, ethical approval is not required to conduct this study.

Competing Interests The authors declare that they have no competing interests.

Funding No funding was received.

References

Arokiasamy P, Pradhan J (2013) Maternal health care in India: access and demand determinants. Prim Health Care Res Dev 14(4):373–393. https://doi.org/10.1017/S1463423612000552
Basant R (2007) Social, economic and educational conditions of Indian Muslims. Econ Polit Wkly 42:828–832
Bhutta ZA, Darmstadt GL, Hasan BS, Haws RA (2005) Community-based interventions for improving perinatal and neonatal health outcomes in developing countries: a review of the evidence. Pediatrics 115(Supplement_2):519–617
Carroli G, Villar J, Piaggio G, Khan-Neelofur D, Gülmezoglu M, Mugford M, Bersgjø P (2001) WHO systematic review of randomised controlled trials of routine antenatal care. Lancet 357(9268):1565–1570
Gandhi S, Dash U, Suresh Babu M (2022) Horizontal inequity in the utilisation of continuum of maternal health care services (CMHS) in India: an investigation of ten years of National Rural Health Mission (NRHM). Int J Equity Health 21(1):7
Ghosh A, Ghosh R (2020) Maternal health care in India: a reflection of 10 years of National Health Mission on the Indian maternal health scenario. Sex Reprod Healthc 25:100530
Gopalakrishnan S, Immanuel AB (2018) Progress of health care in rural India: a critical review of National Rural Health Mission. Int J Commun Med Public Health 5(1):4
Hamal M, Dieleman M, De Brouwere V, de Cock BT (2020) Social determinants of maternal health: a scoping review of factors influencing maternal mortality and maternal health service use in India. Public Health Rev 41(1):1–24
Hill K, Thomas K, AbouZahr C, Walker N, Say L, Inoue M, Suzuki E (2007) Estimates of maternal mortality worldwide between 1990 and 2005: an assessment of available data. Lancet 370(9595):1311–1319
Hogan MC, Foreman KJ, Naghavi M et al (2010) Maternal mortality for 181 countries, 1980–2008: a systematic analysis of progress towards millennium development goal 5. Lancet 375(9726):1609–1623

IIPS and Macro International (2007) National Family Health Survey (NFHS 3) 2005–06; India, vol 1. IIPS, Mumbai

IIPS, ICF (2017) National Family Health Survey (NFHS-4), 2015–16. International Institute for Population Sciences (IIPS)

IIPS, ICF (2021) National Family Health Survey (NFHS-5), 2019–21. International Institute for Population Sciences (IIPS)

Kamal SM, Hassan CH, Alam GM (2015) Determinants of institutional delivery among women in Bangladesh. Asia Pacific J Public Health 27(2):NP1372–NP1388

Koblinsky MA (ed) (2003) Reducing maternal mortality: learning from Bolivia, China, Egypt, Honduras, Indonesia, Jamaica, and Zimbabwe. World Bank Publications. http://documents.worldbank.org/curated/en/262811468771721342/pdf/multi0page.pdf

Kumar G, Choudhary TS, Srivastava A, Upadhyay RP, Taneja S, Bahl R, Mazumder S (2019) Utilisation, equity and determinants of full antenatal care in India: analysis from the National Family Health Survey 4. BMC Pregnancy Childbirth 19(1):1-9

Mistry R, Galal O, Lu M (2009) Women's autonomy and pregnancy care in rural India: a contextual analysis. Soc Sci Med 69(6):926–933

Nayar KR (2007) Social exclusion, caste & health: a review based on the social determinants framework. Indian J Med Res 126(4):355–363

Ng M, Misra A, Diwan V et al (2014) An assessment of the impact of the JSY case transfer program on maternal mortality reduction in Madhya Pradesh, India. Glob Health Action 7:24939

Oguntunde O, Aina O, Ibrahim MS, Umar HS, Passano P (2010) Antenatal care and skilled birth attendance in three communities in Kaduna state, Nigeria. Afr J Reprod Health 14(3):89–96

Pathak PK, Singh A, Subramanian SV (2010) Economic inequalities in maternal health care: prenatal care and skilled birth attendance in India, 1992–2006. PLoS One 5(10):e13593

Ranvive B, Diwan V, De Costa A (2013) India's conditional case transfer programme (the jsy) to promote institutional birth: is there an association between institutional birth proportion and maternal mortality? PLoS One 8:e67452

Rockers PC, Wilson ML, Mbaruku G, Kruk ME (2009) Source of antenatal care influences facility delivery in rural Tanzania: a population-based study. Matern Child Health J 13:879–885

Shahabuddin ASM, De Brouwere V, Adhikari R, Delamou A, Bardaj A, Delvaux T (2017) Determinants of institutional delivery among young married women in Nepal: evidence from the Nepal demographic and health survey, 2011. BMJ Open 7(4):e012446

Shariff A, Singh G (2002) Determinants of maternal health care utilisation in India: evidence from a recent household survey, vol No. 85. National Council of Applied Economic Research, New Dehli

Singh PK, Rai RK, Alagarajan M, Singh L (2012) Determinants of maternity care services utilization among married adolescents in rural India. PLoS One 7(2):e31666

SRS (2019) Special bulletin on maternal mortality in India 2015–17. Office of Registrar General, India: Sample Registration System

SRS (2022) Special bulletin on maternal mortality in India 2018–20. Office of Registrar General, India: Sample Registration System

Tann CJ, Kizza M, Morison L, Mabey D, Muwanga M, Grosskurth H, Elliott AM (2007) Use of antenatal services and delivery care in Entebbe, Uganda: a community survey. BMC Pregnancy Childbirth 7(1):1–11

Tarekegn SM, Lieberman LS, Giedraitis V (2014) Determinants of maternal health service utilization in Ethiopia: analysis of the 2011 Ethiopian demographic and health survey. BMC Pregnancy Childbirth 14(1):1–13

United Nations Children's Fund (UNICEF) 2008 THE State of the world's children 2009: maternal and newborn health. https://www.unicef.org/sowc09/docs/SOWC09-FullReport-EN.pdf

WHO U.N.F.P.A, Unicef I.C.M., Inc F (2018) Definition of skilled health personnel providing care during childbirth: the 2018 joint statement by who. WHO, Geneva

World Health Organization (2015) Trends in estimates of maternal mortality ratio 1990–2015. World Health Organization, Geneva

Yadav AK, Jena PK, Sahni B, Mukhopadhyay D (2021) Comparative study on maternal healthcare services utilisation in selected empowered action group states of India. Health Soc Care Community 29(6):1948–1959

Zaveri A, Paul P, Roy R, Chouhan P (2023) Facilitators and barriers to the utilisation of maternal healthcare services in empowered action group states, India. J Health Manag 25(3):431–447

Zureick-Brown S, Newby H, Chou D, Mizoguchi N, Say L, Suzuki E, Wilmoth J (2013) Understanding global trends in maternal mortality. Int Perspect Sex Reprod Health 39(1):032

Chapter 14
Mental Health of Pregnant Women in Bangladesh During the COVID-19 Pandemic: A Cross-Sectional Study

Sumaia Rahman, Ahammad Hossain, Al MuktadirMunam, Ayesha Akter Lima, Rejvi Ahmed Bhuiya, Jayanta Das , and Md. Kamruzzaman

Abstract Traditionally perceived as a joyful period, pregnancy brings forth a spectrum of emotions for women. However, the advent of the COVID-19 pandemic introduced a myriad of sociodemographic and obstetric challenges for pregnant women in Bangladesh. These complexities had profound implications for both the mental well-being of expectant mothers and the health of their unborn children. This chapter aims to identify the risk factors contributing to antenatal depression, anxiety, and stress during a pandemic situation. A community-based cross-sectional study of 430 pregnant women was performed with the assistance of four recruited nurses. The structured questionnaire contained three sections: demographic and obstetric information; the Depression, Anxiety, and Stress Scale (DASS-21); and the Multidimensional Scale of Perceived Social Support (MSPSS). The chapter's data analysis utilized SPSS-25 and MS Excel, employing Pearson's chi-squared test, bivariate analysis, and multinomial logistic regression to examine correlations between the independent and outcome variables. Multinomial logistic regression analysis disclosed that pregnant women residing in urban areas, those expressing concern about family financial situations, and employed women anxious about caring for their unborn child during the pandemic exhibited higher levels of depression. Similarly, women affected by physical illness or COVID-19 infection during preg-

S. Rahman · A. Hossain · A. MuktadirMunam · A. A. Lima
Department of Computer Science & Engineering, Varendra University, Rajshahi, Bangladesh

R. A. Bhuiya
Department of Crop Science and Technology, University of Rajshahi, Rajshahi, Bangladesh

J. Das
Department of Geography, Rampurhat College, Rampurhat, West Bengal, India

M. Kamruzzaman (✉)
Institute of Bangladesh Studies, University of Rajshahi, Rajshahi, Bangladesh
e-mail: mkzaman@ru.ac.bd

© The Author(s), under exclusive license to Springer Nature Singapore Pte Ltd. 2024
P. Chouhan et al. (eds.), *Sexual and Reproductive Health of Women*, https://doi.org/10.1007/978-981-97-8418-9_14

nancy were more prone to anxiety. Notably, well-educated women and those with planned pregnancies received greater social support. Additionally, financial stability within a woman's family positively correlated with increased social support during pregnancy. This chapter underscores the negative impact of specific demographic and obstetric characteristics on the mental health of pregnant women in Bangladesh during the COVID-19 pandemic. To mitigate prenatal and postpartum complexities, the implementation of mental health promotion programs, such as online campaigns and informative media broadcasts, is imperative. Furthermore, enhancing obstetric knowledge and awareness among pregnant women can contribute significantly to reducing psychological complexities during this challenging period.

Keywords COVID-19 · Pregnant women · DASS-21 · MSPSS · Demographic and obstetric factors

14.1 Introduction

The COVID-19 pandemic has significantly altered daily life throughout the world, and as of September 2022, more than 6.6 million fatalities had occurred worldwide as a result of SARS-CoV-2, the virus that causes COVID-19, which has spread quickly throughout the planet and has infected more than 633 million people (Luo et al. 2022). People's mental health may also be at risk due to the virus's unknowable characteristics and the lack of information on its transmission, reproduction, risk factors, mortality, and disease-causing effects on pregnancy and fetuses (Effati-Daryani et al. 2020). Stress, worry, and depression are some of the most common psychological symptoms that may arise from this (Effati-Daryani et al. 2020). In low-and middle-order countries, anxiety, depression, and stress are prevalent among almost all segments of the population due to socioeconomic discomfort during this pandemic situation. During the COVID-19 pandemic, pregnant women were more prone to experience anxiety and depression (Luo et al. 2022). They could not take any medical treatment, go to open places, eat whatever they wanted, or take meditation because they were afraid of getting contaminated by the novel coronavirus. Pregnant women frequently experienced depression and anxiety, and these two mental illnesses frequently co-occurred (Bante et al. 2021). Around 10% of pregnant women worldwide experience mental health issues, primarily depression; this number is higher (16%) in poor countries than in others (Bante et al. 2021). To prevent adverse health outcomes, addressing the impact of the COVID-19 pandemic on the mental health of childbearing women is a critical public health challenge. This issue, which requires timely and appropriate healthcare support, is a significantly understudied research area (Nwafor et al. 2021).

Concerns about the increased severity of the COVID-19 disease in this demographic, the possibility that a mother's infection will spread to her unborn child, and an elevated risk of negative neonatal outcomes are just a few of the special issues that pregnant and postpartum women face (Basu et al. 2021). Additionally, according to recent studies, more perinatal women during the pandemic had depression, anxiety, dissociation, posttraumatic stress disorder symptoms, loneliness, and isolation than perinatal women did before the epidemic (Basu et al. 2021). If emotional issues, problems with memory and attention, hunger loss, weight loss, early-morning awakenings, and negative self-talk persist for more than 2 weeks, depression during pregnancy may be diagnosed (Karaçam and Ançel 2009). If a woman experiences thoughts of self-harm, a generalized loss of interest and energy, generalized remorse, and hopelessness, depression is likely (Karaçam and Ançel 2009).

The results of these studies could have significant ramifications because antenatal mental health problems are known to be linked to poor maternal psychosocial functioning and undesirable birth outcomes, as well as to neurodevelopmental outcomes for the offspring, postnatal depression, and posttraumatic stress disorder (Zilver et al. 2021). Antenatal depression has been linked to domestic violence, a lack of social support, social conflict, having low income, antenatal anxiety, unwanted pregnancies, a history of depression, and prior lost pregnancies, and antenatal anxiety has been linked to less-positive attitudes toward pregnancy, a lack of education, a lack of marital satisfaction, a lack of social support, a longer duration of infertility, and a history of unsuccessful treatment with assisted reproduction (Waqas et al. 2015). For instance, research conducted in rural Bangladesh in 2011 reported a prevalence of 18% and 29% for prenatal depression and anxiety, respectively (Waqas et al. 2015).

Previous research has consistently shown that having a spouse, being in the top quintile of income, having a medical condition, seeing pregnancy danger signs, experiencing life-threatening situations, and having food insecurity in the home are all significantly linked to co-occurring anxiety and depression (Bante et al. 2021). According to another study, melancholy, worry, and stress are likely involved in the development of hyperemesis gravidarum (HG), as a result of negative physiological repercussions (Tan et al. 2014). According to one study, mothers with peripheral artery disease (PAD) during pregnancy had impaired ANS (Antenatal Screening) function, which was also present in their children (Braeken et al. 2013). Another study examined how common sadness, anxiety, and stress were among expectant mothers during the COVID-19 lockdown (Nwafor et al. 2021). Another study discovered that factors such as the number of pregnancies, a woman's spouse's education level, the support of her spouse, and marital satisfaction were predictive of anxiety symptoms and that factors such as her spouse's education level, adequate household income, her spouse's support, and marital satisfaction were predictive of stress symptoms (Effati-Daryani et al. 2020).

In our research, we have tried to determine the risk components related with antenatal depression, anxiety, and stress. Even though anxiety and depression can be treated, only around one-third and fewer than half of pregnant women have received the proper care for their anxiety and their depression, respectively (Bante et al. 2021). The Rajshahi division of Bangladesh undertook a community-based cross-sectional study to identify the risk variables. Three sections were covered in the questionnaire part. Online and offline, both types of surveys were conducted to collect primary data by four nurses. We conducted a bivariate analysis on the data on pregnant women to document information about depression, anxiety, and stress. We analyzed how COVID-19 prevention became a cause of depression. To fulfill the purpose of this chapter, we emphasized pregnant women's mood disorders, worries about miscarriage, worries about unplanned pregnancy, religious belief in overcoming frustration, financial instability during COVID-19, and worries about their newborn's care during COVID-19.

14.2 Data Sources and Methods

The community-based cross-sectional study was conducted in the Rajshahi division of Bangladesh, spanning October 2021 to March 2022. According to the PHC-2022 census, the total population of Rajshahi division was 20,353,119 in 2022, and among that, 50.44% were female. The health facility in Rajshahi city is highly enriched, so collecting the data to successfully do this research was easy for us.

14.2.1 Sample-Size Determination

A total of 430 pregnant women, aged between 18 and 40 years, participated in our survey. These women were at various stages of pregnancy, encompassing different trimesters. The participants were diverse in their geographic locations, where some were from villages and others from towns. The sample size for our chapter was determined by using the following formula (Hossain and Munam 2022; Naing and Winn 2006):

$$n = \frac{z^2 \times p \times (1-p)}{C^2} \quad (14.1)$$

where z is 1.96, for the 95% confidence level; p is the probability of picking a choice, expressed as a decimal (0.5 is used for highly dispersed populations); and C is the allowed error percentage, expressed as a decimal ($C = 0.04726$). With a 5% level of significance and a 95% confidence interval, Table 14.1 shows the sample size required ($n = 430$).

Table 14.1 Sample-size determination

C	z (5%)	p	α	n
0.04726	1.96	0.5	0.05	430

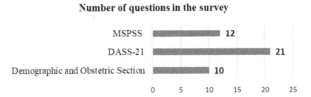

Fig. 14.1 Sections of the survey questionnaire

14.2.2 Measurement

The questionnaire consisted of three sections: (1) demographic and obstetric data, (2) the Depression, Anxiety, and Stress Scale (DASS-21), and (3) the Multidimensional Scale of Perceived Social Support (MSPSS). In the demographic and obstetric section, participants were asked about their age, residence, weight, educational qualification, family financial stability, duration of pregnancy, mood disorders, and miscarriage history; about whether their pregnancy was planned/unplanned; and about the effect that their career had on their unborn child. The DASS-21 is a self-report questionnaire that aims to measure the distinct and independent aspects of anxiety and depression as well as a third construct (called stress). The DASS-21 version contains three scales—depression, anxiety, and stress, each of which consists of seven items. A four-point rating scale is used here, ranging from 0, which means "did not apply to me at all," to 3, which means "applied to me very much or most of the time" (Norton 2007; Saricam 2018; Hossain and Karim 2018; Hossain et al. 2022; Kamruzzaman et al. 2022). The MSPSS was designed to assess perceptions of social support adequacy from three specific sources: family, friends, and significant others. Each of these sources consisted of four items. A seven-point rating scale ranging from very strongly disagree (1) to very strongly agree (7) was implemented (Dahlem et al. 1991) (Fig. 14.1).

14.2.3 Data Collection

For this research, we utilized a primary dataset, which was collected through both online and offline survey questionnaires. The cross-sectional study was carried out at Ma o Shishu Kollayan Kendro (meaning "maternity and child welfare center") in the district of Rajshahi. It is a government organization at which pregnant women receive emergency obstetric services. Dr. Tahsina Shamim Tasu was in charge of this clinic. To obtain women's consent, we first gave them a written request. After their confirmation, we started to collect their data. The survey's goals were explained to the pregnant women, and their anonymity was guaranteed. We collected data only from those women who were interested. Four nurses were recruited to collect the data. They conducted interviews once every two weeks with the participants and filled out the corresponding forms. Prior to the data-collection phase, we engaged in pretesting the survey with three pregnant women. Their feedback was instrumental in refining the questionnaire. Initially prepared in English, the questionnaire was subsequently translated into Bangla to enhance comprehension among the participants. To ensure greater accuracy and consistency, the collected data were reviewed on a daily basis.

14.2.4 Data Analysis

Data were inputted into MS Excel, preprocessed, and analyzed by using SPSS version 25. To determine the relationship between the independent and outcome variables, bivariate analysis was used here (Hossain et al. 2015). Multivariate logistic regression was performed on those variables with a p-value of 0.05 or less in the bivariate analysis (Hossain et al. 2019; Kamruzzaman et al. 2021; Rahman et al. 2023; Hossain et al. 2023). To evaluate the variables, we additionally estimated odds ratios (ORs) with 95% confidence intervals.

14.3 Results

Table 14.2 demonstrates some demographic and obstetric characteristics associated with the depression level of pregnant women. According to Table 14.2, women pregnant for 4–6 months comparatively suffered more from severe (18.6%) and extreme (20.6%) levels of depression than those pregnant for other durations. Pregnant women who lived in towns suffered more from severe (17.8%) and extreme (19.1%) level of depression than those who lived in villages. Interestingly, according to Table 14.2, well-educated pregnant women suffered more from depression than less-educated women did. Pregnant women who experienced mood disorders had higher levels of depression than pregnant women who did not. Among pregnant women (20.9%), more of those who were concerned about miscarriage had extreme depression than did those who were not (16.8%). Pregnant women who had no family financial stability were more likely to suffer from extreme levels of depression (22.7%) than those who had such stability (12.2%). During pregnancy, the women who were always/sometimes worried about their family's financial stability were more likely to suffer from severe (13.4%, 20.0%) or extreme (24.4%, 24.6%) levels of depression than those who never worried about it (17.7%, 8.3%). Pregnant women who suffered from an illness/COVID-19 infection were more likely to be extremely depressed (21.4%) than those who did not (15.5%).

The bivariate analysis indicates that the different levels of depression were significantly associated with residence, belief that religion reduces frustration, family financial stability, worry about family financial situation, expectation or family's expectation, worry about taking care of their unborn child, and suffering from an illness or COVID-19 infection. Depression was not associated with the participants' education, duration of pregnancy, mood disorders, worry about miscarriage,

Table 14.2 Bivariate analysis of demographic and obstetric factors and their association with depression scale classification among pregnant women in the city of Rajshahi, Bangladesh

Variable Categories		Depression Scale Classification					Total	χ2 Test (p-Value)
		Normal	Mild	Moderate	Severe	Extremely Severe		
Duration of Pregnancy	1–3 months	9 (15.8%)	11 (19.3%)	19 (33.3%)	10 (17.5%)	8 (14.0%)	57 (100%)	9.206 (0.325)
	4–6 months	35 (17.6%)	38 (19.1%)	48 (24.1%)	37 (18.6%)	41 (20.6%)	199 (100%)	
	7–9 months	45 (25.9%)	25 (14.4%)	50 (28.7%)	27 (15.5%)	27 (15.5%)	174 (100%)	
Residence	Village	40 (30.3%)	18 (13.6%)	34 (25.8%)	21 (15.9%)	19 (14.4%)	132 (100%)	11.398 (0.022)
	Town	49 (16.4%)	56 (18.8%)	83 (27.9%)	53 (17.8%)	57 (19.1%)	298 (100%)	
Education	Illiterate/class 1–10	39 (22.9%)	33 (19.4%)	44 (25.9%)	24 (14.1%)	30 (17.6%)	170 (100%)	8.570 (0.380)
	SSC-HSC	34 (21.5%)	28 (17.7%)	45 (28.5%)	29 (18.4%)	22 (13.9%)	158 (100%)	
	Honors/master's	16 (15.7%)	13 (12.7%)	28 (27.5%)	21 (20.6%)	24 (23.5%)	102 (100%)	
Patient's Mood Disorder	Yes	51 (18.8%)	49 (18.0%)	72 (26.5%)	47 (17.3%)	53 (19.5%)	272 (100%)	3.160 (0.531)
	No	38 (24.1%)	25 (15.8%)	45 (28.5%)	27 (17.1%)	23 (14.6%)	158 (100%)	
Worried about Miscarriage	Yes	24 (26.4%)	13 (14.3%)	25 (27.5%)	10 (11.0%)	19 (20.9%)	91 (100%)	5.639 (0.228)
	No	65 (19.2%)	61 (18.0%)	92 (27.1%)	64 (18.9%)	57 (16.8%)	339 (100%)	

(continued)

Table 14.2 (continued)

Variable Categories		Depression Scale Classification					Total	χ2 Test (p-Value)
		Normal	Mild	Moderate	Severe	Extremely Severe		
Planned or Unplanned Pregnancy	Planned	60 (19.2%)	55 (17.6%)	85 (27.2%)	54 (17.3%)	58 (18.6%)	312 (100%)	1.844 (0.764)
	Unplanned	29 (24.6%)	19 (16.1%)	32 (27.1%)	20 (16.9%)	18 (15.3%)	118 (100%)	
Belief that Religion Reduces Frustration	Always	61 (18.1%)	58 (17.2%)	85 (25.2%)	66 (19.6%)	67 (19.9%)	337 (100%)	22.031 (0.005)
	Sometimes	12 (30.0%)	3 (7.5%)	15 (37.5%)	4 (10.0%)	6 (15.0%)	40 (100%)	
	Never	16 (30.2%)	13 (24.5%)	17 (32.1%)	4 (7.5%)	3 (5.7%)	53 (100%)	
Family Financial Stability	Yes	47 (22.9%)	28 (13.7%)	65 (31.7%)	40 (19.5%)	25 (12.2%)	205 (100%)	14.586 (0.006)
	No	42 (18.7%)	46 (20.4%)	52 (23.1%)	34 (15.1%)	51 (22.7%)	225 (100%)	
Worried about Family Financial Situation	Always	16 (13.4%)	28 (23.5%)	30 (25.2%)	16 (13.4%)	29 (24.4%)	119 (100%)	31.853 (0.000)
	Sometimes	21 (16.2%)	17 (13.1%)	34 (26.2%)	26 (20.0%)	32 (24.6%)	130 (100%)	
	Never	52 (28.7%)	29 (16.0%)	53 (29.3%)	32 (17.7%)	15 (8.3%)	181 (100%)	
Your or Family's Expectation	Son	6 (8.5%)	17 (23.9%)	19 (26.8%)	15 (21.1%)	14 (19.7%)	71 (100%)	20.894 (0.007)
	Daughter	21 (28.0%)	6 (8.0%)	29 (38.7%)	11 (14.7%)	8 (10.7%)	75 (100%)	
	Anyone	62 (21.8%)	51 (18.0%)	69 (24.3%)	48 (16.9%)	54 (19.0%)	284 (100%)	

Worried about Taking Care of Unborn Child	Always	21 (16.4%)	26 (20.3%)	33 (25.8%)	24 (18.8%)	24 (18.8%)	128 (100%)	34.410 (0.000)
	Sometimes	26 (16.3%)	18 (11.3%)	44 (27.5%)	28 (17.5%)	44 (27.5%)	160 (100%)	
	Never	42 (29.6%)	30 (21.1%)	40 (28.2%)	22 (15.5%)	8 (5.6%)	142 (100%)	
Adverse Effects of Employment on the Unborn Child	Always	5 (18.5%)	5 (18.5%)	7 (25.9%)	5 (18.5%)	5 (18.5%)	27 (100%)	2.643 (0.955)
	Sometimes	6 (13.3%)	7 (15.6%)	14 (31.1%)	10 (22.2%)	8 (17.8%)	45 (100%)	
	Never	78 (21.8%)	62 (17.3%)	96 (26.8%)	59 (16.5%)	63 (17.6%)	358 (100%)	
Suffer from Illness or COVID-19 Infection	Yes	22 (13.8%)	20 (12.6%)	53 (33.3%)	30 (18.9%)	34 (21.4%)	159 (100%)	4.726 (0.005)
	No	67 (24.7%)	54 (19.9%)	64 (23.6%)	44 (16.2%)	42 (15.5%)	271 (100%)	
Patient's Age Group	18–24 years	51 (20.6%)	47 (19.0%)	68 (27.5%)	42 (17.0%)	39 (15.8%)	247 (100%)	2.320 (0.677)
	25–40 years	38 (20.8%)	27 (14.8%)	49 (26.8%)	32 (17.5%)	37 (17.5%)	183 (100%)	
Patient's Weight Group	37–49 kg	12 (15.8%)	16 (21.1%)	18 (23.7%)	14 (18.4%)	16 (21.1%)	76 (100%)	11.766 (0.162)
	50–69 kg	67 (24.5%)	38 (13.9%)	76 (27.7%)	46 (16.8%)	47 (17.2%)	274 (100%)	
	≥ 70 kg	10 (12.5%)	20 (25.0%)	23 (28.7%)	14 (17.5%)	13 (16.3%)	80 (100%)	

planned/unplanned pregnancy, adverse effect of employment on their unborn child, age, or weight.

Table 14.3 shows some of the demographic and obstetric characteristics associated with the stress levels of pregnant women. According to Table 14.3, well-educated pregnant women (52.9%) suffered more from an extreme level of stress than did less-educated women (32.9%). Pregnant women (48.2%) who experienced mood disorders were more likely to have extreme levels of stress than pregnant women who did not (34.2%). Pregnant women (47.6%) who had no family financial stability suffered more from extreme levels of stress than those who had such stability (38.0%). During pregnancy, the women who were always/sometimes worried about their family's financial stability suffered more from an extreme (50.4%, 52.3%) level of stress than those who never worried about it (31.5%). Pregnant women who suffered from an illness/COVID-19 infection were more likely to be extremely stressed (52.2%) than those who did not (37.6%) suffer from an illness/COVID-19 infection.

The bivariate analysis reveals that the different levels of stress were significantly associated with education, belief that religion reduces frustration, worry about family financial situation, worry about taking care of their unborn child, and suffering from an illness or COVID-19 infection. On the contrary, stress was not significantly associated with the participants' residence, duration of pregnancy, mood disorder, worry about miscarriage, planned or unplanned pregnancy, family financial stability, expectation or family expectation, adverse effects of employment on their unborn child, age, or weight.

Table 14.4 demonstrates some demographic and obstetric characteristics associated with the anxiety level of pregnant women. According to Table 14.4, women pregnant for 4–6 months suffered from severe (27.6%) or extreme (20.6%) levels of anxiety. Pregnant women who lived in towns suffered more from severe (26.5%) or extreme (17.8%) levels of anxiety than those who lived in villages. Extreme levels of anxiety were more common in pregnant women (19.5%) who had mood disorders than in those (14.6%) who did not. Pregnant women who had physical illnesses or COVID-19 infections were more likely to experience severe or extreme levels of anxiety (31.4%, 22.6%) during their pregnancies than those who did not (21.0%, 14.8%).

The bivariate analysis reveals that the different levels of anxiety of a pregnant woman were significantly associated with their suffering from an illness or COVID-19 infection ($p = 0.000$). In contrast, according to this analysis, the different levels of anxiety were not significantly associated with other demographic or obstetric characteristics of pregnant women.

Table 14.5 demonstrates some demographic and obstetric characteristics associated with the Multidimensional Scale of Perceived Social Support (significant others). According to Table 14.5, during pregnancy, less-educated pregnant women (18.2%) received much less or moderate social support from their significant others than well-educated pregnant women. During the pregnancy period, the women who had an unplanned pregnancy (20.3%) received much less or moderate social support from their significant others than those who had a planned pregnancy (10.3%). The

Table 14.3 Bivariate analysis of demographic and obstetric factors and their association with Stress Scale Classification among pregnant women in the city of Rajshahi, Bangladesh

Variable Categories		Stress Scale Classification					Total	χ^2 Test (p-Value)
		Normal	Mild	Moderate	Severe	Extremely Severe		
Duration of Pregnancy	1–3 months	5 (8.8%)	5 (8.8%)	15 (26.3%)	8 (14.0%)	24 (42.1%)	57 (100%)	5.124 (0.744)
	4–6 months	9 (4.5%)	14 (7.0%)	48 (24.1%)	43 (21.6%)	85 (42.7%)	199 (100%)	
	7–9 months	11 (6.3%)	14 (8.0%)	33 (19.0%)	40 (23.0%)	76 (43.7%)	174 (100%)	
Residence	Village	12 (9.1%)	13 (9.8%)	33 (25.0%)	28 (21.2%)	46 (34.8%)	132 (100%)	8.260 (0.083)
	Town	13 (4.4%)	20 (6.7%)	63 (21.1%)	63 (21.1%)	139 (46.6%)	298 (100%)	
Education	Illiterate/class 1–10	11 (6.5%)	17 (10.0%)	45 (26.5%)	41 (24.1%)	56 (32.9%)	170 (100%)	15.389 (0.050)
	SSC-HSC	9 (5.7%)	7 (4.4%)	34 (21.5%)	33 (20.9%)	75 (47.5%)	158 (100%)	
	Honors/master's	5 (4.9%)	9 (8.8%)	17 (16.7%)	17 (16.7%)	54 (52.9%)	102 (100%)	
Patient's Mood Disorder	Yes	13 (4.8%)	18 (6.6%)	58 (21.3%)	52 (19.1%)	131 (48.2%)	272 (100%)	8.779 (0.067)
	No	12 (7.6%)	15 (9.5%)	38 (24.1%)	39 (24.7%)	54 (34.2%)	158 (100%)	
Worried about Miscarriage	Yes	7 (7.7%)	5 (5.5%)	28 (30.8%)	18 (19.8%)	33 (36.3%)	91 (100%)	6.431 (0.169)
	No	18 (5.3%)	28 (8.3%)	68 (20.1%)	73 (21.5%)	152 (44.8%)	339 (100%)	

(continued)

Table 14.3 (continued)

Variable Categories		Stress Scale Classification						χ2 Test (p-Value)
		Normal	Mild	Moderate	Severe	Extremely Severe	Total	
Planned or Unplanned Pregnancy	Planned	18 (5.8%)	21 (6.7%)	69 (22.1%)	67 (21.5%)	137 (43.9%)	312 (100%)	1.606 (0.808)
	Unplanned	7 (5.9%)	12 (10.2%)	27 (22.9%)	24 (20.3%)	48 (40.7%)	118 (100%)	
Belief that Religion Reduces Frustration	Always	18 (5.3%)	24 (7.1%)	69 (20.5%)	65 (19.3%)	161 (47.8%)	337 (100%)	20.023 (0.010)
	Sometimes	3 (7.5%)	1 (2.5%)	12 (30.0%)	13 (32.5%)	11 (27.5%)	40 (100%)	
	Never	4 (7.5%)	8 (15.5%)	15 (28.3%)	13 (24.5%)	13 (24.5%)	53	
Family Financial Stability	Yes	12 (5.9%)	21 (10.2%)	54 (26.3%)	40 (19.5%)	78 (38.0%)	205 (100%)	8.959 (0.062)
	No	13 (5.8%)	12 (5.3%)	42 (18.7%)	51 (22.7%)	107 (47.6)	225 (100%)	
Worried about Family Financial Situation	Always	6 (5.0%)	6 (5.0%)	22 (18.5%)	25 (21.0%)	60 (50.4%)	119 (100%)	21.351 (0.006)
	Sometimes	7 (5.4%)	6 (4.6%)	23 (17.7%)	26 (20.0%)	68 (52.3%)	130 (100%)	
	Never	12 (6.6%)	21 (11.6%)	51 (28.2%)	40 (22.1%)	57 (31.5%)	181 (100%)	
Your or Family's Expectation	Son	4 (5.6%)	1 (1.4%)	12 (16.9%)	15 (21.1%)	39 (54.9%)	71 (100%)	12.028 (0.150)
	Daughter	4 (5.3%)	6 (8.0%)	22 (29.3%)	16 (21.3%)	27 (36.0%)	75 (100%)	
	Anyone	17 (6.0%)	26 (9.2%)	62 (21.8%)	60 (21.1%)	119 (41.9%)	284 (100%)	

Category								
Worried about Taking Care of Unborn Child	Always	7 (5.5%)	13 (10.2%)	22 (17.2%)	31 (24.2%)	55 (43.0%)	128 (100%)	25.367 (0.001)
	Sometimes	6 (3.8%)	7 (4.4%)	34 (21.3%)	25 (15.6%)	88 (55.0%)	160 (100%)	
	Never	12 (8.5%)	13 (9.2%)	40 (28.2%)	35 (24.6%)	42 (29.6%)	142 (100%)	
Adverse Effects of Employment on the Unborn Child	Always	0 (0.0%)	2 (7.4%)	6 (22.2%)	7 (25.9%)	12 (44.4%)	27 (100%)	8.201 (0.414)
	Sometimes	1 (2.2%)	3 (6.7%)	7 (15.6%)	9 (20.0%)	25 (55.6%)	45 (100%)	
	Never	24 (6.7%)	28 (7.8%)	83 (23.2%)	75 (20.9%)	148 (41.3%)	358 (100%)	
Suffer from Illness or COVID-19 Infection	Yes	9 (5.7%)	8 (5.0%)	30 (18.9%)	29 (18.2%)	83 (52.2%)	159 (100%)	9.616 (0.047)
	No	16 (5.9%)	25 (9.2%)	66 (24.4%)	62 (22.9%)	102 (37.6%)	271 (100%)	
Patient's Age Group	18–24 years	11 (4.5%)	23 (9.3%)	57 (23.1%)	55 (22.3%)	101 (40.9%)	247 (100%)	4.970 (0.290)
	25–40 years	14 (7.7%)	10 (5.5%)	39 (21.3%)	36 (19.7%)	84 (45.9%)	183 (100%)	
Patient's Weight Group	37–49 kg	5 (6.6%)	8 (10.5%)	12 (15.8%)	19 (25.0%)	32 (42.1%)	76 (100%)	5.901 (0.658)
	50–69 kg	15 (5.5%)	19 (6.9%)	70 (25.5%)	54 (19.7%)	116 (42.3%)	274 (100%)	
	≥ 70 kg	5 (6.3%)	6 (7.5%)	14 (17.5%)	18 (22.5%)	37 (46.3%)	80 (100%)	

Note: Likelihood ratios are used where the self-cell values are less than 5

Table 14.4 Bivariate analysis of demographic and obstetric factors and their association with anxiety scale classification among pregnant women in the city of Rajshahi, Bangladesh

Variable Categories		Anxiety Scale Classification					Total	χ2 Test (p-Value)
		Normal	Mild	Moderate	Severe	Extremely Severe		
Duration of Pregnancy	1–3 months	4 (7.0%)	7 (12.3%)	22 (38.6%)	15 (26.3%)	9 (15.8%)	57 (100%)	6.742 (0.565)
	4–6 months	19 (9.5%)	24 (12.1%)	60 (30.2%)	55 (27.6%)	41 (20.6%)	199 (100%)	
	7–9 months	18 (10.3%)	27 (15.5%)	66 (37.9%)	37 (21.3%)	26 (14.9%)	174 (100%)	
Residence	Village	15 (11.4%)	18 (13.6%)	48 (36.4%)	28 (21.2%)	23 (17.4%)	132 (100%)	1.919 (0.751)
	Town	26 (8.7%)	40 (13.4%)	100 (33.6%)	79 (26.5%)	53 (17.8%)	298 (100%)	
Education	Illiterate/class 1–10	14 (8.2%)	27 (15.9%)	62 (36.5%)	40 (23.5%)	27 (15.9%)	170 (100%)	6.821 (0.556)
	SSC-HSC	20 (12.7%)	19 (12.0%)	50 (31.6%)	43 (27.2%)	26 (16.5%)	158 (100%)	
	Honors/master's	7 (6.9%)	12 (11.8%)	36 (35.3%)	24 (23.5%)	23 (22.5%)	102 (100%)	
Patient's Mood Disorder	Yes	20 (7.4%)	31 (11.4%)	96 (35.3%)	72 (26.5%)	53 (19.5%)	272 (100%)	8.384 (0.078)
	No	21 (13.3%)	27 (17.1%)	52 (32.9%)	35 (22.2%)	23 (14.6%)	158 (100%)	
Worried about Miscarriage	Yes	7 (7.7%)	16 (17.6%)	37 (40.7%)	13 (14.3%)	18 (19.8%)	91 (100%)	8.651 (0.070)
	No	34 (10.0%)	42 (12.4%)	111 (32.7%)	94 (27.7%)	58 (17.1%)	339 (100%)	

Category	Subcategory							
Planned or Unplanned Pregnancy	Planned	25 (8.0%)	44 (14.1%)	105 (33.7%)	78 (25.0%)	60 (19.2%)	312 (100%)	4.838 (0.304)
	Unplanned	16 (13.6%)	14 (11.9%)	43 (36.4%)	29 (24.6%)	16 (13.6%)	118 (100%)	
Belief that Religion Reduces Frustration	Always	32 (9.5%)	39 (11.6%)	124 (36.8%)	79 (23.4%)	63 (18.7%)	337 (100%)	10.814 (0.212)
	Sometimes	3 (7.5%)	7 (17.5%)	13 (32.5%)	12 (30.0%)	5 (12.5%)	40 (100%)	
	Never	6 (11.3%)	12 (22.6%)	11 (20.8%)	16 (30.2%)	8 (15.1%)	53 (100%)	
Family Financial Stability	Yes	19 (9.3%)	29 (14.1%)	69 (33.7%)	51 (24.9%)	37 (18.0%)	205 (100%)	0.252 (0.993)
	No	22 (9.8%)	29 (12.9%)	79 (35.1%)	56 (24.9%)	39 (17.3%)	225 (100%)	
Worried about Family Financial Situation	Always	6 (5.0%)	14 (11.8%)	44 (37.0%)	33 (27.7%)	22 (18.5%)	119 (100%)	9.952 (0.268)
	Sometimes	13 (10.0%)	14 (10.8%)	41 (31.5%)	34 (26.2%)	28 (21.5%)	130 (100%)	
	Never	22 (12.2%)	30 (16.6%)	63 (34.8%)	40 (22.1%)	26 (14.4%)	181 (100%)	
Your or Family's Expectation	Son	5 (7.0%)	4 (5.6%)	34 (47.9%)	13 (18.3%)	15 (21.1%)	71 (100%)	13.325 (0.101)
	Daughter	9 (12.0%)	10 (13.3%)	28 (37.3%)	18 (24.0%)	10 (13.3%)	75 (100%)	
	Anyone	27 (9.5%)	44 (15.5%)	86 (30.3%)	76 (26.8%)	51 (18.0%)	284 (100%)	

(continued)

Table 14.4 (continued)

Variable Categories		Anxiety Scale Classification					Total	χ2 Test (p-Value)
		Normal	Mild	Moderate	Severe	Extremely Severe		
Worried about Taking Care of Unborn Child	Always	13 (10.2%)	14 (10.9%)	40 (31.3%)	33 (25.8%)	28 (21.9%)	128 (100%)	11.141 (0.194)
	Sometimes	15 (9.4%)	16 (10.0%)	57 (35.6%)	41 (25.6%)	31 (19.4%)	160 (100%)	
	Never	13 (9.2%)	28 (19.7%)	51 (35.9%)	33 (23.2%)	17 (12.0%)	142 (100%)	
Adverse Effects of Employment on the Unborn Child	Always	2 (7.4%)	2 (7.4%)	8 (29.6%)	6 (22.2%)	9 (33.3%)	27 (100%)	10.003 (0.265)
	Sometimes	1 (2.2%)	5 (11.1%)	16 (35.6%)	14 (31.1%)	9 (20.0%)	45 (100%)	
	Never	38 (10.6%)	51 (14.2%)	124 (34.6%)	87 (24.3%)	58 (16.2%)	358 (100%)	
Suffer from Illness or COVID-19 Infection	Yes	7 (4.4%)	11 (6.9%)	55 (34.6%)	50 (31.4%)	36 (22.6%)	159 (100%)	22.934 (0.000)
	No	34 (12.5%)	47 (17.3%)	93 (34.3%)	57 (21.0%)	40 (14.8%)	271 (100%)	
Patient's Age Group	18–24 years	23 (9.3%)	34 (13.8%)	84 (34.0%)	66 (26.7%)	40 (16.2%)	247 (100%)	1.598 (0.809)
	25–40 years	18 (9.8%)	24 (13.1%)	64 (35.0%)	41 (22.4%)	36 (19.7%)	183 (100%)	
Patient's Weight Group	37–49 kg	9 (11.8%)	8 (10.5%)	23 (30.3%)	19 (25.0%)	17 (22.4%)	76 (100%)	7.990 (0.434)
	50–69 kg	27 (9.9%)	36 (13.1%)	97 (35.4%)	73 (26.6%)	41 (15.0%)	274 (100%)	
	≥ 70 kg	5 (6.3%)	14 (17.5%)	28 (35.0%)	15 (18.8%)	18 (22.5%)	80 (100%)	

Table 14.5 The bivariate analysis of the demographic and obstetric characteristics and Multidimensional Scale of Perceived Social Support (significant others)

Variable Categories		Multidimensional Scale of Perceived Social Support (Significant Others)		Total	χ2 test (p-Value)
		Low Support/ Moderate Support	High Support		
Duration of Pregnancy	1–3 months	6 (10.5%)	51 (89.5%)	57 (100%)	0.327 (0.830)
	4–6 months	27 (13.6%)	172 (86.4%)	199 (100%)	
	7–9 months	23 (13.2%)	151 (86.8%)	174 (100%)	
Residence	Village	20 (15.2%)	112 (84.8%)	132 (100%)	0.762 (0.383)
	Town	36 (12.1%)	262 (87.9%)	298 (100%)	
Education	Illiterate/class 1–10	31 (18.2%)	139 (81.8%)	170 (100%)	6.836 (0.033)
	SSC-HSC	16 (10.1%)	142 (89.9%)	158 (100%)	
	Honors/ master's	9 (8.8%)	93 (91.2%)	102 (100%)	
Patient's Mood Disorder	Yes	36 (13.2%)	236 (86.8%)	272 (100%)	0.029 (0.864)
	No	20 (12.7%)	138 (87.3%)	158 (100%)	
Worried about Miscarriage	Yes	12 (13.2%)	79 (86.8%)	91 (100%)	0.003 (0.958)
	No	44 (13.0%)	295 (87.0%)	339 (100%)	
Planned or Unplanned Pregnancy	Planned	32 (10.3%)	280 (89.7%)	312 (100%)	7.684 (0.006)
	Unplanned	24 (20.3%)	94 (79.7%)	118 (100%)	
Belief that Religion Reduces Frustration	Always	38 (11.3%)	299 (88.7%)	337 (100%)	4.226 (0.121)
	Sometimes	8 (20.0%)	32 (80.0%)	40 (100%)	
	Never	10 (18.9%)	43 (81.1%)	53 (100%)	
Family Financial Stability	Yes	23 (11.2%)	182 (88.8%)	205 (100%)	1.125 (0.289)
	No	33 (14.7%)	192 (85.3%)	225 (100%)	

(continued)

Table 14.5 (continued)

Variable Categories		Multidimensional Scale of Perceived Social Support (Significant Others)		Total	χ2 test (p-Value)
		Low Support/ Moderate Support	High Support		
Worried about Family Financial Situation	Always	18 (15.1%)	101 (84.9%)	119 (100%)	0.788 (0.675)
	Sometimes	17 (13.1%)	113 (86.9%)	130 (100%)	
	Never	21 (11.6%)	160 (88.4%)	181 (100%)	
Your or Family's Expectation	Son	12 (16.9%)	59 (83.1%)	71 (100%)	3.287 (0.193)
	Daughter	13 (17.3%)	62 (82.7%)	75 (100%)	
	Anyone	31 (10.9%)	253 (89.1%)	284 (100%)	
Worried about Taking Care of Unborn Child	Always	19 (14.8%)	109 (85.2%)	128 (100%)	0.576 (0.750)
	Sometimes	19 (11.9%)	141 (88.1%)	160 (100%)	
	Never	18 (12.7%)	124 (87.3%)	142 (100%)	
Adverse Effects of Employment on the Unborn Child	Always	4 (14.8%)	23 (85.2%)	27 (100%)	0.396 (0.820)
	Sometimes	7 (15.6%)	38 (84.4%)	45 (100%)	
	Never	45 (12.6%)	313 (87.4%)	358 (100%)	
Suffer from Illness or COVID-19 Infection	Yes	22 (13.8%)	137 (86.2%)	159 (100%)	0.147 (0.701)
	No	34 (12.5%)	237 (87.5%)	271 (100%)	
Patient's Age Group	18–24 years	33 (13.4%)	214 (86.6%)	247 (100%)	0.058 (0.809)
	25–40 years	23 (12.6%)	160 (87.4%)	183 (100%)	
Patient's Weight Group	37–49 kg	9 (11.8%)	67 (88.2%)	76 (100%)	0.489 (0.783)
	50–69 kg	38 (13.9%)	236 (86.1%)	274 (100%)	
	≥ 70 kg	9 (11.3%)	71 (88.8%)	80 (100%)	

Note: Low support and moderate support are merged here because the self-cell values are less than 5 for some attributes

bivariate analysis indicates that the Multidimensional Scale of Perceived Social Support (significant others) was significantly associated with participants' education and their planned/unplanned pregnancy. It also reveals that the MSPSS (significant others) was not significantly associated with other demographic or obstetric characteristics of pregnant women.

Table 14.6 demonstrates the association between the MSPSS (family) and some demographic and obstetric characteristics among pregnant women. According to Table 14.6, pregnant women (31.9%) who were worried about their family financial situation during their pregnancy received much less or moderate social support from their family than those who were not (21.0%). The bivariate analysis indicates that the MSPSS (family) was significantly associated ($p = 0.044$) with the worrying about their or their family's financial situation. However, other demographic and obstetric characteristics were not significantly associated with the Multidimensional Scale of Perceived Social Support (family).

Table 14.6 The bivariate analysis of the demographic and obstetric characteristics and Multidimensional Scale of Perceived Social Support (family)

Variable	Categories	Multidimensional Scale of Perceived Social Support (Family)		Total	χ^2 Test (p-Value)
		Low Support/ Moderate Support	High Support		
Duration of Pregnancy	1–3 months	44 (25.3%)	130 (74.7%)	174 (100%)	0.609 (0.738)
	4–6 months	56 (28.1%)	143 (71.9%)	199 (100%)	
	7–9 months	17 (29.8%)	40 (70.2%)	57 (100%)	
Residence	Village	32 (24.2%)	100 (75.8%)	132 (100%)	0.847 (0.358)
	Town	85 (28.5%)	213 (71.5%)	298 (100%)	
Education	Illiterate/class 1–10	52 (30.6%)	118 (69.4%)	170 (100%)	3.270 (0.195)
	SSC-HSC	44 (27.8%)	114 (72.2%)	158 (100%)	
	Honors/master's	21 (20.6%)	81 (79.4%)	102 (100%)	
Patient's Mood Disorder	Yes	75 (27.6%)	197 (72.4%)	272 (100%)	0.050 (0.824)
	No	42 (26.6%)	116 (73.4%)	158 (100%)	
Worried about Miscarriage	Yes	29 (31.9%)	62 (68.1%)	91 (100%)	1.265 (0.261)
	No	88 (26.0%)	251 (74.0%)	339 (100%)	

(continued)

Table 14.6 (continued)

Variable Categories		Multidimensional Scale of Perceived Social Support(Family)		Total	χ2 Test (p-Value)
		Low Support/ Moderate Support	High Support		
Planned or Unplanned Pregnancy	Planned	79 (25.3%)	233 (74.7%)	312 (100%)	2.048 (0.152)
	Unplanned	38 (32.2%)	80 (67.8%)	118 (100%)	
Belief that Religion Reduces Frustration	Always	86 (25.5%)	251 (74.5%)	337 (100%)	2.345 (0.310)
	Sometimes	14 (35.0%)	26 (65.9%)	40 (100%)	
	Never	17 (32.1%)	36 (67.9%)	53 (100%)	
Family Financial Stability	Yes	51 (24.9%)	154 (75.1%)	205 (100%)	1.075 (0.300)
	No	66 (29.3%)	159 (70.7%)	225 (100%)	
Worried about Family Financial Situation	Always	38 (31.9%)	81 (68.1%)	119 (100%)	6.100 (0.044)
	Sometimes	41 (31.5%)	89 (68.5%)	130 (100%)	
	Never	38 (21.0%)	143 (79.0%)	181 (100%)	
Your or Family's Expectation	Son	24 (33.8%)	47 (66.2%)	71 (100%)	2.429 (0.297)
	Daughter	22 (29.3%)	53 (70.7%)	75 (100%)	
	Anyone	71 (25.0%)	213 (75.0%)	284 (100%)	
Worried about Taking Care of Unborn Child	Always	38 (29.7%)	90 (70.3%)	128 (100%)	1.229 (0.541)
	Sometimes	45 (28.1%)	115 (71.9%)	160 (100%)	
	Never	34 (23.9%)	108 (76.1%)	142 (100%)	
Adverse Effects of Employment on the Unborn Child	Always	10 (37.0%)	17 (63.0%)	27 (100%)	2.581 (0.275)
	Sometimes	15 (33.3%)	30 (66.7%)	45 (100%)	
	Never	92 (25.7%)	266 (74.3%)	358 (100%)	
Suffer from Illness or COVID-19 Infection	Yes	48 (30.2%)	111 (69.8%)	159 (100%)	1.131 (0.288)
	No	69 (25.5%)	202 (74.5%)	271 (100%)	

Table 14.6 (continued)

Variable Categories		Multidimensional Scale of Perceived Social Support(Family)		Total	χ2 Test (p-Value)
		Low Support/ Moderate Support	High Support		
Patient's Age Group	18–24 years	66 (26.7%)	181 (73.3%)	247 (100%)	0.070 (0.791)
	25–40 years	51 (27.9%)	132 (72.1%)	183 (100%)	
Patient's Weight Group	37–49 kg	18 (23.7%)	58 (76.3%)	76 (100%)	2.933 (0.231)
	50–69 kg	82 (29.9%)	192 (70.1%)	274 (100%)	
	≥ 70 kg	17 (21.3%)	63 (78.8%)	80 (100%)	

Note: Low support and moderate support are merged here because the self-cell values are less than 5 for some attributes

Table 14.7 illustrates the relationship between the MSPSS (friends) and the obstetric and demographic traits among pregnant women. According to Table 14.7, women who were 7–9 months pregnant (60.9%) received less social support from their friends than those who were 1–3 (45.6%) or 4–6 (49.7%) months pregnant. During the pregnancy period, less-educated pregnant women (60.6%) received less social support from their friends than well-educated pregnant women did (35.3%). Pregnant women (59.1%) whose family financial situation was not good during the COVID-19 period received less social support from their friends than those who whose family financial situation was good (47.8%). In addition, pregnant women who always (71.4%) worried about their family financial situation received less social support from their friends than those who were sometimes (46.9%) or never (47.0%) worried about it. Employed pregnant women who were always (64.8%) worried about taking care of their unborn child received less social support from their friends than those who sometimes (45.0%) or never (53.5%) worried about it.

The bivariate analysis indicates that the MSPSS (friends) was significantly associated with participants' education, duration of pregnancy, family financial stability, worry about family financial situation, worry about taking care of their unborn child, and adverse effects of employment on their unborn child. On the contrary, according to Table 14.7, the MSPSS (friends) was not statistically significant for other characteristics.

Table 14.8 presents a summary of the multinomial logistic regression of participants' Depression Scale Classification and its associated factors. Pregnant women who lived in towns were 2.05 times more likely to suffer from an extreme level of depression than were pregnant women who lived in villages (OR = 2.05; 95% CI: 1.08–16.25; $p = 0.00$). Pregnant women who always worried about their family's financial situation throughout the COVID-19 era experienced an extreme level of depression 3.53 times more often than those who never worried about it (OR = 3.53;

Table 14.7 The bivariate analysis of the demographic and obstetric characteristics and Multidimensional Scale of Perceived Social Support (friends)

Variable Categories		Multidimensional Scale of Perceived Social Support (Friends)			Total	χ2 Test (p-Value)
		Low Support	Moderate Support	High Support		
Duration of Pregnancy	1–3 months	26 (45.6%)	19 (33.3%)	12 (21.1%)	57 (100%)	10.077 (0.039)
	4–6 months	99 (49.7%)	50 (25.1%)	50 (25.1%)	199 (100%)	
	7–9 months	106 (60.9%)	28 (16.1%)	40 (23.0%)	174 (100%)	
Residence	Village	79 (59.8%)	23 (17.4%)	30 (22.7%)	132 (100%)	3.636 (0.162)
	Town	152 (51.0%)	74 (24.8%)	72 (24.2%)	298 (100%)	
Education	Illiterate/ class 1–10	103 (60.6%)	33 (19.4%)	34 (20.0%)	170 (100%)	19.743 (0.001)
	SSC-HSC	92 (58.2%)	35 (22.2%)	31 (19.6%)	158 (100%)	
	Honors/ master's	36 (35.3%)	29 (28.4%)	37 (36.3%)	102 (100%)	
Patient's Mood Disorder	Yes	152 (55.9%)	63 (23.2%)	57 (21.0%)	272 (100%)	3.149 (0.207)
	No	79 (50.0%)	34 (21.5%)	45 28.5%	158 (100%)	
Worried about Miscarriage	Yes	54 (59.3%)	18 (19.8%)	19 (20.9%)	91 (100%)	1.466 (0.480)
	No	177 (52.2%)	79 (23.3%)	83 (24.5%)	339 (100%)	
Planned or Unplanned Pregnancy	Planned	171 (54.8%)	70 (22.4%)	71 (22.8%)	312 (100%)	0.703 (0.703)
	Unplanned	60 (50.8%)	27 (22.9%)	31 (26.3%)	118 (100%)	
Belief that Religion Reduces Frustration	Always	182 (54.0%)	75 (22.3%)	80 (23.7%)	337 (100%)	1.756 (0.780)
	Sometimes	18 (45.0%)	11 (27.5%)	11 (27.5%)	40 (100%)	
	Never	31 (58.5%)	11 (20.8%)	11 (20.8%)	53 (100%)	
Family Financial Stability	Yes	98 (47.8%)	44 (21.5%)	63 (30.7%)	205 (100%)	10.878 (0.004)
	No	133 (59.1%)	53 (23.6%)	39 (17.3%)	225 (100%)	

(continued)

Table 14.7 (continued)

Variable Categories		Multidimensional Scale of Perceived Social Support (Friends)			Total	χ2 Test (p-Value)
		Low Support	Moderate Support	High Support		
Worried about Family Financial Situation	Always	85 (71.4%)	17 (14.3%)	17 (14.3%)	119	25.667 (0.000)
	Sometimes	61 (46.9%)	40 (30.8%)	29 (22.3%)	130	
	Never	85 (47.0%)	40 (22.1%)	56 (30.9%)	181	
Your or Family's Expectation	Son	42 (59.2%)	13 (18.3%)	16 (22.5%)	71 (100%)	2.104 (0.717)
	Daughter	36 (48.0%)	20 (26.7%)	19 (25.3%)	75 (100%)	
	Anyone	153 (48.0%)	64 (22.5%)	67 (23.6%)	284 (100%)	
Worried about Taking Care of Unborn Child	Always	83 (64.8%)	17 (13.3%)	28 (21.9%)	128 (100%)	18.453 (0.001)
	Sometimes	72 (45.0%)	52 (32.5%)	36 (22.5%)	160 (100%)	
	Never	76 (53.5%)	28 (19.7%)	38 (26.8%)	142 (100%)	
Adverse Effects of Employment on the Unborn Child	Always/sometimes	27 (38.0%)	19 (26.8%)	25 (35.2%)	71 (100%)	9.298 (0.010)
	Never	204 (56.8%)	78 (21.7%)	77 (21.4%)	359 (100%)	
Suffer from Illness or COVID-19 Infection	Yes	84 (52.8%)	40 (25.2%)	35 (22.0%)	159 (100%)	1.103 (0.576)
	No	147 (54.2%)	57 (21.0%)	67 (24.7%)	271 (100%)	
Patient's Age Group	18–24 years	121 (49.0%)	61 (24.7%)	65 (26.3%)	247 (100%)	5.244 (0.073)
	25–40 years	110 (60.1%)	36 (19.7%)	37 (20.2%)	183 (100%)	
Patient's Weight Group	37–49 kg	39 (51.3%)	18 (23.7%)	19 (25.0%)	76 (100%)	1.674 (0.795)
	50–69 kg	145 (52.9%)	65 (23.7%)	64 (23.4%)	274 (100%)	
	≥ 70 kg	47 (58.8%)	14 (17.5%)	19 (23.8%)	80 (100%)	

95% CI: 1.21–10.27; $p = 0.02$). Pregnant women or their families who had always expected a son were 2.31 times more likely to experience an extreme level of depression than those who did not (OR = 2.31; 95% CI: 0.79–6.78; $p = 0.13$). Employed pregnant women who were always worried about taking care of their unborn child were 3.43 times more likely to suffer from an extreme level of depression than those

Table 14.8 Multinomial logistic regression analysis of Depression Scale Classification and its associated factors among pregnant women

Variable	Depression Scale Classification (ref = normal)											
	Mild			Moderate			Severe			Extremely Severe		
	OR	p-Value	95% CI for OR	OR	p-Value	95% CI for OR	OR	p-Value	95% CI for OR	OR	p-Value	95% CI for OR
Residence (ref: Village)												
Town	2.58	0.92	1.27–5.26	1.93	0.03	1.05–3.50	2.07	0.04	1.03–4.16	2.05	0.00	1.08–16.25
Belief that Religion Reduces Frustration (ref: Never)												
Always	1.04	0.92	0.43–2.51	1.13	0.75	0.50–2.55	3.93	0.02	1.19–12.95	4.20	0.03	1.08–16.25
Sometimes	0.31	0.13	0.06–1.45	1.13	0.82	0.38–3.39	1.25	0.79	0.24–6.51	2.22	0.36	0.40–12.32
Family Financial Stability (ref: No)												
Yes	0.90	0.79	0.41–1.95	1.88	0.07	0.95–3.74	1.86	0.11	0.85–4.06	1.35	0.47	0.60–3.06
Worried about Family Financial Situation (ref: Never)												
Always	2.19	0.11	0.82–5.85	2.06	0.11	0.83–5.10	1.80	0.17	0.46–3.67	3.53	0.02	1.21–10.27
Sometimes	1.32	0.54	0.53–3.30	1.49	0.30	0.68–3.26	1.80	0.17	0.76–4.28	3.03	0.02	1.18–7.79
Your or Family's Expectation (ref: Anyone)												
Son	3.20	0.02	1.14–9.01	2.63	0.05	0.96–7.21	2.95	0.04	1.03–8.46	2.31	0.13	0.79–6.78
Daughter	0.36	0.05	0.13–1.01	1.12	0.74	0.56–2.24	0.54	0.16	0.28–1.29	0.38	0.05	0.15–1.00
Worried about Taking Care of Unborn Child (ref: Never)												
Always	0.99	0.98	0.40–2.42	1.06	0.88	0.42–2.39	1.85	0.18	0.75–4.56	3.43	0.02	1.18–9.99
Sometimes	0.73	0.47	0.31–1.72	1.38	0.37	0.67–2.87	1.55	0.29	0.68–3.54	5.04	0.00	1.91–13.31
Suffer from Illness or COVID-19 Infection (ref: No)												
Yes	0.91	0.82	0.43–1.94	2.25	0.01	1.19–4.26	1.71	0.14	0.83–3.46	1.81	0.11	0.88–3.73

who never worried about it (OR = 3.43; 95% CI: 1.18–9.99; $p = 0.02$). Women who were pregnant and had a physical illness or COVID-19 infection were 1.81 times more likely to have depression than women who had not experienced a physical illness or COVID-19 infection (OR = 1.81; 95% CI: 0.88–3.73; $p = 0.11$).

Table 14.9 displays a summary of the multinomial logistic regression of participants' Stress Scale Classification and its associated factors. According to Table 14.9, during the COVID-19 era, pregnant women who always worried about their family's financial situation were 1.47 times more likely to experience acute stress than those who never worried about it (OR = 1.47; 95% CI: 0.45–4.76; $p = 0.52$). Employed pregnant women who were always or sometimes worried about taking care of their unborn child were 1.85 times or 3.46 times more likely to suffer from extreme levels of stress. During the pregnancy period, women who were affected by a physical illness or COVID-19 infection were 1.19 times more likely to suffer from an extreme level of stress than those who were more affected by a physical illness or COVID-19 infection (OR = 1.19; 95% CI: 0.48–2.93; $p = 0.71$).

Table 14.10 represents a summary of the multinomial logistic regression of participants' Anxiety Scale Classification and its associated factors. According to Table 14.10, pregnant women who were affected by a physical illness or COVID-19 infection during their pregnancy were 4.37 times more likely to suffer from an extreme level of anxiety than those who were not affected by a physical illness or COVID-19 infection (OR = 4.37; 95% CI: 1.73–11.07; $p = 0.002$).

The multinomial logistic regression analysis of MSPSS (significant others) and its associated factors is shown in Table 14.11. According to Table 14.11, during the pregnancy period, well-educated pregnant women were 1.83 times more likely to receive a high level of social support from their significant others than less-educated women (OR = 1.83; 95% CI: 0.94–3.51; $p = 0.07$). In comparison to women who had unplanned pregnancies, those who had planned pregnancies were 2.06 times more likely to experience a high level of social support from their significant others (OR = 2.06; 95% CI: 1.15–3.71; $p = 0.02$).

Table 14.12 displays the multinomial logistic regression analysis of MSPSS (family) and its associated factors. According to Table 14.12, pregnant women who were always worried about their family financial situation were 0.56 times less likely to receive a high level of social support from their family than those who were never worried about it (OR = 0.56; 95% CI: 0.34–0.95; $p = 0.03$). But this attribute contains a statistically significant value, where $p < 0.05$.

Table 14.13 displays the multinomial logistic regression analysis of MSPSS (Friends) and its associated factors. According to Table 14.13, pregnant women who passed the SSC-HSC were 2.13 times more likely to receive a high level of social support from their friends (OR = 2.48; 95% CI: 1.30–4.72; $p = 0.005$). In addition, pregnant women who had achieved a degree with honors or a master's degree were 1.08 times more likely to receive a moderate level of social support from their friends than less-educated women were (OR = 1.08; 95% CI: 0.59–1.94; $p = 0.80$). Pregnant women who had family financial stability were 1.35 times more likely to receive a high level of social support from their family than those who did not have family financial stability.

Table 14.9 Multinomial logistic regression analysis of Stress Scale Classification and its associated factors among pregnant women

Variable		Stress Scale Classification (ref = normal)									
		Mild			Moderate			Severe			Extremely Severe		
		OR	p-Value	95% CI for OR	OR	p-Value	95% CI for OR	OR	p-Value	95% CI for OR	OR	p-Value	95% CI for OR
Belief that Religion Reduces Frustration (ref: Never)	Always	0.69	0.59	0.17–2.14	0.92	0.90	0.26–3.20	1.07	0.91	0.30–3.76	2.17	0.23	0.62–7.63
	Sometimes	0.16	0.17	0.01–2.14	0.91	0.91	0.16–5.05	1.27	0.78	0.23–7.08	0.93	0.94	0.16–5.34
Worried about Family Financial Situation (ref: Never)	Always	0.36	0.18	0.08–1.58	0.85	0.80	0.25–2.91	1.03	0.95	0.30–3.58	1.47	0.52	0.45–4.76
	Sometimes	0.48	0.28	0.12–1.87	0.65	0.45	0.21–1.99	1.02	0.96	0.34–3.14	1.30	0.63	0.45–3.78
Worried about Taking Care of Unborn Child (ref: Never)	Always	2.92	0.13	0.73–11.64	1.05	0.93	0.31–3.51	1.58	0.45	0.48–5.22	1.85	0.29	0.58–5.80
	Sometimes	1.75	0.45	0.41–7.34	2.02	0.23	0.63–6.43	1.44	0.54	0.45–4.70	3.46	0.03	1.13–10.57
Suffer from Illness or COVID-19 Infection (ref: No)	Yes	0.47	0.21	0.14–1.54	0.81	0.66	0.31–2.10	0.77	0.60	0.29–2.01	1.19	0.71	0.48–2.93

Table 14.10 Multinomial logistic regression analysis of Anxiety Scale Classification and its associated factors among pregnant women

	Anxiety Scale Classification (ref = normal)											
	Mild			Moderate			Severe			Extremely Severe		
Variable	OR	p-Value	95% CI for OR	OR	p-Value	95% CI for OR	OR	p-Value	95% CI for OR	OR	p-Value	95% CI for OR
Suffer from Illness or COVID-19 Infection (ref: No) Yes	1.14	0.81	0.40–3.23	2.87	0.02	1.19–6.91	4.26	0.002	1.74–10.45	4.37	0.002	1.73–11.07

Table 14.11 Multinomial logistic regression analysis of Multidimensional Scale of Perceived Social Support (significant others) and its associated factors among pregnant women

Variable		Multidimensional Scale of Perceived Social Support (Significant Others) *Ref: Low Support/ Moderate Support*		
		High Support		
		OR	*p*-Value	95% CI for OR
Education (ref: illiterate/class 1–10)	SSC-HSC	2.14	0.06	0.96–4.74
	Honors/master's	1.83	0.07	0.94–3.51
Planned or Unplanned Pregnancy (ref: Unplanned)	Planned	2.06	0.02	1.15–3.71

Table 14.12 Multinomial logistic regression analysis of Multidimensional Scale of Perceived Social Support (family) and its associated factors among pregnant women

Variable		Multidimensional Scale of Perceived Social Support (Family) (Ref: Low Support/Moderate Support)		
		High Support		
		OR	*p*-Value	95% CI for OR
Worried About Family Financial Situation (ref: Never)	Always	0.56	0.03	0.34–0.95
	Sometimes	0.57	0.04	0.35–0.97

Table 14.13 Multinomial logistic regression analysis of Multidimensional Scale of Perceived Social Support (friends) and its associated factors among pregnant women

Variable		Multidimensional Scale of Perceived Social Support (Friends) (Ref: Low Support)					
		Moderate Support			High Support		
		OR	*p*-Value	95% CI for OR	OR	*p*-Value	95% CI for OR
Duration of Pregnancy (ref: 1–3 months)	4–6 months	0.36	0.01	0.17–0.75	0.81	0.61	0.37–1.77
	7–9 months	0.70	0.28	0.35–1.36	1.09	0.81	0.51–2.34
Education (ref: Illiterate/Class 1–10)	SSC-HSC	2.13	0.03	1.08–4.21	2.48	0.005	1.30–4.72
	Honors/master's	1.08	0.80	0.59–1.94	0.92	0.79	0.51–1.66
Family Financial Stability (ref: No)	Yes	0.83	0.54	0.45–1.51	1.35	0.31	0.75–2.44
Worried about Family Financial Situation (ref: Never)	Always	0.43	0.04	0.19–0.96	0.38	0.02	0.17–0.83
	Sometimes	0.93	0.83	0.48–1.80	0.68	0.26	0.35–1.32
Worried about Taking Care of Unborn Child (ref: Never)	Always	0.71	0.38	0.33–1.53	0.95	0.89	0.48–1.86
	Sometimes	1.98	0.03	1.06–3.70	1.24	0.50	0.66–2.31
Adverse Effects of Employment on the Unborn Child (ref: Never)	Always	0.71	0.38	0.33–1.53	1.50	0.44	0.54–4.16
	Sometimes	1.98	0.03	1.06–3.70	2.03	0.08	0.91–4.53

14.4 Discussion

The main focus of our study is to determine antenatal depression, anxiety, and stress and their associated factors. According to the bivariate analysis in this study, pregnant women who lived in towns suffered more from severe and extreme levels of depression and anxiety. But rural residence was significantly associated with antenatal depression (Fisher et al. 2012; Zahidie et al. 2011; Kazi et al. 2006). Our study shows that well-educated pregnant woman suffered more from extreme levels of depression and stress. But interestingly, less-educated pregnant women or less-educated homemakers suffered more from antenatal depression during their pregnancy period (Zahidie et al. 2011; Waqas et al. 2015; Luo et al. 2022; Husain et al. 2011). According to this study, pregnant women who experienced mood disorders had higher levels of depression, stress, and anxiety. Bipolar I disorder is rapidly increasing among pregnant women, leading to prenatal depression (Di Florio et al. 2013; Noble 2005). Women with bipolar I disorder reportedly have an approximately 50% risk of having a perinatal major affective episode per pregnancy/postpartum period (Di Florio et al. 2013). According to our study, pregnant women who were concerned about their miscarriage had extreme levels of depression. This study verified that miscarriage represents a significant emotional burden for pregnant women, one that increases their depression and anxiety (Cumming et al. 2007). Previous studies have also claimed that after a miscarriage, a woman's anxiety symptoms increase, which is related to reproductive loss (Klier et al. 2002; Geller et al. 2004). Miscarriage was significantly associated with antenatal anxiety and depression (Westdahl et al. 2008; Lancaster et al. 2010; Koleva et al. 2011). Our study shows that during the COVID-19 pandemic, pregnant women who did not have family financial stability and who were worried about their family financial situation suffered from extreme levels of depression. The study found that pregnant women who belonged to low-income families suffered more depression, anxiety, and stress during the COVID-19 period (Fan et al. 2021; Bryson et al. 2021). The study also revealed that pregnant women's belonging to a low-income family was strongly associated with their having prenatal depression, anxiety, and stress (Gurung et al. 2005; Leigh and Milgrom 2008; Di Florio et al. 2013; Luo et al. 2022). In other studies, pregnant women who suffered from an illness or COVID-19 infection during the outbreak experienced extreme levels of depression, anxiety, and stress (Durankuş and Aksu 2022). Our study also has the same result. In addition, this study's bivariate analysis yielded some results about the MSPSS. According to our study, less-educated pregnant women received a low level of social support from their friends and significant others. For this reason, less-educated pregnant women suffered more from depression, anxiety, and stress during their pregnancy period. Our study found that women who received more social support during their pregnancy had fewer symptoms of depression, anxiety, and stress during the peripartum period (Fisher et al. 2012; Racine et al. 2019; Biaggi et al. 2016; Niesche and Haase 2012). Our study shows that pregnant women who had an unplanned pregnancy received a low level of social support from their significant others. Unintended/unplanned pregnancy was a strong predictor of increased levels of antenatal anxiety and depression among pregnant women (Fisher et al. 2012; Westdahl et al. 2008; Getinet et al. 2018; Lancaster et al. 2010; Blackmore et al. 2011; Rich-Edwards et al. 2006). According to this study, pregnant women who had poor family financial circumstances and who frequently worried about it did not receive much social assistance from their families or friends during their pregnancies. Previous studies' results have found that low income and a low level of social support are significantly associated with antenatal depression and anxiety (Westdahl et al. 2008; Leigh and Milgrom 2008; Brooks et al. 2020; Dayan et al. 2010). The research findings in our study show that employed pregnant women who always worried about taking care of their unborn child received a low level of social support from their friends. As a result, they suffered from depression, anxiety, and stress during their pregnancy period. Previous research has also revealed that due to work stress, employed pregnant women suffered from more anxiety and stress (Melchior et al. 2007; Waqas et al. 2015). We also noted some key findings from the results of our multinomial logistic regression analysis. Pregnant women who lived in towns suffered from more depression than those who lived in villages. Pregnant women who were worried about their family financial situation suffered from more depression and stress during their pregnancy period. Employed pregnant women had higher levels of depression and stress than homemakers/unemployed women did. Pregnant women who had a physical illness/COVID-19 infection suffered more anxiety, stress, and depression. We also found that well-educated pregnant women who had family financial stability received much more social support from their friends and family. Whereas no significant link was found between prenatal depression and social support in our study (Humayun et al. 2013), other studies have claimed that social support may reduce the negative effects of stressful life situations or may prevent depression directly (Cohen and Wills 1985; Cannuscio et al. 2004; Stewart et al. 2014; Nasreen et al. 2011).

14.4.1 Limitations

Given that the prevalence of COVID-19 was high during data collection, working with a large dataset was challenging for us. Moreover, hospitals in this area do not maintain patient databases, so past records could not be collected. We guarantee that an investigation with a large population will be conducted in the future, and we believe that the findings of this chapter will have far-reaching implications for future health studies.

14.4.2 Recommendations

The cross-sectional study on the mental health of pregnant women in Bangladesh during the COVID-19 pandemic illuminates critical factors influencing antenatal depression, anxiety, and stress. The identified risk factors, including urban residence, financial concerns, and employment-related anxieties, provide valuable insights for targeted interventions. The findings here underscore the necessity for comprehensive mental health–promotion programs tailored to the unique challenges faced by expectant mothers, particularly those residing in urban areas or expressing financial apprehensions. The correlation between social support and the well-being of well-educated women and those with planned pregnancies highlights the importance of community-driven initiatives. This chapter's emphasis on online campaigns and media broadcasts as tools for dissemination further establishes the need for innovative approaches. In conclusion, this chapter recommends a devising multipronged strategy encompassing mental health awareness, obstetric education, and social support initiatives to alleviate the mental health complexities faced by pregnant women in Bangladesh amid the COVID-19 pandemic.

14.5 Conclusions

The World Health Organization predicts that depressive disorders would rank as the second-most-common global cause of disease. Anxiety, depression, and stress during pregnancy can have devastating effects on children in Bangladesh, including stunted development, low birth weight, and even death. According to this chapter, pregnant women who worried about their miscarriage, experienced mood disorders, had no family financial stability, had low family income, lacked social support, and experienced a physical illness during the COVID-19 period suffered more from depression, anxiety, and stress. Adequate antenatal care should be provided to pregnant women to reduce prenatal and postpartum complexities. Finally, mothers need to be provided with practical support to improve their mental health.Declaration

Availability of Data and Material The data analyzed in this chapter are available from the corresponding author upon reasonable request. The corresponding author takes responsibility for the integrity and accuracy of the data analysis.

Ethics Approval and Consent to Participate The Research Ethical Committee (REC) of Varendra University, Bangladesh, gave its approval for this chapter, which was conducted in accordance with the Helsinki Declaration's rules (Ref: 1.07.2021/REC/VU). Verbal consent was obtained from all adult study participants.

Competing Interests The authors declare that they have no competing interests.

Funding No funding was received.

References

Bante A, Mersha A, Zerdo Z, Wassihun B, Yeheyis T (2021) Comorbid anxiety and depression: prevalence and associated factors among pregnant women in Arba Minch zuria district, Gamo zone, Southern Ethiopia. PLoS One 16(3):e0248331. https://doi.org/10.1371/journal.pone.0248331

Basu A, Kim HH, Basaldua R, Choi KW, Charron L, Kelsall N, Hernandez-Diaz S, Wyszynski DF, Koenen KC (2021) A cross-national study of factors associated with women's perinatal mental health and wellbeing during the COVID-19 pandemic. PLoS One 16(4):e0249780. https://doi.org/10.1371/journal.pone.0249780

Biaggi A, Conroy S, Pawlby S, Pariante CM (2016) Identifying the women at risk of antenatal anxiety and depression: a systematic review. J Affect Disord 191:62–77. https://doi.org/10.1016/j.jad.2015.11.014

Blackmore ER, Côté-Arsenault D, Tang W, Glover V, Evans J, Golding J, O'Connor TG (2011) Previous prenatal loss as a predictor of perinatal depression and anxiety. Br J Psychiatry J Ment Sci 198(5):373–378. https://doi.org/10.1192/bjp.bp.110.083105

Braeken MAKA, Kemp AH, Outhred T, Otte RA, Monsieur GJYJ, Jones A, Van den Bergh BRH (2013) Pregnant mothers with resolved anxiety disorders and their offspring have reduced heart rate variability: implications for the health of children. PLoS One 8(12):e83186. https://doi.org/10.1371/journal.pone.0083186

Brooks SK, Weston D, Greenberg N (2020) Psychological impact of infectious disease outbreaks on pregnant women: rapid evidence review. bioRxiv 189:26. https://doi.org/10.1101/2020.04.16.20068031

Bryson H, Mensah F, Price A, Gold L, Mudiyanselage SB, Kenny B, Dakin P, Bruce T, Noble K, Kemp L, Goldfeld S (2021) Clinical, financial and social impacts of COVID-19 and their associations with mental health for mothers and children experiencing adversity in Australia. PLoS One 16(9):e0257357. https://doi.org/10.1371/journal.pone.0257357

Cannuscio CC, Colditz GA, Rimm EB, Berkman LF, Jones CP, Kawachi I (2004) Employment status, social ties, and caregivers' mental health. Soc Sci Med 58(7):1247–1256. https://doi.org/10.1016/S0277-9536(03)00317-4

Cohen S, Wills TA (1985) Stress, social support, and the buffering hypothesis. Psychol Bull 98(2):310–357. https://doi.org/10.1037/0033-2909.98.2.310

Cumming GP, Klein S, Bolsover D, Lee AJ, Alexander DA, Maclean M, Jurgens JD (2007) The emotional burden of miscarriage for women and their partners: trajectories of anxiety and depression over 13 months. BJOG 114(9):1138–1145. https://doi.org/10.1111/j.1471-0528.2007.01452.x

Dahlem NW, Zimet GD, Walker RR (1991) The multidimensional scale of perceived social support: a confirmation study. J Clin Psychol 47(6):756–761. https://doi.org/10.1002/1097-4679(199111)47:6<756::aid-jclp2270470605>3.0.co;2-1

Dayan J, Creveuil C, Dreyfus M, Herlicoviez M, Baleyte J-M, O'Keane V (2010) Developmental model of depression applied to prenatal depression: role of present and past life events, past emotional disorders and pregnancy stress. PLoS One 5(9):e12942. https://doi.org/10.1371/journal.pone.0012942

Di Florio A, Forty L, Gordon-Smith K, Heron J, Jones L, Craddock N, Jones I (2013) Perinatal episodes across the mood disorder spectrum. JAMA Psychiatry (Chicago, Ill) 70(2):168–175. https://doi.org/10.1001/jamapsychiatry.2013.279

Durankuş F, Aksu E (2022) Effects of the COVID-19 pandemic on anxiety and depressive symptoms in pregnant women: a preliminary study. J Matern Fetal Neonatal Med 35(2):205–211. https://doi.org/10.1080/14767058.2020.1763946

Effati-Daryani F, Zarei S, Mohammadi A, Hemmati E, Ghasemi Yngyknd S, Mirghafourvand M (2020) Depression, stress, anxiety and their predictors in Iranian pregnant women during the outbreak of COVID-19. BMC Psychol 8(1):99. https://doi.org/10.1186/s40359-020-00464-8

Fan S, Guan J, Cao L, Wang M, Zhao H, Chen L, Yan L (2021) Psychological effects caused by COVID-19 pandemic on pregnant women: a systematic review with meta-analysis. Asian J Psychiatr 56(102533):102533. https://doi.org/10.1016/j.ajp.2020.102533

Fisher J, Cabral de Mello M, Patel V, Rahman A, Tran T, Holton S, Holmes W (2012) Prevalence and determinants of common perinatal mental disorders in women in low-and lower-middle-income countries: a systematic review. Bull World Health Organ 90(2):139G–149G. https://doi.org/10.2471/BLT.11.091850

Geller PA, Kerns D, Klier CM (2004) Anxiety following miscarriage and the subsequent pregnancy: a review of the literature and future directions. J Psychosom Res 56(1):35–45. https://doi.org/10.1016/S0022-3999(03)00042-4

Getinet W, Amare T, Boru B, Shumet S, Worku W, Azale T (2018) Prevalence and risk factors for antenatal depression in Ethiopia: systematic review. Depress Res Treat 2018:1

Gurung RAR, Dunkel-Schetter C, Collins N, Rini C, Hobel CJ (2005) Psychosocial predictors of prenatal anxiety. J Soc Clin Psychol 24(4):497–519. https://doi.org/10.1521/jscp.2005.24.4.497

Hossain A, Karim MS (2018) Prevalence of depression, anxiety and stress: a case study among Varendra University Students. Scholars' Press, Atlanta

Hossain A, Munam AM (2022) Factors influencing facebook addiction among Varendra university students in the lockdown during the COVID-19 outbreak. Comput Hum Behav Rep 6(100181):100181. https://doi.org/10.1016/j.chbr.2022.100181

Hossain A, Kamruzzaman M, Ali MA (2015) ARIMA with GARCH family modeling and projection on share volume of DSE. Economics World 3(4):171. https://doi.org/10.17265/2328-7144/2015.0708.003

Hossain A, Mahamud R, Bishwas MR, Kamruzzaman M (2019) Evaluation of Facebook addiction and its associated factors among Varendra university students: a cross sectional survey study. In: 7th International Conference on Data Science and SDGs, pp 677–684

Hossain A, Bhuiya RA, Zulficar Ali M (2022) The association between obesity and depression, anxiety, and stress disorders among university students at Rajshahi city in Bangladesh. J Psychiatr Psychiatr Disorder 06(05):263. https://doi.org/10.26502/jppd.2572-519x0172

Hossain A, Munam AM, Bhuiya RA, Amin MR, Ali MZ (2023) Socio-demographic factors influencing physical health among youth during the COVID-19 pandemic in Bangladesh. SN Soc Sci 3(7):115. https://doi.org/10.1007/s43545-023-00700-z

Humayun A, Haider II, Imran N, Iqbal H, Humayun N (2013) Antenatal depression and its predictors in Lahore, Pakistan. La revue de Sante de La Mediterranee Orientale [Eastern Mediterranean Health Journal] 19(4):327–332. https://doi.org/10.26719/2013.19.4.327

Husain N, Parveen A, Husain M, Saeed Q, Jafri F, Rahman R, Tomenson B, Chaudhry IB (2011) Prevalence and psychosocial correlates of perinatal depression: a cohort study from urban Pakistan. Arch Womens Ment Health 14(5):395–403. https://doi.org/10.1007/s00737-011-0233-3

Kamruzzaman M, Hossain A, Kabir E (2021) Smoker's characteristics, general health and their perception of smoking in the social environment: a study of smokers in Rajshahi City, Bangladesh. Z Gesundh [Journal of Public Health] 30(6):1501–1512. https://doi.org/10.1007/s10389-020-01413-w

Kamruzzaman M, Hossain A, Islam MA, Ahmed MS, Kabir E (2022) Prevalence of depression, anxiety, stress, and their associated factors among University students in Bangladesh. Research Square, Durham. https://doi.org/10.21203/rs.3.rs-1530510/v1

Karaçam Z, Ançel G (2009) Depression, anxiety and influencing factors in pregnancy: a study in a Turkish population. Midwifery 25(4):344–356. https://doi.org/10.1016/j.midw.2007.03.006

Kazi A, Fatmi Z, Hatcher J, Kadir MM, Niaz U, Wasserman GA (2006) Social environment and depression among pregnant women in urban areas of Pakistan: importance of social relations. Soc Sci Med 63(6):1466–1476. https://doi.org/10.1016/j.socscimed.2006.05.019

Klier CM, Geller PA, Ritsher JB (2002) Affective disorders in the aftermath of miscarriage: a comprehensive review. Arch Womens Ment Health 5(4):129–149. https://doi.org/10.1007/s00737-002-0146-2

Koleva H, Stuart S, O'Hara MW, Bowman-Reif J (2011) Risk factors for depressive symptoms during pregnancy. Arch Womens Ment Health 14(2):99–105. https://doi.org/10.1007/s00737-010-0184-0

Lancaster CA, Gold KJ, Flynn HA, Yoo H, Marcus SM (2010) Risk factors for depressive symptoms during pregnancy: a systematic review. Am J Obs Gynecol 202:5–14. https://doi.org/10.1016/j.ajog.2009.09.007

Leigh B, Milgrom J (2008) Risk factors for antenatal depression, postnatal depression and parenting stress. BMC Psychiatry 8(1):24. https://doi.org/10.1186/1471-244X-8-24

Luo Y, Zhang K, Huang M, Qiu C (2022) Risk factors for depression and anxiety in pregnant women during the COVID-19 pandemic: evidence from meta-analysis. PLoS One 17(3):e0265021. https://doi.org/10.1371/journal.pone.0265021

Melchior M, Caspi A, Milne BJ, Danese A, Poulton R, Moffitt TE (2007) Work stress precipitates depression and anxiety in young, working women and men. Psychol Med 37(8):1119–1129. https://doi.org/10.1017/s0033291707000414

Naing L, Winn T (2006) Practical issues in calculating the sample size for prevalence studies. Arch Orofac Sci 1:9–14

Nasreen HE, Kabir ZN, Forsell Y, Edhborg M (2011) Prevalence and associated factors of depressive and anxiety symptoms during pregnancy: a population based study in rural Bangladesh. BMC Womens Health 11(1):22. https://doi.org/10.1186/1472-6874-11-22

Niesche R, Haase M (2012) Emotions and ethics: a Foucauldian framework for becoming an ethical educator. Educ Philos Theory 44(3):276–288. https://doi.org/10.1111/j.1469-5812.2010.00655.x

Noble RE (2005) Depression in women. Metab Clin Exp 54(5):49–52. https://doi.org/10.1016/j.metabol.2005.01.014

Norton PJ (2007) Depression anxiety and stress scales (DASS-21): psychometric analysis across four racial groups. Anxiety Stress Coping 20(3):253–265. https://doi.org/10.1080/10615800701309279

Nwafor JI, Okedo-Alex IN, Ikeotuonye AC (2021) Prevalence and predictors of depression, anxiety, and stress symptoms among pregnant women during COVID-19-related lockdown in Abakaliki, Nigeria. Malawi Med J 33(1):54–58. https://doi.org/10.4314/mmj.v33i1.8

Racine N, Plamondon A, Hentges R, Tough S, Madigan S (2019) Dynamic and bidirectional associations between maternal stress, anxiety, and social support: the critical role of partner and family support. J Affect Disord 252:19–24. https://doi.org/10.1016/j.jad.2019.03.083

Rahman S, Munam AM, Hossain A, Hossain ASMD, Bhuiya RA (2023) Socio-economic factors affecting the academic performance of private university students in Bangladesh: a cross-sectional bivariate and multivariate analysis. SN Soc Sci 3(2):26. https://doi.org/10.1007/s43545-023-00614-w

Rich-Edwards JW, Kleinman K, Abrams A, Harlow BL, McLaughlin TJ, Joffe H, Gillman MW (2006) Sociodemographic predictors of antenatal and postpartum depressive symptoms among women in a medical group practice. J Epidemiol Community Health 60(3):221–227. https://doi.org/10.1136/jech.2005.039370

Saricam H (2018) The psychometric properties of Turkish version of depression anxiety stress scale-21 (DASS-21) in health control and clinical samples. J Cognit Behav Psychother Res 7(1):19–30

Stewart RC, Umar E, Tomenson B, Creed F (2014) Validation of the multi-dimensional scale of perceived social support (MSPSS) and the relationship between social support, intimate partner violence and antenatal depression in Malawi. BMC Psychiatry 14:180. https://doi.org/10.1186/1471-244X-14-180

Tan PC, Zaidi SN, Azmi N, Omar SZ, Khong SY (2014) Depression, anxiety, stress and hyperemesis gravidarum: temporal and casecontrolled correlates. PLoS One 9(3):e92036. https://doi.org/10.1371/journal.pone.0092036

Waqas A, Raza N, Lodhi HW, Muhammad Z, Jamal M, Rehman A (2015) Psychosocial factors of antenatal anxiety and depression in Pakistan: is social support a mediator? PLoS One 10(1):e0116510. https://doi.org/10.1371/journal.pone.0116510

Westdahl C, Milan S, Magriples U, Kershaw TS, Rising SS (2008) Social support and social conflict as predictors of prenatal depression. Obstet Gynecol 110:134–140

Zahidie A, Kazi A, Fatmi Z, Bhatti MT, Dureshahwar S (2011) Original article social environment and depression among pregnant women in rural areas of Sind, Pakistan. J Pak Med Assoc 61:1–3

Zilver SJM, Broekman BFP, Hendrix YMGA, de Leeuw RA, Mentzel SV, van Pampus MG, de Groot CJM (2021) Stress, anxiety and depression in 1466 pregnant women during and before the COVID-19 pandemic: a Dutch cohort study. J Psychosom Obstet Gynaecol 42(2):108–114. https://doi.org/10.1080/0167482X.2021.1907338

Chapter 15
Individual-and Community-Level Determinants of Maternal Healthcare Utilization in Afghanistan

Aditya Singh, Sayed Ataullah Saeedzai, Ajit Kumar Jaiswal, Shivani Singh, and Rakesh Chandra

Abstract To increase the utilization of maternal healthcare services, the factors that affect must first be identified. However, national-level studies on this topic in the country are lacking. Therefore, this chapter aims to identify and examine the factors affecting maternal healthcare utilization in Afghanistan. This chapter uses data from the first Demographic and Health Survey conducted in Afghanistan in 2015 to examine the factors associated with the utilization of maternal healthcare services among ever-married women (aged 15–49) who have had at least one birth during the 5 years preceding the survey. Multilevel binary logistic regression analyses were carried out to understand the net effect of predictor variables on the utilization of maternity care. The results show that the utilization of maternal health services is considerably low in Afghanistan. Only about 18%, 48%, and 33% Afghan mothers had availed themselves of antenatal care (ANC), safe delivery, and postnatal care (PNC) services, respectively. Findings have indicated a considerable amount of variation in the use of maternity care depending on education, wealth, ethnicity, parity, and place of residence. Maternal care in Afghanistan is associated with a woman and her partner's education, ethnicity, wealth, parity, exposure to mass media, and place of residence. The chapter finds a strong association between the utilization of antenatal care and both safe delivery and postnatal care. Exposure to mass media and mothers' participation in health expenditure decision-making are

---

A. Singh (✉)
Banaras Hindu University, Varanasi, India

S. A. Saeedzai
Ministry of Public Health, Kabul, Afghanistan

A. K. Jaiswal
International Institute for Population Sciences, Mumbai, India

S. Singh
Independent Researcher, Lucknow, India

R. Chandra
Tata Institute of Social Sciences, Mumbai, India

© The Author(s), under exclusive license to Springer Nature Singapore Pte Ltd. 2024
P. Chouhan et al. (eds.), *Sexual and Reproductive Health of Women*, https://doi.org/10.1007/978-981-97-8418-9_15

positively associated with maternal care utilization in Afghanistan. These results suggest the need to adopt a targeted approach to reduce differentials in the utilization of maternal care in Afghanistan. In the short term, the government should focus on promoting antenatal care and the use of mass media. In the long term, the government should promote girl's education and reduce wealth inequalities.

Keywords Maternal healthcare · Determinants · Women · India

15.1 Introduction

After the Afghan Civil War (1992–1996), an Islamic fundamentalist political movement, the Taliban, gained control over the country and continued to hold the power until 2001. They forced a strict interpretation of sharia (Islamic law), which put several restrictions on women's rights, including their movement in public spaces (Ghasemi 1998). This significantly curtailed their access to healthcare services. A prohibition on receiving care from male health workers, the destruction of existing health infrastructure, and a dwindling health workforce due to continuous war, conflict, and insurgency left many pregnant women without the assistance of skilled health personnel such as doctors, nurses, and midwives (Acerra et al. 2009).

As a result, Afghanistan's maternal mortality ratio by the year 2002 was one of the highest in the world, about 1600 maternal deaths per 100,000 live births (Ministry of Economy 2013). In the post-Taliban era (2002 onwards), maternal mortality in the country has declined significantly, as it has anywhere else in the world. As of 2015, according to a United Nations estimate, it stood at close to 400 maternal deaths per 100,000 live births (Akseer et al. 2016). Though much lower than it was during Taliban regime, it is still one of the highest in the world, and millions of mothers are dying due to pregnancy-related causes.

Growing evidence from around the world suggests that an overwhelming majority of these deaths can be prevented if mothers are provided with essential emergency obstetric care during pregnancy, childbirth, and the postpartum period (WHO 2016). Being a signatory to the United Nations' Millennium Development Goals and Sustainable Development Goals (Ministry of Foreign Affairs 2017), the government of Afghanistan has a legal duty to make sure that women do not die or suffer complications from preventable pregnancy-related causes (Reproductive Health Task Force 2012). Unfortunately, in a country that has suffered war and conflict for decades, both access to and the utilization of maternal healthcare services are extremely poor (Acerra et al. 2009; Akseer et al. 2016).

A review of previous studies reveals a dearth of literature on a couple of points, namely large-scale national-level studies examining the factors that affect maternal healthcare service utilization in Afghanistan; the ones that do exist are not truly nationally representative. For instance, a study based on the Afghan Mortality Survey in 2010 cannot be said to be truly nationally representative, because the survey did not capture information from several conflict-ridden and insecure areas in the southern part of the country (Singh et al. 2013). Another study did not include important variables such as region/province of residence, women's autonomy, ethnicity, etc. and employed simple regression techniques to deal with the hierarchical dataset that it used (Shahram et al. 2015). To fill this gap and to better understand the factors associated with the utilization of maternal healthcare services in Afghanistan and the additional risk factors stemming from the communities in which women live, a multilevel analytical framework using the most recent data from the Demographic and Health Survey (2015) is needed. By examining the healthcare needs of mothers and identifying the barriers in access to maternal healthcare services, this chapter aims to help the government in designing appropriate, context-relevant programs and policy responses.

15.2 Data and Methods

The data for this chapter come from the first Afghanistan Demographic and Health Survey (DHS), conducted during 2015–2016. The survey is a nationally representative cross-sectional survey carried out in all 34 provinces of the country. It collected information on a host of issues, including the knowledge and practice of family planning, fertility levels, the nutritional status of children and women, childhood mortality, maternal and child health, and domestic violence. The survey uses a stratified two-stage sampling design. The second stage involved the systematic sampling of households. After a house-listing operation in all of the selected clusters, a fixed number of 27 households per cluster was selected through an equal probability systematic selection process, yielding a total sample size of 25,650 households (Central Statistics Organization 2015). Readers interested in the deeper details on sampling can refer to the national report of 2015 Afghanistan DHS, available at the website of the DHS Program (www.dhsprogram.com). The response rate for household and individual surveys was 98% and 97%, respectively. Among the chapter population, only 19,787 ever-married women who had a delivery in the 5 years preceding the survey period were included in the analysis. Missing values were excluded from the analysis (Central Statistics Organization 2015).

15.2.1 Ethical Statement

The Afghanistan Demographic and Health Survey of 2015 was conducted under the supervision of the Ministry of Public Health (MoPH), a ministry of the government of Afghanistan. The survey protocol and the questionnaires were approved by the ICF International's Institutional Review Board (IRB) and the Ministry of Public Health of Afghanistan. Before interviewing the respondents to the survey, formal written consent was obtained, and ethical issues were taken care of. Moreover, this chapter is based on anonymous public use datasets with no identifiable information on the survey participants.

15.2.2 Outcome Variables

The chapter measured three outcome variables, namely ≥ four antenatal care (ANC) visits, institutional delivery, and a postnatal checkup within 24 h of delivery, as indicators of maternal healthcare utilization. Delivery conducted either in a medical institution/health facility/hospital is referred to as institutional delivery. All outcome variables were binary in nature: They had only two response categories—yes or no. Henceforth, in this article, the terms *antenatal care* and *postnatal care* are defined as ≥ four ANC visits and a postnatal checkup within 24 h of delivery, respectively.

15.2.3 Exposure Variables

Maternal healthcare utilization is a result of a complex mesh of factors (Anderson 1973). Back in 1994, Thaddeus and Maine grouped these factors according to the kind of delays that they caused: delay in decision-making, delay in reaching the facility, and delay in receiving adequate care (Thaddeus and Maine 1994). According to the health behavior model of Anderson, healthcare utilization is determined by the dynamics of three type of factors: predisposing factors, enabling factors, and need. Predisposing factors include sociodemographic variables such as age, gender, occupation, ethnicity, religion, attitudes, and beliefs, among others. Enabling factors include an individual's income, health insurance, access to care, quality of social networks, etc. The need factor motivates service use and may include perceived health status (Anderson 1973). Several individual- and community-level variables were considered for determining associations between the three outcome variables and different determining factors.

15.2.3.1 Individual Level

This chapter considered a host of socioeconomic and demographic predictors, such as a woman and her spouse's education, women's household economic status, their exposure to mass media, their employment status, parity (the number of children born alive to a woman), their affiliation with an ethnic group, their participation in health expenditure decision-making, and their place of residence. The selection of these variables was guided by existing literature on maternal healthcare utilization in developing countries.

A woman and her spouse's education is based on their total number of years of schooling. The variable has four categories: no education, primary, secondary, and higher. A mother's occupation falls into one of four categories: not working, agriculture, services, or manual labor (both high-skill and low-skill labor). The wealth index is a composite index of household amenities that is often used as a proxy for the economic status of a household. The wealth index is already given in the dataset. It has five categories: poorest, poorer, middle, richer, and richest. This chapter also includes a variable representing the autonomy of women. The survey asks about who decides to spend on maternal care, whose original responses include the following: the respondent alone, the respondent and their spouse/partner together, the spouse/partner alone, someone else, and other. In this chapter, the variable has been recoded by merging the first two categories into "both" and the last two categories into "other." Thus, the variable now has three categories: both, only spouse, and other. The variable representing exposure to mass media has three categories: full exposure, partial exposure, and no exposure. Full exposure refers to a woman's exposure to all three types of mass media—namely TV, radio, and newspapers—at least once a week. Partial exposure refers to a woman's exposure to at least one medium once a weak. No exposure refers to a woman's lack of exposure to any of these media. The ethnicity variable refers to which of the many ethnic groups in Afghanistan that a woman belongs to. The eight categories in this variable represent Afghanistan's major ethnicities. All other minority ethnic groups fall into the category "other." The place-of-residence variable is determined by whether a mother lives in a rural or urban area. To capture regional variation, this chapter has grouped the 34 provinces of the country into six regions on the basis of their geographical location: either the central (Kabul, Kapisa, Parwan, Wardak, Logar, Panjsher, and Bamyan), northeastern (Baghlan, Kunduz, Badkhashan, and Takhar), eastern (Nangarhar, Laghman, Kunarha, and Nuristan provinces), northwestern (Balkh, Sar-e-pul, Samangan, Jawzjan, and Faryab), southern (Ghazni, Paktika, Paktya, Khost, Daykundi, Urozgan, Zabul, and Kandahar), or western region (Badghis, Ghor, Herat, Farah, and Nimroz).

15.2.3.2 Community-Level Variables

The analysis in this chapter included some primary sampling unit (PSU) factors (i.e., contextual determinants), such as the proportion of illiterate respondents, proportion of poor respondents, and proportion of the respondents who had three or fewer ANC visits.

15.2.4 Statistical Analysis

We used contingency table analysis and multilevel logistic regression to understand the factors associated with postnatal care in Afghanistan. Cross-tabulation was carried out to understand the differentials in the utilization of postnatal care across selected background characteristics. Multilevel logistic regression was used to understand the contextual determinant of antenatal care, safe delivery, and postnatal care in the country.

Multilevel models allow data to be clustered and put into a hierarchy, and if they are ignored, they could generate improper standard errors for the coefficients of the predictor variables and error terms. Due to the sampling procedures used, DHS datasets have a hierarchical structure, where women and men are nested within the household, which itself is nested in a PSU or village, followed nesting within districts and within states. This structure produces a dataset in which observations are not fully independent, due to their origin in the same household or PSU. This violates the assumption of the independence of observations made in a simple regression analysis. Multilevel models allow for such datasets and produce standard errors adjusted for the clustering of observations. The second reason for using multilevel logistic regression in this chapter was that we wanted to estimate the effects of contextual–/village–/community-level variables on the utilization of maternal healthcare services [45]. These variables do not vary from person to person in a single community but do produce a clustering effect that can be dealt with only when they fit a multilevel regression model. A four-level logit model can be written as follows:

$$logit \pi_{ijkl} = \beta_0 + BX'ijkl + (u0l + v0kl + w0kl)$$

where i, j, k, and l are the level-1 (individual); level-2 (village or PSU); level-3 (district) and level-4 (state)—or community-level—units, respectively, and π_{ij} is the probability of using ANC, safe delivery, and PNC for the ith women in the jth, k^{th}, and l^{th} PSUs, districts, and states.

Before multilevel models are applied, the extent to which the outcome of interest varies at a high level should be assessed. We applied three models to determine the binary outcome of model 0 (i.e., the null model), model 1, and model 2. The null model is fitted without any variable because we wish to assess the need for a multilevel model. Model 1 includes only contextual determinants by modifying some of the variables at the PSU level to assess the extent of variability in the outcomes across the levels after controlling for the individual predictors that were omitted from the model. In model 2, also a full model, we include all the individual sociodemographic factors. The intraclass correlation (ICC) can be calculated and is formulated as follows:

$$\frac{\sigma_j^2}{\left(\sigma_j^2 + 3.29\right)}$$

where σ_j^2 represents the community-level variance. The results of the multilevel logistic regression are presented as odds ratios. A statistical analysis is performed on Stata 12 SE (Stata Corporation, College Station, Texas, USA) [47].

15.3 Results

15.3.1 Profile of the Respondents

Table 15.1 presents the unweighted percentage distribution of the mothers who had experienced their last childbirth during the 5 years preceding the survey. A considerable proportion of mothers enjoyed high parity. For instance, about 8% of all mothers had between 8 and 16 children, whereas about 33% had between five and seven children. The proportion of poorest mothers was about 18.8%. On ethnicity, about 43.1% of mothers were Pashtun and 29.5% Tajik. Other dominant ethnic groups included Hazara and Uzbek.

Most mothers were uneducated (85.1%). Only 1.5% of mothers had higher education. The level of education among the spouses was slightly better, where about 43.5% of them had at least some education. On the employment status of the mother, most of them were unemployed. About 38.8% mothers were completely unexposed to mass media. About 47.3% of mothers reported that the decision to spend money on their health-related care was taken only by their spouse. About 76% of mothers lived in rural areas. About 17.3% of mothers lived in the central region, where the national capital, Kabul, is.

Table 15.1 Distribution of mothers who had at least one live birth during the 5 years preceding the survey, according to background characteristics in Afghanistan, DHS 2015

Background characteristics	%	N^a
Parity		
1–2	30.5	6031
3–4	28.3	5598
5–8	33.3	6579
8–16	8.0	1579
Wealth quintile		
Poorest	18.8	3727
Poorer	22.7	4495
Middle	22.1	4378
Richer	21.6	4280
Richest	14.7	2907
Ethnic group		
Pashtun	43.1	8522
Tajik	29.5	5827
Hazara	8.7	1717
Uzbek	6.8	1345
Turkmen	2.1	414
Nuristani	5.2	1031
Baloch	1.2	240
Pashai	1.9	381
Other	1.4	275

(continued)

Table 15.1 (continued)

Background characteristics	%	N^a
Mother's education		
No education	85.1	16,834
Primary	7.1	1404
Secondary	6.3	1246
Higher	1.5	303
Spouse's education		
No education	56.5	11,039
Primary	13.9	2718
Secondary	22.5	4386
Higher	7.1	1383
Employment status of mother		
Not working	86.7	17,138
Agriculture	5.3	1049
Services	4.7	920
Manual labor	3.4	662
Mass-media exposure		
Full exposure	2.3	443
No exposure	38.8	7643
Partial exposure	58.9	11,609
Decision to spend on mother's health		
Both	43.9	8575
Only spouse	47.3	9228
Other	8.9	1729
Place of residence		
Urban	24.0	4742
Rural	76.0	15,045
Region		
Northeast	10.5	2078
Central	17.3	3415
East	15.3	3025
Northwest	13.6	2691
South	27.5	5435
West	15.9	3143
Total	100	19,787

[a]The total n for each variable may not always be 19,787, because some values are missing

15.3.2 Differentials in Maternal Healthcare Service Utilization

Table 15.2 shows the percentage of women who utilized maternal healthcare services according to selected background characteristics. Nationally, about 18.3% of all mothers in Afghanistan had four or more antenatal care visits. About 48.4% of mothers delivered in health facilities, and about 32.7% received a postnatal checkup within 48 hours of delivery.

Table 15.2 Utilization of maternal healthcare services according to selected background characteristics of mothers in Afghanistan, DHS 2015

Background characteristics	≥ 4 ANC visits (%)	Institutional delivery (%)	Postnatal checkup within 2 days (%)
Parity			
01–02	20.4	55.9	37.1
03–04	18.1	47.2	32.6
05–07	17.0	43.4	29.2
08–16	15.9	44.1	31.2
Wealth quintile			
Poorest	12.4	26.7	26.9
Poorer	11.9	35.8	25.2
Middle	16.2	45.3	29.9
Richer	21.4	61.9	37.2
Richest	34.2	80.1	49.5
Ethnic group			
Pashtun	14.6	49.9	30.8
Tajik	24.8	55.4	41.4
Hazara	22.3	45.1	28.5
Uzbek	24.0	55.7	41.4
Turkmen	18.1	54.1	39.1
Nuristani	0.3	2.0	1.4
Baloch	9.6	37.8	14.2
Pashai	9.7	19.4	13.1
Other	28.0	53.3	42.9
Mother's education			
No education	15.5	44.0	29.2
Primary	28.6	67.2	48.9
Secondary	35.1	76.0	52.3
Higher	53.8	89.4	72.0
Spouse's education			
No education	14.1	38.7	27.0
Primary	19.9	55.9	38.5
Secondary	22.9	60.8	38.8
Higher	34.9	73.0	49.1
Employment status of mother			
Not working	19.1	50.8	34.2
Agriculture	3.6	10.9	5.2
Services	25.4	59.0	39.7
Manual labor	10.4	30.3	26.6
Mass-media exposure			
Full exposure	41.6	86.7	64.8
No exposure	10.5	29.8	21.2
Partial exposure	22.4	59.1	39.1
Decision to spend on mother's health			

(continued)

Table 15.2 (continued)

Background characteristics	≥ 4 ANC visits (%)	Institutional delivery (%)	Postnatal checkup within 2 days (%)
Both	22.4	52.7	36.5
Only spouse	14.3	42.9	28.5
Other	19.8	57.7	37.1
Place of residence			
Urban	29.6	72.1	44.4
Rural	14.7	40.8	29.0
Region			
Northeast	22.2	48.4	31.9
Central	32.8	64.3	43.3
East	10.5	36.3	23.1
Northwest	26.3	55.5	46.0
South	11.0	47.5	20.2
West	13.1	37.8	41.3
Total	18.3	48.4	32.7

Note: This table features unweighted percentages

Among those women who had only one or two children, the rates of adequate antenatal care visits and safe delivery care were 20.4% and 55.9%, respectively. The rate of antenatal care (15.5%) and that of postnatal care (29.2%) were very low among uneducated women. Similarly, the rate of institutional delivery was 44.0% among women with no formal education, and the same was found to be high, at 89.4%, for those with higher education. A similar pattern was found for the educational level of a woman's spouse. The proportion of women using adequate antenatal care was 34.9% among women whose spouse had a higher education, much higher than the women whose spouses were uneducated. The same held true for institutional delivery and postnatal care.

The utilization of antenatal care was highest among Tajik mothers (24.8%) and lowest among Nuristanis (0.3%). Nuristani mothers lagged behind mothers from other ethnicities in the utilization of institutional delivery care (2.0%) and of postnatal care (1.4%). The utilization of antenatal care (3.6%), institutional delivery care (10.9%), and postnatal care (5.2) was considerably lower among women who worked in agriculture.

The utilization of all three services was lower among women who were unexposed or underexposed to mass media and lived in rural areas. For instance, although only 40.8% of mothers in rural areas delivered in health facilities, the proportion of such women in urban areas was about 72.1%. According to regions, the utilization of services was highest in the central region, where about 32.8% and 64.3% of mothers utilized antenatal care and went to a health facility for delivery, respectively.

15.3.3 Factors Associated with the Utilization of Maternal Healthcare Services

15.3.3.1 Four or More Antenatal Care Visits (≥ Four ANC Visits)

Table 15.3 presents the results from the multilevel regression analysis conducted to examine the association between the number of ANC visits and other factors, such as women's age, their place of residence, and some of their other socioeconomic characteristics. The results of the null model show that about 27%, 35%, and 42% of the variance in the utilization of ANC visits was attributable to differences across states, districts, and villages, respectively.

Table 15.3 Odds ratios and 95% confidence intervals (CIs) for four or more antenatal care visits among mothers in Afghanistan, DHS 2015 ($n = 19{,}137$)

Covariates	Model 0	Model 1	Model 2
Community characteristics			
Community poverty			
Low®			
Middle		0.754***(0.637 0.893)	1.028 (0.863 1.224)
High		0.403***(0.329 0.494)	0.762**(0.604 0.961)
Community illiteracy			
Low®			
Middle		0.608***(0.520 0.712)	0.749***(0.638 0.880)
High		0.400***(0.323 0.496)	0.543***(0.435 0.678)
Individual characteristics			
Age			
15 to 19 years®			
20 to 24 years			1.013 (0.897 1.144)
25 to 29 years			1.108 (0.948 1.296)
Place of residence			
Urban®			
Rural			0.908 (0.752 1.095)
Parity			
Two®			
Three			1.017 (0.888 1.164)
Four and above			0.857**(0.753 0.976)
Educational level of mother			

(continued)

Table 15.3 (continued)

Covariates	Model 0	Model 1	Model 2
No education®			1.183**(1.018 1.374)
Primary			1.248***(1.058 1.472)
Secondary			1.846***(1.363 2.5)
Higher			
Educational level of spouse			
No education®			
Primary			1.008 (0.889 1.143)
Secondary			1.152**(1.032 1.286)
Higher			1.375***(1.175 1.608)
Wealth Index			
Poorest®			
Poorer			1.143 (0.972 1.345)
Middle			1.456***(1.225 1.731)
Richer			1.566***(1.303 1.883)
Richest			2.265***(1.817 2.823)
Ethnicity			
Pashtun®			
Tajik			0.973 (0.835 1.133)
Hazara			0.955 (0.744 1.226)
Uzbek			0.92 (0.718 1.178)
Turkmen			0.938 (0.629 1.4)
Nuristani			0.099**(0.017 0.585)
Baloch			0.761 (0.432 1.343)
Pashai			0.455***(0.281 0.736)
Other			1.035 (0.732 1.464)
Media exposure			
All sources®			
None of the sources			0.507***(0.389 0.662)
At least any one source			0.733**(0.573 0.937)
Respondent's occupation			
Not working®			
Self-employed			0.82 (0.545 1.234)

(continued)

Table 15.3 (continued)

Covariates	Model 0	Model 1	Model 2
Professional/managerial			1.28**(1.049 1.562)
High-skill/low-skill manual labor			1.003 (0.736 1.366)
Variance (_cons) [state]	1.543***(0.907 2.626)	1.257***(0.746 2.118)	0.984***(0.579 1.674)
ICC (%)	0.27	0.25	0.21
Variance (_cons) [state > district]	0.482***(0.337 0.689)	0.116***(0.054 0.249)	0.096***(0.043 0.212)
ICC (%)	0.35	0.27	0.23
Variance (_cons) [state > district > PSU]	0.387***(0.304 0.493)	0.303***(0.231 0.397)	0.263***(0.195 0.353)
ICC (%)	0.42	0.33	0.28

Note: ® = reference category; ICC = intraclass correlation; and *** = $p < 0.01$, ** = $p < 0.05$, and * = $p < 0.10$; Values in the parenthesis are lower and upper values of 95% confidence interval associated with odds ratio.

Model 2 includes all the individual- and community- level factors. Its results show that women with four or more children are 15% less likely to go for ANC visits than women with one or two children were. The likelihood of going for ANC visits increases with increases in education. Women belonging to the middle, richer, and richest wealth classes are 45%, 56%, and 126% more likely to go to ANC visits, respectively, than those belonging to the poorest quintile. Nuristani and Pashai women are 90% and 55% less likely to go for ANC visits than their Pashtun counterparts. Further, women who are not exposed to media are about 50% less likely to go for the required number of ANC visits. Women in professional/managerial occupations are 28% more likely to go for ANC visits. The variation in the use of ANC across all three levels reduced in model 2. A considerable reduction in the ICC (from 42% to 28%) occurred when community-level variables were added to the model.

15.3.3.2 Institutional Delivery

Table 15.3 presents the results from the regression models applied to examine the association between safe delivery and factors such as women's age, their place of residence, and some of their other socioeconomic characteristics. The results of the null model show a significant variation in safe delivery across the three levels. The intraclass correlation of the null model reveals that the PSU level accounted for about 47% of the total variation in safe delivery, followed by district (36%) and state levels (20%). When community-level variables were added to the model, the ICC was reduced to 15%, 20%, and 29% for the state, district, and PSU levels, respectively. The ICC was further reduced to 9%, 14%, and 23%, respectively, when individual-level variables were added to the model. In the full model, rural women were 22% less likely to opt for institutional delivery than their urban counterparts.

An inverse relationship between parity and safe delivery was noticed. Tajik women were 28% more likely to opt for a safe delivery than Pashtun women were. Surprisingly, self-employed women were about 29% less likely to opt for a safe delivery than nonworking women were (Table 15.4).

Table 15.4 Odds ratios and 95% confidence intervals (CIs) for institutional delivery among mothers in Afghanistan, DHS 2015 ($n = 19{,}106$)

Covariates	Model 0	Model 1	Model 2
Constant	0***(0 0)	3.685***(2.627 5.169)	4.405***(2.696 7.196)
Community characteristics			
Community poverty			
Low®		0.583***(0.487 0.697)	0.786***(0.657 0.941)
Middle		0.268***(0.216 0.333)	0.460***(0.365 0.578)
High			
Community illiteracy			
Low®		0.662***(0.56 0.782)	0.865*(0.733 1.021)
Middle		0.49***(0.395 0.609)	0.749***(0.603 0.929)
High			
Community antenatal care			
High®			
Middle		0.641***(0.542 0.757)	0.700***(0.596 0.822)
Low		0.337***(0.271 0.42)	0.398***(0.323 0.492)
Individual characteristics			
Age			
15 to 19 years®			
20 to 24 years			0.957 (0.86 1.066)
25 to 29 years			0.966 (0.842 1.108)
Place of residence			
Urban®			
Rural			0.785**(0.644 0.957)
Parity			
Two®			
Three			0.696***(0.617 0.784)
Four and above			0.602***(0.537 0.674)
Educational level of mother			
No education®			

(continued)

Table 15.4 (continued)

Covariates	Model 0	Model 1	Model 2
Primary			1.326***(1.141 1.541)
Secondary			1.596***(1.331 1.913)
Higher			2.23***(1.435 3.468)
Educational level of spouse			
No education®			
Primary			1.245***(1.118 1.385)
Secondary			1.303***(1.183 1.436)
Higher			1.484***(1.263 1.743)
Wealth index			
Poorest®			
Poorer			1.28***(1.125 1.456)
Middle			1.315***(1.143 1.512)
Richer			1.61***(1.383 1.874)
Richest			2.204***(1.804 2.692)
Ethnicity			
Pashtun®			
Tajik			1.28***(1.103 1.486)
Hazara			1.114 (0.865 1.433)
Uzbek			1.132 (0.883 1.451)
Turkmen			1.345 (0.907 1.993)
Nuristani			0.195***(0.067 0.563)
Baloch			0.817 (0.507 1.316)
Pashai			0.365***(0.239 0.556)
Other			1.129 (0.804 1.585)
Mass-media exposure			
All sources®			
None of the sources			0.382***(0.271 0.54)
At lest anyone source			0.55***(0.393 0.77)
Respondent's occupation			
Not working®			

(continued)

Table 15.4 (continued)

Covariates	Model 0	Model 1	Model 2
Self-employed			0.71**(0.525 0.96)
Professional/managerial			1.064 (0.883 1.281)
High-skill/low-skill manual labor			0.888 (0.691 1.142)
Variance (_cons) [state]	1.284***(0.738 2.234)	0.692***(0.404 1.185)	0.424***(0.235 0.765)
ICC (%)	0.20	0.15	0.09
Variance (_cons) [state > district]	1.015***(0.78 1.32)	0.261***(0.172 0.398)	0.218***(0.139 0.341)
ICC (%)	0.36	0.20	0.14
Variance (_cons) [state > district > PSU]	0.643***(0.539 0.767)	0.416***(0.338 0.512)	0.351***(0.28 0.441)
ICC (%)	0.47	0.29	0.23

Note: ® = reference category; ICC = intraclass correlation; and *** = $p < 0.01$, ** = $p < 0.05$, and * = $p < 0.10$

15.3.3.3 Postnatal Care

Table 15.5 depicts our findings on the effect of different independent predictors on postnatal care among women. The proportion of women who went for three or fewer ANC visits at the PSU level were also included in Table 15.5. In model 1, the women living in PSUs where the average number of ANC visits fell within the middle and lower categories were 29% and 52% less likely, respectively, to go for postnatal checkups. About 22%, 26%, and 31% of the variance in the use of PNC was attributed to state, district, and PSU levels, respectively. In the full model, women whose spouses had received secondary and higher levels of education were around 21% and 35% more likely to go to PNC checkups, respectively, than those with illiterate spouses. The measures of variation remained significant across communities. The ICC associated with safe delivery was estimated at only 18%, 23%, and 27% across state, district, and PSU levels, respectively.

Table 15.5 Odds ratios and 95% confidence intervals (CIs) for postnatal checkup within 48 hours after delivery among mothers in Afghanistan, DHS 2015 (n = 19,137)

Covariates	Model 0	Model 1	Model 2
Constant	0.342***(0.228 0.512)	0.883 (0.604 1.29)	0.806 (0.501 1.294)
Community characteristics			
Community poverty			
Low®			
Middle		0.822**(0.704 0.96)	0.978 (0.834 1.147)
High		0.539***(0.446 0.65)	0.797**(0.646 0.985)
Community illiteracy			
Low®			
Middle		0.771***(0.666 0.892)	0.931 (0.803 1.081)
High		0.657***(0.541 0.797)	0.887 (0.728 1.081)
Community antenatal care			
High®			
Middle		0.711***(0.616 0.821)	0.752***(0.653 0.865)
Low		0.487***(0.399 0.593)	0.542***(0.447 0.659)
Individual characteristics			
Age group			
15 to 19 years®			
20 to 24 years			1.123**(1.012 1.247)
25 to 29 years			1.116 (0.975 1.278)
Place of residence			
Urban®			
Rural			0.994 (0.833 1.186)
Parity			
Two®			
Three			0.883**(0.786 0.992)
Four and above			0.75***(0.671 0.838)
Educational level of mother			
No education®			
Primary			1.409***(1.228 1.617)
Secondary			1.373***(1.173 1.608)
Higher			2.204***(1.601 3.034)

(continued)

Table 15.5 (continued)

Covariates	Model 0	Model 1	Model 2
Educational level of spouse			
No education®			
Primary			1.21***(1.088 1.346)
Secondary			1.216***(1.106 1.338)
Higher			1.358***(1.172 1.574)
Wealth index			
Poorest®			
Poorer			1.161**(1.019 1.323)
Middle			1.348***(1.17 1.553)
Richer			1.4***(1.201 1.631)
Richest			1.695***(1.4 2.052)
Ethnicity			
Pashtun®			
Tajik			1.086 (0.95 1.241)
Hazara			0.872 (0.687 1.107)
Uzbek			0.907 (0.721 1.14)
Turkmen			0.805 (0.561 1.154)
Nuristani			0.263**(0.07 0.989)
Baloch			0.776 (0.47 1.28)
Pashai			0.495***(0.319 0.77)
Other			0.951 (0.695 1.301)
Mass-media exposure			
All sources®			
None of the sources			0.466***(0.358 0.607)
At least any one source			0.651***(0.506 0.836)
Respondent's occupation			
Not working®			
Self-employed			0.654**(0.461 0.928)
Professional/managerial			1.099 (0.918 1.315)
High-skill/low-skill manual labor			1.012 (0.793 1.292)
Variance (_cons) [state]	1.341***(0.801 2.243)	1.05***(0.629 1.752)	0.817***(0.479 1.395)

(continued)

Table 15.5 (continued)

Covariates	Model 0	Model 1	Model 2
ICC (%)	0.25	0.22	0.18
Variance (_cons) [state > district]	0.42***(0.308 0.572)	0.215***(0.145 0.32)	0.217***(0.148 0.319)
ICC (%)	0.32	0.26	0.23
Variance (_cons) [state > district > PSU]	0.327***(0.261 0.409)	0.246***(0.19 0.318)	0.207***(0.155 0.276)
ICC (%)	0.38	0.31	0.27

Note: ® = reference category; ICC = intraclass correlation; and *** = $p < 0.01$, ** = $p < 0.05$, and * = $p < 0.10$

15.4 Discussion

Afghanistan has been riddled with war and misrule for decades, resulting into poor healthcare infrastructure and one of the highest maternal and child mortality rates in the world (Acerra et al. 2009). Although maternal mortality has improved in manifold ways since the fall of the Taliban, it is still considerably high (United Nations Population Fund 2015) because maternal health services are either nonexistent or underutilized. In the post-Taliban era, the government has made several efforts to increase the number of healthcare workers and to improve health infrastructure with whatever limited resources they have had at their disposal. In the wake of limited financial resources, two basic packages, the Basic Package of Health Services (BPHS) and the Essential Package of Hospital Services (EPHS), were decided to be delivered through nongovernmental organizations (NGOs) working throughout the country, primarily in rural areas (Newbrander et al. 2014). As a result, maternity services in the country have improved to a considerable extent, and their impact can be seen in the lower maternal mortality ratio the recent years (Frost et al. 2016).

However, the utilization of maternal health services is considerably low in Afghanistan. Only about 18%, 48%, and 33% of Afghan mothers had availed themselves of antenatal care, safe delivery, and postnatal care services, respectively. Hence, this chapter assessed the factors affecting the utilization of maternal health services among Afghan mothers (who had their last childbirth during the 5 years preceding the survey) by using the latest Demographic and Health Survey, conducted in 2015. This chapter identified several socioeconomic, sociodemographic, and geographic factors that have had considerable influences on maternal healthcare utilization in Afghanistan.

In this chapter, the education of women and their spouses remained strong predictors of maternal healthcare service utilization, and these results are consistent with the findings from studies conducted in many other developing countries (Shahram et al. 2015; Singh et al. 2014a, b; Worku et al. 2013). Arguably, education transforms women's attitudes toward their traditional gender roles, which in turn allows women to achieve greater decision-making autonomy within their household (Jejeebhoy 1995). A woman's increased authority to make decisions enables her to move about her community more freely and to actively seek maternal health services as needed (Hobcraft 1993). Formal education also encourages and enables woman to use modern maternity services by providing her with knowledge about modern healthcare and by challenging her traditional beliefs about maternity (Greenaway et al. 2012).

Wealth also turned out to be a strong predictor of maternal healthcare utilization in Afghanistan. This aligns with the results of previous studies, which have found wealth to positively influence the use of health services (Singh et al. 2014a, b; Worku et al. 2013; Mustafa and Mukhtar 2015; Zakar et al. 2017). Household wealth is expected to have a positive relationship with maternal health service use because the service user often incurs many direct costs (e.g., the cost of consultation and the purchase of recommended medication) and indirect costs, such as transportation (Arthur 2012). The higher use of healthcare services among wealthier women signifies their ability to afford the costs and other expenses (including bribes) that come with using these services (McIntyre et al. 2006).

Our results also revealed that some ethnic groups, especially Nuristanis and Pashais, are significantly less likely to receive maternal care than are Pashtuns, the largest and most dominant ethnic group in Afghanistan. Low maternal healthcare utilization among these ethnic groups could be because the terrain of the areas that they live in is highly undulating with limited possibilities for road development, meaning limited or no access to health facilities (Mashal 2015). Nuristanis live mainly in the province of Nuristan, which is in the heart of the Hindu Kush mountains, which are characterized by steep valleys, thousands of streams, and almost no motorable roads to connect with the regional capital, Parun (BBC 2013). The province has only one 50-bed hospital, in Parun, which is still under construction. The government has a minimal presence in the regional capital, and none of the districts in the province is yet connected by a metaled road to the capital Parun. In fact, one of the districts, Barg-e Matal, remained under Taliban control until recently). Security concerns prevent many trained female healthcare professionals from working in Nuristan and other isolated regions (United Nations Develpoment Program 2016). The Pashais are also scattered mainly in the provinces of Laghman and Nangahar, in eastern Afghanistan, where the government presence is still minimal. This part of the country is also highly inaccessible, neglected, and underdeveloped compared to the reference province, the central region (Jolliffe 2010).

An important finding of this chapter is that the utilization of maternal healthcare is likely to be lower for those women for whom the decision to spend on their healthcare needs is generally made by their spouses. Given that the society in Afghanistan is a strongly patriarchal, orthodox, and religious, where the lives of women are largely controlled by men who are generally unaware of women's healthcare needs, this is not surprising (Singh et al. 2013). This finding becomes all the more important because the proportion of households where the decision to spend on a woman's healthcare is made solely by her spouse is close to 50% of the sample.

Women with partial or no exposure to mass media were far less likely to utilize maternal health services than women with full exposure to mass media. Studies in the past have also found a similar relationship between the use of services and exposure to mass media. Mass media is an effective and inexpensive tool to persuade target audiences to adopt new beliefs and behaviors or to expose them to critical health information. However, in Afghanistan, access to mass media is still considerably poor, especially in rural areas. About 52% of households do not have a radio, and about 60% of households do not have a television. To increase the utilization of health services by women, the government should take steps to increase access to mass media, especially in rural and remote areas, where most Afghans live.

The findings of this chapter suggest that the use of antenatal care has a remarkable effect on the likelihood of undergoing institutional delivery care and postnatal care. Two national-level studies from India have recorded similar findings (Dixit et al. 2013; Singh et al. 2014a, b). The use of antenatal care increases the likelihood of subsequent care in many ways. It not only provides confidence in the subsequent use of services by familiarizing a woman with the healthcare system but also shakes her inherent beliefs, attitudes, and motivations about the risk and effectiveness of delivering in an institution (Sugathan et al. 2001). The counseling by healthcare workers makes women more aware of the possible complications during home delivery and the benefits of delivering at a health facility and encourages them to deliver at a healthcare facility and avail themselves of postnatal care (Mishra and Retherford 2008).

Our study revealed that rural women are less likely to receive care than are their urban counterparts. This finding aligns with that of many previous studies conducted in different settings (Singh et al. 2013; Shahram et al. 2015). Previous studies have recorded a huge rural–urban divide in the availability and accessibility of health services (Frost et al. 2016). According to one report, rural areas had only 16.7 public health workers (including unqualified support staff) per 10,000 people, compared with 36 per 10,000 people in urban areas (Ministry of Public Health, 2005a, b). Although the MoPH in the BPHS pledged that it would train 5000 female health workers for rural areas and claims to have succeeded in training about 3000 female workers, an overall shortage of community health workers remains in rural areas (Mansoor et al. 2012). Also, the attrition rate of female workers is very high, and hiring workers to work in rural areas has been extremely difficult, even though the government pays a hardship allowance of up to 250% of the base salary (Ministry of Public Health 2005a, b).

As for the coverage of health facilities in rural areas, it has certainly increased since 2003; however, the quality of services provided in these rural facilities is still very poor because of the chronic shortage of health workers, pharmaceuticals, and equipment (Cockcroft et al. 2011; Nic Carthaigh et al. 2015; Onis et al. 2007). A lack of effective transportation and communication infrastructure and insecurity along many of the routes in rural areas are two more reasons why people in rural areas are less likely to utilize healthcare services (Carvalho et al. 2013). Moreover, the fact that women in rural areas are on average poorer, less educated, and more readily influenced by traditional beliefs about health than are their urban counterparts could also be contributing to the rural–urban divide in maternal healthcare service utilization.

Contrary to common belief, considerable region variation in the use of maternal healthcare persists in Afghanistan. In this content, the southern, eastern, and northeastern regions turn out to lag behind the central region, which is also home the national capital, Kabul. The level of socioeconomic and infrastructure development in the southern, eastern, and northeastern provinces is relatively low. For instance, the highest poverty rates in Afghanistan are found in the eastern, southern, and northeastern provinces of Paktita, Paktya, Laghman, Badkhashan, and Kunaraha (Jolliffe 2010). The highest literacy rate, on the other hand, is found in the provinces of the central region, namely Kabul, Wadrak, Kapisa, Logar, and Panjsher (Jolliffe 2010).

15.5 Conclusion

The present chapter showed that the utilization of maternal healthcare services among Afghan women is unacceptably low. Such poor coverage of these services could be detrimental to maternal and child health indicators in the country. The National Reproductive Health Policy released in 2012 reiterates that all women have a right to the best possible care before and during pregnancy and childbirth and during the postpartum period at all levels of the health system (Reproductive Health Task Force 2012). To ensure that this right is exercised by every woman, the government should focus on disadvantaged groups.

The findings of this chapter underscore the need to address the social determinants of health, such as education, wealth, and ethnicity. If rapid strides are to be made in reducing maternal mortality, the government needs to enhance the level of girls' education in Afghan society. However, in a war-torn, highly orthodox, and patriarchal society where women's movement outside the four walls of their home is highly regulated, promoting girls' education is a herculean task. The results of this chapter suggest that the education of women's partners, especially male ones, should also be encouraged because they have the societal upper hand in decision-making at the household level. Poverty forces millions of people around the world to forgo treatment or healthcare. The same is true in Afghan society as well. Poorer mothers are far less likely to avail themselves of maternal care. The poorest segment of Afghan mothers should therefore be identified and given special assistance to encourage them to utilize maternal healthcare services. Exposure to mass media messages can have a significant impact on the level of service utilization; therefore, the government should focus on promoting maternal healthcare services through mass media, especially in rural areas.

This chapter has shown that antenatal care visits can have remarkable effects on women's utilization of institutional delivery and postnatal care services. Afghan policy should focus on improving the coverage of antenatal care by increasing the number of community healthcare workers in rural areas—where most of the population lives, without proper access to healthcare services. Unfortunately, a severe shortage of trained female community healthcare workers persists due to a lack of nurse-training schools. The results of this chapter also suggest that the reach of the government's health department in rural, remote, and difficult-to-access areas in the country, such as the province of Nuristan, is still far from satisfactory. The government needs to design targeted interventions for such areas while keeping local problems in view. Currently, the coverage of services in the provinces surrounding Kabul is much better than that of other, far-off provinces; hence, the government needs to devise strategies to reduce regional differentials as well.

Declaration

Availability of Data and Material The datasets and materials used in this study are available upon reasonable request to the corresponding author, or the data can be requested from the DHS website (www.measuredhs.com).

Ethics Approval and Consent to Participate The survey protocol and the questionnaires were approved by the ICF Institutional Review Board (IRB) and the Ministry of Public Health of Afghanistan. Before the respondents to the survey were interviewed, formal written consent was obtained, and ethical issues were taken care of.

Competing Interests The authors declare that they have no competing interests.

Funding The authors didn't receive funding for this work.

References

Acerra JR, Iskyan K, Qureshi ZA, Sharma RK (2009) Rebuilding the healthcare system in Afghanistan: an overview of primary care and emergency services. Int J Emerg Med 2:77–82

Akseer N, Salehi AS, Hossain SM, Mashal MT, Rasooly MH, Bhatti Z, Bhutta ZA (2016) Achieving maternal and child health gains in Afghanistan: a countdown to 2015 country case study. Lancet Glob Health 4(6):e395–e413

Anderson JG (1973) Health services utilization: framework and review. Health Serv Res 8(3):184

Arthur E (2012) Wealth and antenatal care use: implications for maternal healthcare utilisation in Ghana. Heal Econ Rev 2:1–8

BBC (2013) Afghanistan's Nuristan province at mercy of the Taliban. Bristich Broadcasting Corporation, London. http://www.bbc.co.uk/news/world-asia-21035695

Carvalho N, Salehi AS, Goldie SJ (2013) National and sub-national analysis of the health benefits and cost-effectiveness of strategies to reduce maternal mortality in Afghanistan. Health Policy Plan 28(1):62–74

Central Statistics Organization (CSO) Ministry of Public Health (MoPH) and ICF (2015) Afghanistan demographic and health survey 2015 [internet]. Kabul, Afghanistan. 2017. http://dhsprogram.com/pubs/pdf/FR323/FR323.pdf

Cockcroft A, Khan A, Md Ansari N, Omer K, Hamel C, Andersson N (2011) Does contracting of healthcare in Afghanistan work? Public and service-users' perceptions and experience. BMC Health Serv Res 11(2):1–10

Dixit P, Dwivedi LK, Ram F (2013) Estimating the impact of antenatal care visits on institutional delivery in India: a propensity score matching analysis, vol 8, p 3192517

Frost A, Wilkinson M, Boyle P, Patel P, Sullivan R (2016) An assessment of the barriers to accessing the basic package of health services (BPHS) in Afghanistan: was the BPHS a success? Glob Health 12(1):1–11

Ghasemi ME (1998) Islam, international human rights & (and) women's equality: afghan women under taliban rule. S Cal Rev L & Women's Stud 8:445

Greenaway ES, Leon J, Baker DP (2012) Understanding the association between maternal education and use of health services in Ghana: exploring the role of health knowledge. J Biosoc Sci 44(6):733–747

Hobcraft J (1993) Women's education, child welfare and child survival: a review of the evidence. Health Transit Rev 3:159–175

Jejeebhoy SJ (1995) Women's education, autonomy, and reproductive behaviour: experience from developing countries. Oxford University Press, Oxford

Jolliffe DM (2010) Poverty status in Afghanistan-a profile based on the National Risk and vulnerability assessment (NRVA) 2007–08, vol No. 63180. The World Bank, Herndon, pp 1–71

Mansoor GF, Hill PS, Barss P (2012) Midwifery training in post-conflict Afghanistan: tensions between educational standards and rural community needs. Health Policy Plan 27(1):60–68

Mashal M (2015). Afghan Province tucked in mountains lies beyond reach of aid and time. New York Times. https://www.nytimes.com/2015/12/26/world/asia/nuristan-afghanistan-taliban.html

McIntyre D, Thiede M, Dahlgren G, Whitehead M (2006) What are the economic consequences for households of illness and of paying for healthcare in low-and middle-income country contexts? Soc Sci Med 62(4):858–865

Ministry of Foreign Affairs. Afghanistan's Sustainable Development Goals (SDGs) (2017) [cited 2017 Apr 27]. http://mfa.gov.af/en/page/6547/afghanistans-sustainable-development-goals-sdgs

Ministry of Public Health (2005a) A basic package of health services for Afghanistan. Ministry of Public Health, New Delhi. http://apps.who.int/medicinedocs/documents/s21746en/s21746en.pdf

Ministry of Public Health (2005b) Revised National Salary Policy for NGOs Working in Health Sector. Ministry of Public Health, New Delhi. https://webgate.ec.europa.eu/europeaid/online-services/index.cfm?ADSSChck = 1375069165553&do = publi.getDoc&documentId = 94460&pubID = 128652

Minsitry of Economy (2013) Islamic Republic of Afghanistan: the millennium development goals 2012 [internet]. Kabul, Afghanistan; 2013. http://www.af.undp.org/content/dam/afghanistan/docs/MDGs/Afghanistan MDGs 2012 Report.pdf

Mishra V, Retherford RD (2008) The effect of antenatal care on professional assistance at delivery in rural India. Popul Res Policy Rev 27:307–320

Mustafa MH, Mukhtar AM (2015) Factors associated with antenatal and delivery care in Sudan: analysis of the 2010 Sudan household survey. BMC Health Serv Res 15:1–9

Newbrander W, Ickx P, Feroz F, Stanekzai H (2014) Afghanistan's basic package of health services: its development and effects on rebuilding the health system. Glob Public Health 9(sup1):S6–S28

Nic Carthaigh N, De Gryse B, Esmati AS, Nizar B, Van Overloop C, Fricke R, Philips M (2015) Patients struggle to access effective healthcare due to ongoing violence, distance, costs and health service performance in Afghanistan. Int Health 7(3):169–175

Onis MD, Onyango AW, Borghi E, Siyam A, Nishida C, Siekmann J (2007) Development of a WHO growth reference for school-aged children and adolescents. Bull World Health Organ 85(9):660–667

Reproductive Health Task Force (2012) National reproductive health policy: 2012-2016. Islamic Republic of Afghanistan Ministry of Public Health. chrome-extension://efaidnbmnnnibpcajpcgl-clefindmkaj/https://extranet.who.int/countryplanningcycles/sites/default/files/planning_cycle_repository/afghanistan/reproductive_health_policyenglish15120131426710553325325.pdf

Shahram MS, Hamajima N, Reyer JA (2015) Factors affecting maternal healthcare utilization in Afghanistan: secondary analysis of Afghanistan health survey 2012. Nagoya J Med Sci 77(4):595

Singh PK, Rai RK, Alagarajan M (2013) Report: addressing maternal and child health in post-conflict Afghanistan: the way forward. East Mediterr Health J 19:826

Singh A, Kumar A, Pranjali P (2014a) Utilization of maternal healthcare among adolescent mothers in urban India: evidence from DLHS-3. PeerJ 2:e592

Singh PK, Kumar C, Rai RK, Singh L (2014b) Factors associated with maternal healthcare service utilization in nine high focus states in India: a multilevel analysis based on 14 385 communities in 292 districts. Health Policy Plan 29(5):542–559

Sugathan KS, Mishra VK, Retherford RD (2001) Promoting institutional deliveries in rural India: the role of antenatal-care services. International Institute for Population Sciences, Mumbai

Thaddeus S, Maine D (1994) Too far to walk: maternal mortality in context. Soc Sci Med 38(8):1091–1110

United Nations Develpoment Program (2016) Female nurses in demand: UNDP trains 200 + young women to save lives in rural areas. United Nations Develpoment Program. http://www.af.undp.org/content/afghanistan/en/home/ourwork/womenempowerment/successstories/FemaleNursesinDemand.html

United Nations Population Fund (2015) Midwives help lower Afghanistan's towering maternal death rate [Internet]. United Nations Population Fund, Washington. http://www.unfpa.org/news/midwives-help-lower-afghanistans-towering-maternal-death-rate

Worku AG, Yalew AW, Afework MF (2013) Factors affecting utilization of skilled maternal care in Northwest Ethiopia: a multilevel analysis. BMC Int Health Hum Rights 13(1):1–11

World Health Organization (2016) Maternal Mortality: Factsheet 2016. World Health Organization, Geneva. http://www.who.int/mediacentre/factsheets/fs348/en/

Zakar R, Zakar MZ, Aqil N, Chaudhry A, Nasrullah M (2017) Determinants of maternal healthcare service utilization in Pakistan: evidence from Pakistan demographic and health survey, 2012-13. J Obstet Gynaecol 37(3):330–337

Chapter 16
Full Antenatal Care Service Utilization Among Tribal Mothers in India: A Multilevel Analysis

Aditya Singh 🅘, Mahashweta Chakrabarty 🅘, Sourav Chowdhury 🅘, Vineet Kumar 🅘, Rakesh Chandra 🅘, and Shivani Singh 🅘

Abstract Scheduled Tribes (ST) are one of the most disadvantaged socioeconomic groups in India, with a significant maternal mortality and morbidity burden. The coverage of full antenatal care (ANC) is low among ST mothers, leading to poor maternal and child health outcomes.

We analyzed the data from the fourth round of the National Family Health Surveys (NFHS-4), conducted in 2015–2016. A multilevel binary logistic regression model was used to examine the factors associated with full ANC among ST mothers in India. Only one in every six tribal mothers in India received full ANC. Although 46% of ST mothers had four or more ANC visits and about 88% received one or more tetanus toxoid (TT) injections, only 27% consumed 100 or more iron–folic acid (IFA) tablets/equivalent amount of IFA in syrup during their pregnancy. Household wealth, maternal education, pregnancy registration, and spouse's presence at the last ANC visit were associated with higher odds of receiving full ANC. High parity and undergoing the first ANC visit in the second or third trimester were associated with lower odds of receiving full ANC. India's northern and central regions reveal a deplorable condition compared to southern and western regions in terms of the utilization of full ANC. To improve the coverage of full

A. Singh (✉)
Banaras Hindu University, Varanasi, Uttar Pradesh, India
e-mail: adityasingh@bhu.ac.in

M. Chakrabarty · V. Kumar
Department of Geography, Banaras Hindu University, Varanasi, Uttar Pradesh, India
e-mail: vkgeog@bhu.ac.in

S. Chowdhury
Department of Geography, Raiganj University, Raiganj, West Bengal, India
Department of Geography, Shishuram Das College, Bhusna, West Bengal, India

R. Chandra
School of Health System Studies, Tata Institute of Social Sciences, Mumbai, India

S. Singh
Independent Researcher, Lucknow, India

ANC, the government should prioritize reaching out to poor, illiterate, and high-parity ST women and encourage early registration of preganacy and a timely first ANC visit.

Keywords Scheduled tribes · Antenatal care · NFHS · India · Pregnancy care · Maternal health

16.1 Introduction

India is the home to the world's second-largest Indigenous population, after Africa (Bahuguna et al. 2016). The tribal population of the country, as per the 2011 census, was 104 million, constituting about 9% of the total population, nearly four times larger than the total population of Australia (Office of the Registrar General and Census Commissioner 2011). About 90% of this population lives in rural areas and only 10% in urban areas, with significant variations in the distribution across states (Fig. 16.1). These communities have been officially recognized and listed in the Constitution of India as Scheduled Tribes (STs) (Chowdhury et al. 2022a; Tribal Cultural Heritage in India Foundation 2017). The Government of India acknowledges STs as a socially and economically disadvantaged group that needs protective arrangements and affirmative action (Chowdhury et al. 2022a, b; Government of India 1949). The Central and State governments, therefore, have introduced several schemes to improve their socioeconomic standing and have enacted several laws to protect them from discrimination and exploitation. Nevertheless, STs remain India's most socially and spatially excluded social group (Srivastava 2018). This

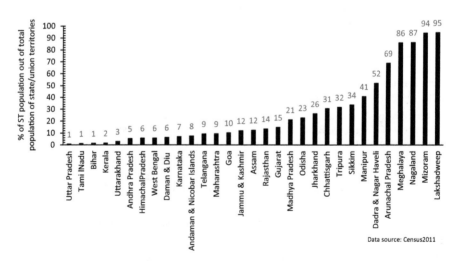

Fig. 16.1 Percentage of Scheduled Tribe (ST) population in Indian states and union territories, 2011. (Data source: Census of India, 2011)

disadvantage is evident in their health outcomes, particularly maternal mortality and morbidity (Narain 2019).

Although India has witnessed a decline in maternal mortality over the past 2 decades, primarily attributed to various initiatives taken by the central and state governments (Ministry of Health and Family Welfare 2013; Register General of India 2020), the rate of reduction in maternal mortality and morbidity has been sluggish (Adhikari et al. 2016). Previous studies have noted glaring inequalities in maternal mortality across social groups, with ST mothers more likely to die of maternity-related causes than mothers belonging to other social groups (Haddad et al. 2012; Kumar and Singh 2016; Singh et al. 2012).

Evidence suggests that the provision of affordable and accessible maternal healthcare services can lead to a significant reduction in maternal mortality and morbidity. India has implemented numerous programs and schemes over the years to increase the coverage of maternal health services and reduce maternal mortality and morbidity (Banerjee et al. 2014; Chaudhary et al. 2017; Lim et al. 2010; Reddy 2019; Sinha et al. 2019). The emphasis, however, has been on getting pregnant women to give birth in hospitals and clinics through conditional cash transfer programs. That is why four out of five mothers deliver in hospitals these days. Antenatal care (ANC) coverage, however, remains relatively low in India (International Institute for Population Sciences (IIPS) and ICF 2017). This low coverage of ANC could be one of the reasons why one-fourth of maternal deaths in India are still attributable to pre-eclampsia, eclampsia, and antepartum hemorrhage, all of which could be easily identified and managed during ANC visits (Kumar et al. 2019a).

ANC coverage is generally defined in terms of the number and timing of ANC visits, but these indicators do not provide a comprehensive picture. Many prefer "full antenatal care" instead, which considers the receipt of three components, namely the number of ANC visits, number of tetanus toxoid (TT) injections received, and number of iron–folic acid (IFA) tablets or equivalent amount of syrup consumed (International Institute for Population Sciences (IIPS) and ICF 2017). These three components of full ANC are essential for a pregnant mother. ANC visits ensure proper health screenings and the allocation of necessary care services for pregnant women (Ali et al. 2020). The consumption of 100 IFA tablets or equivalent syrup is associated with a lower risk of anemia among mothers and children, reducing the risk of poor birth outcomes (Kapil et al. 2019). Similarly, TT vaccination helps mothers and children fight against tetanus infection (Verma et al. 2016).

Estimates from the fourth round of the National Family Health Surveys (NFHS-4) show that full ANC coverage is just 21% nationally, with significant variations across geographies and socioeconomic groups (International Institute for Population Sciences (IIPS) and ICF 2017). For example, only 16% of ST women receive complete ANC, compared to 26% of the General caste category women. Despite the low utilization of ANC services among ST mothers, none of the existing research on the use of maternal healthcare in India has examined the coverage of full ANC among these mothers in detail at the national or state level (Adhikari et al. 2016; John et al. 2019; Kumar et al. 2019a; Negi et al. 2010; Nongdhar et al. 2018; Ogbo et al. 2019; Roy 2017; Sathiya Susuman 2012; Singh et al. 2014; Varma et al. 2011). Although many earlier studies have used caste or social group as an explanatory variable, they have typically focused on the distinctions between the four groups rather than the disparities or variations within them (Jat et al. 2011; Kumar et al. 2019b).

Although reducing intergroup disparities between India's four official social groups is crucial, recognizing that these groups are not homogeneous and are composed of various subgroups/communities with varying social and economic standings is equally important. Many academics, planners, and politicians consider the ST category a single entity, although this is not the case. It comprises numerous tribal communities of varied social and economic standing, giving rise to heterogeneity within this social group. To improve overall coverage and reduce within-group disparities in full ANC, the various factors affecting full ANC in ST women must be investigated and the vulnerable groups of women within this heterogeneous community need to be identified. This research, therefore, examines the socioeconomic and biodemographic factors that affect ST mothers' use of full ANC in India.

This research work differs from earlier research in four significant ways. First, it employs full ANC as a measure of ANC coverage, in contrast to the most of previous studies undertaken in India. Second, this research focuses exclusively on ST women, a significant yet neglected subgroup of India's population. Third, recognizing the variation within the ST category, it examines within-ST differentials in full ANC coverage to identify vulnerable groups that could be targeted for further improvement in the coverage of full ANC. Fourth and finally, it employs multilevel modeling to obtain correct standard errors (SEs) adjusted for the clustering of observations rather than the single-level modeling approach used by the majority of previous studies.

16.2 Data and Methods

16.2.1 Data

This research used data from the fourth round of the NFHS, conducted during 2015–2016. The NFHS is a series of cross-sectional, nationally representative surveys that collect information on a wide range of topics related to population health, including birth outcomes for mothers and children, sexual and reproductive health, and family planning (International Institute for Population Sciences (IIPS) and ICF 2017). The NFHS-4 was approved by the Ministry of Health and Family Welfare of the government of India. The anonymous data of this survey are available for public use and can be obtained from the Demographic and Health Surveys website www.measuredhs.com.

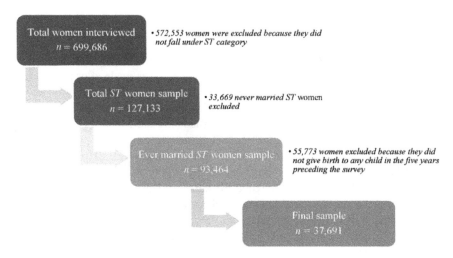

Fig. 16.2 Process of sample selection

16.2.2 Sampling Design and Study Size

In the fourth round of the NFHS, about 699,686 women between the ages of 15 and 49 were interviewed from 601,509 households, after a two-stage stratified sampling method with a response rate of 97% was used. Detailed information about the sampling procedure used in this survey can be obtained from the national report of NFHS-4 (International Institute for Population Sciences (IIPS) and ICF 2017). Fig. 16.2 shows that the survey interviewed 699,686 women nationwide. Out of them, 127,133 belonged to STs. Among all ST women, 93,464 were ever married. Out of 93,464 ever-married ST women, only 37,691 from 9366 public sector undertakings (PSUs), 589 districts, and 36 states had at least one child in the 5 years preceding the survey. Thus, in total, 37,691 ST women form the basis of our analysis.

16.2.3 Dependent Variables

We have used full ANC as our primary dependent or outcome variable. The outcome variable was defined on the basis of the NFHS-4 national report (International Institute for Population Sciences (IIPS) and ICF 2017). A pregnant mother is considered to have full ANC only when she had received all of the following during her pregnancy: at least four ANC visits, at least one TT injection, and 100 or more IFA tablets/equivalent amount of syrup. In NFHS-4, the data for all the three components of full ANC are available only for the current child or the last child. That is why only one child per woman is considered in the analysis.

16.2.4 Independent Variables

We considered a host of socioeconomic and biodemographic predictors for this analysis. The selection of these independent variables was made after a thorough review of existing models and frameworks for the study of healthcare utilization, such as Andersen's healthcare utilization model and Thaddeus and Maine's three-delay model (Andersen and Newman 1973; Thaddeus and Maine 1994). We also examined the variables used and the rationale behind their use in the previous studies conducted in India and elsewhere in the world (Adhikari et al. 2016; Afaya et al. 2020; Chowdhury et al. 2022b; Gage and Calixte 2006; Kumar and Singh 2016; Kumar et al. 2019a; Nwosu and Ataguba 2019; Paul and Chouhan 2020; Singh et al. 2014). The inclusion of a variable in the analysis was also dependent on whether it was available in the NFHS-4 dataset.

At the first level—i.e., the individual level—we considered the following variables: "wealth index," "maternal age at last conception," "parity (the number of live births a woman has had in the past)," "maternal education," "mass-media exposure," "health insurance coverage," "previous miscarriage/abortion/stillbirth," "pregnancy registration," "timing of first ANC visit," and "the presence of spouse at last ANC visit." Previous studies have reported regional differences in the utilization of maternity care (Ogbo et al. 2019; Singh et al. 2014). Therefore, we used "region" as an explanatory variable to account for the geographical difference in the usage of full ANC among ST mothers. At level two—i.e., the community level—we assessed the role of mothers' place of residence and the proportion of poor people in PSUs.

16.2.5 Statistical Analysis

First, we described the characteristics of the sample used in this chapter. We then calculated the proportion of ST mothers with full ANC for each category of the explanatory variables. To assess the factors affecting the utilization of full ANC, we decided to use multivariable logistic regression because our dependent variable was binary in nature. However, prior to applying multivariable logistic regression, we assessed the statistical significance of each independent variable by running a logistic regression model with only one independent variable at a time and calculating crude/unadjusted odds ratios (ORs). Unadjusted odds ratio is called unadjusted because the model has only one variable and the odds ratio thus obtained has not been adjusted for other independent variables. Only those variables that were statistically significant at this stage were included in the further analysis—i.e., multivariable logistic regression.

Because NFHS-4 has a hierarchical or clustered structure, where individuals are nested within communities/villages, communities within districts, and districts within states, we cannot use simple multivariable logistic regression, because it would lead to the underestimation of standard errors and the overestimation of statistical significance. For hierarchical datasets such as the NFHS, multilevel models are appropriate because they produce correct standard errors (SEs) adjusted for the clustering of observations in the dataset. Therefore, in this analysis, a four-level multivariable logistic regression has been fitted. The four levels are: individual, PSU, district, and state.

Two models were estimated: the null model and the full model. In model 1, the null model, no explanatory variables were included, whereas model 2 included all the explanatory variables. The final multilevel multivariable logistic regression included only those predictor variables whose unadjusted odds ratios were statistically significant. The results of multilevel multivariable logistic regression are presented in the form of ORs with 95% confidence intervals (CIs). We did not any sample weight in the multilevel model used in this study, because the use of weight in multilevel models could sometimes be problematic (Frank 2008). Because this study uses several explanatory variables that could be correlated with one another, a multicollinearity assessment was also carried out by using the means of variance inflation factors (VIFs). We used MLwiN and Stata statistical software to carry out the statistical analysis for this research (Afaya et al. 2020; Leckie and Charlton 2013; Rasbash et al. 2012). We utilized the *runmlwin* command available in Stata. This module fits multilevel models in MLwiN from within Stata. Three steps are involved in executing the *runmlwin* command. The desired model is first specified by the researcher by using the *runmlwin* command syntax in Stata. The model is then submitted to MLwiN, where it is fitted. MLwiN then returns the results to Stata, where they are displayed and can be accessed for additional analysis.

16.3 Results

Table 16.1 presents the utilization of full ANC according to the background characteristics of ST mothers aged 15–49. Over two-thirds of all ST mothers in India belonged to the poorest and poorer categories of the wealth index. About 41% were illiterate, and only 5% of ST mothers had finished their higher education. About half of ST mothers had received their first ANC within the first trimester of their pregnancy. About 39% of ST mothers were regularly exposed to mass media. About one-tenth of ST mothers lived in urban areas, and about 84% registered their pregnancies with the Anganwadi Centre. Only 20% were covered by health insurance, and over two-thirds went for ANC with their spouse/partner.

Figure 16.3 shows that about 88% of ST mothers had one or more TT injection coverage. The utilization of full ANC among Indian ST mothers was just 16%, due to the lower utilization of four or more ANC visits (46%) and a lower intake of 100 or more IFA tablets/equivalent syrup (27%).

Table 16.2 shows that India's northern and central regions have rather deplorable conditions compared to India's southern and western regions in terms of the utilization of full ANC. Only 9–10% of ST mothers in the northern and central regions had received full ANC, which was lower than the national average. In contrast, about

Table 16.1 Distribution of ST mothers according to background characteristics, India, NFHS-4 (2015–2016)

Background characteristics	n = 37691	%
Wealth quintile		
Poorest	17,657	47
Poor	9659	26
Middle	5508	15
Richer	3160	8
Richest	1708	5
Maternal age at last conception (years)		
15–24	14,302	38
25–34	19,398	51
> 34	3991	11
Parity		
1	11,786	31
2	11,821	31
3	6875	18
> 3	7208	19
Maternal education		
Illiterate	15,593	41
Primary	6089	16
Secondary	14,261	38
Higher	1748	5
Mass-media exposure		
Full exposure	14,763	39
Partial exposure	9090	24
No exposure	13,839	37
Health insurance coverage		
No	30,134	80
Yes	7557	20
Previous miscarriage/abortion/still birth		
Yes	2575	7
No	35,116	93
Pregnancy registration		
No	6095	16
Yes	31,596	84
Timing of first ANC visit		
1st trimester	20,180	54
2nd trimester	8231	22
3rd trimester	1719	5
Presence of spouse at last ANC visit		
No	13,315	35
Yes	24,376	65
Place of residence		
Urban	4880	13

(continued)

Table 16.1 (continued)

Background characteristics	n = 37691	%
Rural	32,811	87
% of poor people in PSU		
Low (0–33)	7424	20
Medium (33–66)	5462	14
High (> 66)	24,805	66
Region		
Northern	3853	10
Central	9303	25
Eastern	9863	26
Western	7085	19
Southern	3762	10
Northeastern	3826	10
Full ANC		
Yes	6170	16
No	31,521	84
≥ 4 ANC visits		
Yes	17,215	46
No	20,475	54
≥ 1 TT injections		
Yes	33,349	88
No	4341	12
≥ 100 IFA tablets/syrup equivalent		
Yes	10,112	27
No	27,578	73

Note: n = number of women (frequency), and all % are weighted

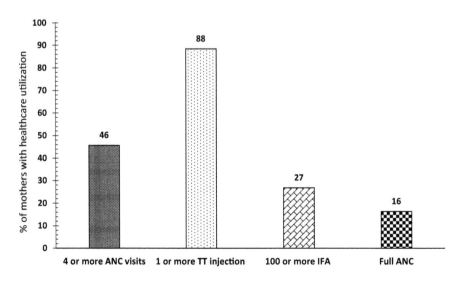

Fig. 16.3 Antenatal care utilization among ST mothers in India, NFHS-4 (2015–2016)

Table 16.2 Utilization of full ANC across regions of India, NFHS-4, 2015–2016

Region	Full ANC		≥ 4 ANC visits		≥ 1 TT injections		≥ 100 IFA tablets/syrup equivalent	
	n	%	n	%	n	%	n	%
Northern	362	9	1385	36	3405	88	692	18
Central	937	10	2970	32	8222	88	1959	21
Eastern	1367	14	4381	44	9054	92	2353	24
Western	1665	24	4186	59	6272	89	2200	31
Southern	1173	31	2579	69	3194	85	1779	47
Northeastern	665	17	1714	45	3202	84	1128	30
India	6170	16	17,215	46	33,350	88	10,112	27

Note: n = number of women (frequency), and all percentages are weighted

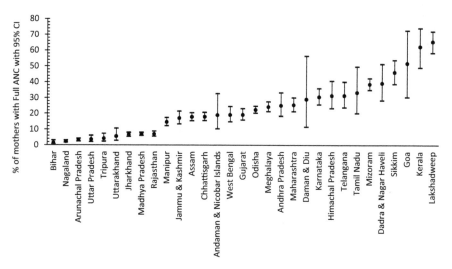

Fig. 16.4 Coverage of full ANC across Indian States and Union Territories, NFHS-4 (2015–2016). The *p*-values associated with the unadjusted odds ratio showed that all explanatory variables were statistically significant, and therefore, all the variables were included in the final model.

31% of ST mothers had full ANC in the southern region, higher than the national average. The coverage of full ANC in the western region was above the national average, with about 25% of women reporting to have received full ANC. The northeastern and eastern regions of India were close to the national average. State-wise coverage of full ANC is provided in Fig. 16.4. Table 16.3 presents unadjusted odds ratios for full ANC utilization among ST mothers.

Table 16.3 Unadjusted odds ratios (with 95% confidence intervals) for receiving full ANC among ST mothers in India

Independent variables	OR	CI (95%) Lower	Upper	p-value
Individual-level variables				
Wealth quintile				
Poorest®				
Poor	1.656	1.529	1.793	<0.001***
Middle	2.665	2.455	2.892	<0.001***
Richer	4.093	3.747	4.471	<0.001***
Richest	6.556	5.922	7.257	<0.001***
Maternal age at last conception (years)				
15–24®				
25–34	1.112	1.045	1.183	0.001***
> 34	0.902	0.826	0.985	0.022**
Parity				
1®				
2	0.854	0.799	0.914	<0.001***
3	0.701	0.647	0.759	<0.001***
> 3	0.456	0.420	0.495	<0.001***
Maternal education				
Illiterate®				
Primary	1.645	1.498	1.806	<0.001***
Secondary	2.762	2.572	2.965	<0.001***
Higher	5.409	4.843	6.041	<0.001***
Mass-media exposure				
Full exposure®				
Partial exposure	0.497	0.466	0.531	<0.001***
No exposure	0.270	0.251	0.291	<0.001***
Health insurance coverage				
No®				
Yes	1.299	1.220	1.382	<0.001***
Previous miscarriage/abortion/still birth				
Yes®				
No	0.859	0.774	0.953	0.004***
Pregnancy registration				
No®				
Yes	8.438	7.382	9.644	<0.001***
Timing of first ANC visit				
1st trimester®				
2nd trimester	0.481	0.449	0.516	<0.001***
3rd trimester	0.263	0.215	0.320	<0.001***

(continued)

Table 16.3 (continued)

Independent variables	OR	CI (95%)		p-value
		Lower	Upper	
Presence of spouse at last ANC visit				
No®				
Yes	3.410	3.195	3.641	<0.001***
PSU-level variables				
Place of residence				
Urban®				
Rural	0.423	0.396	0.452	<0.001***
% of poor people in PSU				
Low (0–33)®				
Medium (33–66)	0.549	0.507	0.593	<0.001***
High (> 66)	0.309	0.291	0.329	<0.001***
Region				
Northern region®				
Central region	0.714	0.634	0.805	<0.001***
Eastern region	1.004	0.892	1.131	0.946
Western region	2.154	1.894	2.449	<0.001***
Southern region	3.395	2.945	3.914	<0.001***
Northeastern region	1.247	1.124	1.383	<0.001***

Note: ® = reference category; OR = odds ratio; CI = confidence interval; and *** $p < 0.01$, ** $p < 0.05$, and * $p < 0.10$

Table 16.4 Empty model, without covariates

Random effects	Full ANC
State random variance (SE)	0.690 (0.184)
State VPC (%)	16
District random variance (SE)	0.131 (0.017)
District VPC (%)	19
Community (PSU) random variance (SE)	0.162 (0.019)
Community (PSU) VPC (%)	23

Note: *SE* stands for standard error and *VPC* stands for variance partition coefficient

16.3.1 Results of Multilevel Logistic Regression

The first step in the multilevel analysis was to examine whether our data justified the decision to apply a multilevel model. We ran a null model and carried out a statistical test to determine whether residuals at higher levels were statistically significant.

The results from the empty model revealed that a significant portion of the total variation in the coverage of full ANC was attributable to the differences across communities, districts, and states, implying that fitting a multilevel model made sense in this context (Table 16.4). The adjusted odds ratios derived from the full model are presented in Table 16.5. The results show that several individual-level variables

Table 16.5 Adjusted odd ratios obtained from the multilevel model showing factors affecting the utilization of full ANC among ST mothers in India

Independent variables	n (37,691)	%	OR	CI (95%) Lower	CI (95%) Upper	p-Value
Individual level variables						
Wealth quintile						
Poorest®	1761	10				
Poor	1613	17	1.184	1.067	1.314	0.002***
Middle	1384	25	1.327	1.159	1.520	<0.001***
Rich	856	27	1.618	1.382	1.894	<0.001***
Richest	555	33	2.002	1.665	2.407	<0.001***
Maternal age at last conception (years)						
15–24®	2431	17				
25–34	3321	17	1.088	1.004	1.179	0.041**
>34	418	10	1.096	0.968	1.242	0.146
Parity						
1®	2324	20				
2	2171	18	0.914	0.843	0.992	0.03**
3	1029	15	0.873	0.789	0.966	0.008***
>3	647	9	0.735	0.654	0.826	<0.001***
Maternal education						
Illiterate®	1460	9				
Primary	962	16	1.035	0.924	1.160	0.551
Secondary	3185	22	1.191	1.077	1.317	0.001***
Higher	564	32	1.596	1.369	1.862	<0.001***
Mass-media exposure						
Full exposure®	3563	24				
Partial exposure	1313	14	0.932	0.856	1.015	0.104
No exposure	1293	9	0.917	0.822	1.023	0.120
Health insurance coverage						
No®	4601	15				
Yes	1569	21	1.100	1.007	1.202	0.034**
Previous miscarriage/abortion/still birth						
Yes®	452	18				
No	5718	16	1.027	0.910	1.159	0.668
Pregnancy registered						
No®	196	3				
Yes	5974	19	1.667	1.452	1.913	<0.001***
Timing of first ANC visit						
1st trimester®	4813	24				
2nd trimester	1046	13	0.637	0.588	0.689	<0.001***
3rd trimester	307	18	0.363	0.295	0.445	<0.001***
Presence of spouse at last ANC visit						
No®	868	7				
Yes	5302	22	1.441	1.325	1.568	<0.001***

(continued)

Table 16.5 (continued)

Independent variables	n (37,691)	%	OR	CI (95%) Lower	Upper	p-Value
PSU-level variables						
Place of residence						
Urban®	1233	25				
Rural	4937	15	0.947	0.844	1.063	0.356
% of poor people in PSU						
Low (0–33)®	1981	27				
Medium (33–66)	1243	23	1.036	0.910	1.179	0.594
High (> 66)	2945	12	0.959	0.832	1.104	0.557
Region						
Northern region®	362	9				
Central region	937	10	0.516	0.229	1.165	0.111
Eastern region	1367	14	0.702	0.314	1.571	0.389
Western region	1665	24	1.761	0.776	3.995	0.176
Southern region	1173	31	1.707	0.823	3.540	0.151
Northeastern region	665	17	0.804	0.401	1.614	0.540
Random effects						
State random variance (SE)	0.310 (0.092)					
State VPC (%)	7					
District random variance (SE)	0.154 (0.025)					
District VPC (%)	10					
Community (PSU) random variance (SE)	0.683 (0.041)					
Community (PSU) VPC (%)	26					

Note: n^* = number of ST mothers from specific subcategories who received full ANC; % = weighted % of n; ® = reference category; OR = odds ratio; CI = confidence interval; SE = standard error; VPC = variance partition coefficient; and *** $p < 0.01$, ** $p < 0.05$, and * $p < 0.10$

included in the analysis turned out to be statistically significant predictors of the utilization of full ANC among ST mothers in India. Some individual-level variables, such as maternal age at the last conception, mass-media exposure, and previous miscarriage/abortion/stillbirth, were statistically significant in the unadjusted model but turned out to be insignificant in the adjusted model. Wealth index, maternal education, pregnancy registration, the timing of the first ANC visit, the spouse's presence at the last ANC visit, and parity were strongly associated with receiving full ANC among ST mothers.

The results show that ST mothers belonging to the top two wealth quintiles were nearly two times more likely (OR = 2.002, CI = 1.665–2.407; OR = 1.618, CI = 1.382–1.894) and that those belonging to the middle quintile were nearly one and half times more likely (OR = 1.327, CI = 1.159–1.520) to receive full ANC than those from the poorest wealth quintile were. Mothers with higher education were around one and half times (OR = 1.596, CI = 1.369–1.862) more likely to receive full ANC than illiterate mothers were.

Mothers who registered their pregnancy were 1.7 times (OR = 1.667, CI = 1.452–1.913) more likely to receive full ANC than mothers who did not. Mothers who had their first ANC visit in either the second or third trimester or later were less likely (OR = 0.637, CI = 0.588–0.689; OR = 0.363, CI = 0.295–0.445) to receive full ANC than those who had their first ANC in the first trimester of their pregnancy. Pregnant women whose spouses accompanied them for ANC were nearly one and half times (OR = 1.441, CI = 1.325–1.568) more likely to receive full ANC than those whose spouses did not accompany them when they went for ANC.

Mothers with two, three, and more than three parities were less likely to receive full ANC than mothers with one parity (OR = 0.914, CI = 0.843–0.992; OR = 0.873, CI = 0.789–0.966; OR = 0.735, CI = 0.654–0.826). ST mothers who were covered by health insurance schemes were about 10% more likely to utilize full ANC than those who were not.

16.4 Discussion

For the past few decades, governments, World Health Organization, and other development organizations have advocated for a continuum of care (CoC) to reduce maternal and child mortality and improve maternal, newborn, and child health (Kothavale and Meher 2021). The central and state governments have been redesigning and revamping the health systems with CoC as the core principle. Since 1996, when the Safe Motherhood and Child Health Program was integrated into the Reproductive and Child Health Program (RCH), maternal healthcare has been at the top of the agenda of the government of India. A growing emphasis on delivering healthcare has arisen to address women's health requirements before, during, and after pregnancy, along with infant and childcare throughout the life cycle to ensure a holistic healthcare experience. This includes ANC coverage, institutional deliveries, postnatal care, and full immunization. Though many of these indicators have improved considerably over the past several years (International Institute for Population Sciences (IIPS) and ICF 2017), the reduction in maternal and neonatal mortality has been slow and inequitable (Bhatia et al. 2021). Though ANC and institutional deliveries have significantly improved, less than one-fifth of women complete the care continuum (Usman et al. 2021). Moreover, the highest number of dropouts (38%) in CoC occur at the first stage—i.e., during ANC (Kothavale and Meher 2021).

In this light, the problem of the low utilization of full ANC among Indian ST mothers becomes more important. This study attempted to examine the factors associated with full ANC among Indian ST mothers. The results of this research revealed that wealth index, maternal education, health insurance coverage, pregnancy registration, and spouse's presence at the last ANC visit were associated with higher odds of receiving full ANC. On the other hand, higher parity and second and third trimester ANC visits were associated with lower odds of receiving full ANC among ST mothers.

Our research found that although the coverage of TT was satisfactory and nearly universal, the consumption or intake of 100 or more IFA tablets or an equivalent amount of syrup was considerably low. Only about 25% of women reported having adequate IFA. During an ANC visit, a skilled healthcare provider generally provides IFA tablets/syrup for only 1 month (Kumar et al. 2019a). This means that if a woman had fewer ANC visits, she would be more likely to have an inadequate intake of IFA. Because the number of ANC visits among ST women is considerably lower than among women belonging to other social groups, this could likely be one of the reasons behind the inadequate coverage of full ANC among ST women. IFA deficiency during pregnancy may have a detrimental effect on the mother's health, the fetus, and fetal growth (Kumar et al. 2019b). IFA consumption during pregnancy decreases the risk of iron deficiency and anemia (Peña-Rosas and Viteri 2006). Hence, appropriate interventions need to be adopted to increase access to and the consumption of IFA supplements among ST mothers.

The disparity in the use of maternal healthcare across economic groups has been a concern of many (Fulpagare et al. 2019; Kumar and Singh 2016; Ogbo et al. 2019). Several studies have recorded that the income of households has a positive impact on maternal healthcare utilization (Adhikari et al. 2016; Jat et al. 2011; Kumar et al. 2019a; Sanneving et al. 2013; Singh et al. 2014, 2022). Our study confirms the same in the case of Indian ST mothers. Mothers from the upper wealth quintiles are usually more educated than those from the lowest wealth quintiles, which has a bearing on their knowledge of available health services. Moreover, mothers from prosperous households often have more disposable income to pay for their healthcare expenses. In contrast, poor mothers are mostly less educated and unemployed and have trouble affording adequate healthcare. Their incomes are often so poor that they are left with little to no money for healthcare after spending on their basic needs (Singh et al. 2014). Our model illustrates that full ANC coverage varied from 15% among ST mothers with primary education to 60% among ST mothers with higher education. This suggests the need for more-inclusive and -equitable higher-education opportunities for adolescent girls from marginalized groups.

Pregnancy registration was associated with higher odds of using full ANC among ST mothers. Previous studies have also corroborated this finding (Adhikari et al. 2016). The registration of pregnant women with health workers, such as anganwadi workers or auxiliary nurse midwives, is one of the earliest and most crucial stages in introducing maternal health services to them. Registration allows expectant mothers to meet these health professionals and learn about the significance of ANC and its long-term health benefits for both the mother and child. Also, once women have registered, they are more likely to communicate with these health workers during their pregnancies, increasing the likelihood that that they will follow health workers' advice on regular ANC visits, IFA consumption, and vaccinations. Furthermore, pregnancy registration is linked to conditional cash transfer schemes such as Janani Suraksha Yojana (JSY) and Pradhan Mantri Matru Vandana Yojana (PMMVY). A pregnant woman is eligible for cash benefits under PMMVY only if she registers her pregnancy within 4 months of conception, attends at least one prenatal care session, and uses IFA tablets and a TT injection (Gautam n.d.; Kumar et al. 2015). Therefore, the reason why early registration is positively associated with utilizing full antenatal care is not surprising. Health workers should focus their information, education, and communication (IEC) activities on teaching women and their families about the significance of registering pregnancies during the first trimester.

ST mothers who received their first ANC during the second or third trimester were less likely to receive full ANC than those who received their first ANC during the first trimester of their pregnancy. Given that pregnancy lasts for 9 months, a pregnant woman who waits too long to receive ANC services is likely to fall short of two of the three criteria for full ANC: 100 or more IFA tablets or equivalent syrup and four or more ANC visits during the prenatal period. Early registration and ANC visits can provide a larger time frame to frontline health workers and healthcare providers to identify vulnerable women and high-risk pregnancies early, reinforce the messages on proper antenatal care, and provide nutrition supplements (IFA, calcium, etc.), which can reduce the risks in the advanced stages of pregnancy and childbirth (Sharma et al. 2020).

Compared to ST mothers whose spouses were not present at their ANC, those whose spouses were present had a higher likelihood of receiving full ANC. This is in line with the findings of previous studies on this issue (Chattopadhyay and Govil 2021; Falade-Fatila and Adebayo 2020). In a patriarchal society like India, where pregnancy and childbirth are usually seen as entirely female concerns, a future mother's prenatal care-seeking behavior is primarily decided by her spouse because, in most cases, they are the household's primary breadwinner, gatekeeper, and decision-maker (Chattopadhyay and Govil 2021; Dahake and Shinde 2020). Involving spouses in maternal care-related decision-making can therefore play a crucial role in eliminating the three delays suggested by Thaddeus and Maine, allowing women easier access to ANC services (Thaddeus and Maine 1994).

In line with the findings of earlier studies, the odds of having full ANC in this study also decreased substantially with increasing parity (Birmeta et al. 2013; Singh et al. 2014; Tikmani et al. 2019). Some have argued that the experience, knowledge, and confidence that mothers with higher parity gain from previous births may be one of the key reasons behind this trend (Singh et al. 2012). Women with multiple children typically rely heavily on their prior experiences. They frequently foster the idea that they do not require maternal healthcare services. Community health workers should be trained to recognize these moms and give them effective counseling to alter their perspectives on the necessity of prenatal care services. A lack of time could also be one of the reasons why women with larger families are less likely to receive full antenatal care. Poor healthcare quality experienced during previous pregnancies might also prevent higher-parity women from seeking timely ANC (Paudel et al. 2017).

An important finding of this chapter is that considerable heterogeneity was found in the coverage of full ANC across different regions in India. The odds of utilizing full ANC in the relatively more developed southern and western regions were almost two times higher than those in the northern region. These results are consistent with findings from previous studies that have noted substantial north–south differences in ANC coverage (Varma et al. 2011). The odds of full ANC coverage for the central region were lower than those for the northern region. This could be due to inadequate provision and poor access to healthcare services in the central region (Singh et al. 2012; Sri et al. 2012).

As for the strengths of this research, we exclusively focused on ST mothers to identify disadvantaged and vulnerable groups within them, which is rarely done because many researchers are under the impression that the ST category is a monolith and that differences and diversity within ST women do not exist. In addition, we used multilevel modeling, which considers the hierarchical structure of NFHS data and provides standard errors corrected for clustering, which is vital for making correct inferences. This research has some limitations also. The data related to healthcare services in NFHS is self-reported. Although the NFHS-4 has taken several steps to tackle the issue of false reporting in healthcare services due to the inability to recall, we must not assume the data to be always perfectly accurate. Because the data used in this research comes from a cross-sectional survey, the association between dependent and independent variables in this research cannot always be interpreted as causality. We searched for relevant variables representing tribal behavior and healthcare availability in the NFHS data, but we could not find any. Therefore, we were unable to include these variables in the model. We suggest that the association between these variables be investigated in future studies. Further research is also needed to explore the factors behind the low level of IFA consumption among ST women.

16.5 Conclusion

Though India has seen a substantial increase in the coverage of safe delivery among ST women, the limited utilization of full ANC is still a cause of concern given that it has implications for further reduction in maternal mortality and morbidity in the country. The coverage of full ANC among ST mothers is considerably low, yet this issue has not received due attention in academic and policy discussions. This research examined the factors associated with full ANC coverage among ST mothers and identified disadvantaged groups that can be targeted in future program interventions to reduce inequities for these ST mothers. Maternal education and household wealth strongly influence the utilization of full ANC. Because most ST mothers are underemployed and uneducated, targeting these disadvantaged women should be a priority for the government's maternal health programs and policies. Apart from these, young first-time mothers should be targeted for counseling to improve their awareness of the importance of full ANC. Ensuring early pregnancy registration and ensuring a timely first ANC visit should be top priorities because these two factors provide women an opportunity to meet health providers and learn the importance of the different components of pregnancy care early in their pregnancy. Additionally, spousal involvement seems to raise the likelihood of a pregnant woman's receiving full ANC. Therefore, any future efforts to improve the coverage of full ANC in the country should also consider implementing innovative strategies to encourage spousal participation in maternal care.

Declaration

Availability of Data and Material The data and materials for this chapter are sourced from publicly available secondary sources accessible at https://dhsprogram.com/methodology/survey/survey-display-541.cfm. Interested individuals can register at the provided link to freely download the necessary data.

Ethics Approval and Consent to Participate This research is based on secondary data, which are available in the public domain. Therefore, ethical approval is not required to conduct this study.

Competing Interests The authors declare that they have no competing interests.

Funding This research did not receive any specific grant from funding agencies in the public, commercial, or not-for-profit sectors.

References

Adhikari T, Sahu D, Nair S, Saha K, Sharma R, Pandey A (2016) Factors associated with utilization of antenatal care services among tribal women: a study of selected states. Indian J Med Res 144(1):58. http://www.ijmr.org.in/text.asp?2016/144/1/58/193284

Afaya A, Azongo TB, Dzomeku VM, Afaya RA, Salia SM, Adatara P, Kaba Alhassan R, Amponsah AK, Atakro CA, Adadem D, Asiedu EO, Amuna P, Amogre Ayanore M (2020) Women's knowledge and its associated factors regarding optimum utilisation of antenatal care in rural Ghana: a cross-sectional study. PLoS One 15(7):e0234575. https://doi.org/10.1371/journal.pone.0234575

Ali N, Elbarazi I, Alabboud S, Al-Maskari F, Loney T, Ahmed LA (2020) Antenatal care initiation among pregnant women in The United Arab Emirates: the Mutaba'ah study. Front Public Health 0:211. https://doi.org/10.3389/FPUBH.2020.00211

Andersen R, Newman JF (1973) Societal and individual determinants of medical care utilization in the United States. Milbank Mem Fund Q Health Soc 51:95–124

Bahuguna K, Ramnath M, Shrivastava KS, Mahapatra R, Suchitra M and Chakravartty A (2016) Indigenous people in India and the web of indifference. DownToEarth. https://www.downtoearth.org.in/coverage/governance/indigenous-people-in-india-and-the-web-of-indifference-55223

Banerjee SK, Andersen KL, Baird TL, Ganatra B, Batra S, Warvadekar J (2014) Evaluation of a multi-pronged intervention to improve access to safe abortion care in two districts in Jharkhand. BMC Health Serv Res 14(1):1–12. https://doi.org/10.1186/1472-6963-14-227

Bhatia M, Dwivedi LK, Banerjee K, Bansal A, Ranjan M, Dixit P (2021) Pro-poor policies and improvements in maternal health outcomes in India. BMC Pregnancy Childbirth 21(1):1–13. https://doi.org/10.1186/S12884-021-03839-W/TABLES/3

Birmeta K, Dibaba Y, Woldeyohannes D (2013) Determinants of maternal health care utilization in Holeta town, Central Ethiopia. BMC Health Serv Res 13(1):256. https://doi.org/10.1186/1472-6963-13-256

Chattopadhyay A, Govil D (2021) Men and maternal health care utilization in India and in selected less-developed states: evidence from a large-scale survey 2015–16. J Biosoc Sci 53(5):724–744. https://doi.org/10.1017/S0021932020000498

Chaudhary S, Rohilla R, Kumar V, Kumar S (2017) Evaluation of Janani Shishu Suraksha Karyakram scheme and out of pocket expenditure in a rural area of northern India. J Family Med Prim Care 6(3):477. https://doi.org/10.4103/2249-4863.222010

Chowdhury S, Singh A, Kasemi N, Chakrabarty M (2022a) Economic inequality in intimate partner violence among forward and backward class women in India: a decomposition analysis. Vict Offenders 1–27:1003. https://doi.org/10.1080/15564886.2022.2080312

Chowdhury S, Singh A, Kasemi N, Chakrabarty M, Roy Pakhadhara T (2022b) Intimate partner violence among scheduled caste women in India: a cross-sectional study. Vict Offenders 19:1030. https://doi.org/10.1080/15564886.2022.2069897

Dahake, Shinde R (2020) Exploring husband's attitude towards involvement in his wife's antenatal care in urban slum community of Mumbai. Indian J Community Med 45(3):320. https://doi.org/10.4103/IJCM.IJCM_344_19

Falade-Fatila O, Adebayo AM (2020) Male partners' involvement in pregnancy related care among married men in Ibadan, Nigeria. Reprod Health 17(1):1–12. https://doi.org/10.1186/S12978-020-0850-2/TABLES/7

Frank J (2008) Multilevel analysis with informative weights. In: Proceedings of the joint statistical meeting, ASA Section on Survey Research Methods, pp 2225–2233. http://www.asasrms.org/Proceedings/y2008/Files/301419.pdf

Fulpagare PH, Saraswat A, Dinachandra K, Surani N, Parhi RN, Bhattacharjee S, Somya S, Purty A, Mohapatra B, Kejrewal N, Agrawal N, Bhatia V, Ruikar M, Gope RK, Murira Z, De Wagt A, Sethi V (2019) Antenatal care service utilization among adolescent pregnant women–evidence from Swabhimaan Programme in India. Front Public Health 7:369. https://doi.org/10.3389/fpubh.2019.00369

Gage AJ, Calixte MG (2006) Effects of the physical accessibility of maternal health services on their use in rural Haiti. Popul Stud 60(3):271–288. https://doi.org/10.1080/00324720600895934

Gautam A (n.d.) A Critical Evaluation of Pradhan Mantri Matru Vandana Yojana. Accessed 22 Sept 2020. https://jgu.edu.in/jsgp/a-critical-evaluation-of-pradhan-mantri-matru-vandana-yojana/

GOI (n.d.) Zonal Council. https://www.mha.gov.in/zonal-council

Government of India (1949) Special representation in sevice for SC/ST. https://dopt.gov.in/sites/default/files/ch-11.pdf

Haddad S, Mohindra KS, Siekmans K, Mk G, Narayana D (2012) "Health divide" between indigenous and non-indigenous populations in Kerala, India: population based study. BMC Public Health 12(1):1–10. https://doi.org/10.1186/1471-2458-12-390

International Institute for Population Sciences (IIPS) and ICF (2017) National Family Health Survey (NFHS-4), 2015–16: India. IIPS, Mumbai

Jat TR, Ng N, San Sebastian M (2011) Factors affecting the use of maternal health services in Madhya Pradesh state of India: A multilevel analysis. Int J Equity Health 10(1):59. https://doi.org/10.1186/1475-9276-10-59

John AE, Nilima, Binu VS, Unnikrishnan B (2019) Determinants of antenatal care utilization in India: a spatial evaluation of evidence for public health reforms. Public Health 166:57–64. https://doi.org/10.1016/j.puhe.2018.09.030

Kapil U, Kapil R, Gupta A (2019) National iron plus initiative: current status & future strategy. Indian J Med Res 150(3):239. https://doi.org/10.4103/IJMR.IJMR_1782_18

Kothavale A, Meher T (2021) Level of completion along continuum of care for maternal, newborn and child health services and factors associated with it among women in India: a population-based cross-sectional study. BMC Pregnancy Childbirth 21(1):1–12. https://doi.org/10.1186/S12884-021-04198-2/TABLES/5

Kumar A, Singh A (2016) Explaining the gap in the use of maternal healthcare services between social groups in India. J Public Health 38(4):771–781. https://doi.org/10.1093/pubmed/fdv142

Kumar V, Misra SK, Kaushal SK, Gupta SC, Khan AM (2015) A study on the effect of Janani Suraksha Yojana on antenatal registration and institutional deliveries in the Agra district of Uttar Pradesh. Indian J Public Health 59(1):54–57. https://doi.org/10.4103/0019-557X.152865

Kumar G, Choudhary TS, Srivastava A, Upadhyay RP, Taneja S, Bahl R, Martines J, Bhan MK, Bhandari N, Mazumder S (2019a) Utilisation, equity and determinants of full antenatal care in India: analysis from the National Family Health Survey 4. BMC Pregnancy Childbirth 19(1):327. https://doi.org/10.1186/s12884-019-2473-6

Kumar G, Choudhary TS, Srivastava A, Upadhyay RP, Taneja S, Bahl R, Martines J, Bhan MK, Bhandari N, Mazumder S (2019b) Utilisation, equity and determinants of full antenatal care in India: analysis from the National Family Health Survey 4. BMC Pregnancy Childbirth 19(1):1–9. https://doi.org/10.1186/S12884-019-2473-6

Leckie G, Charlton C (2013) Runmlwin: A program to run the MLwiN multilevel modeling software from within Stata. J Stat Softw 52(11):1–40. https://doi.org/10.18637/jss.v052.i11

Lim SS, Dandona L, Hoisington JA, James SL, Hogan MC, Gakidou E (2010) India's Janani Suraksha Yojana, a conditional cash transfer programme to increase births in health facilities: an impact evaluation. Lancet 375(9730):2009–2023. https://doi.org/10.1016/S0140-6736(10)60744-1

Ministry of Health & Family Welfare (2013) A strategic approach to reproductive, maternal, newborn, child and adolescent health (RMNCH+A) in India. https://nhm.gov.in/images/pdf/RMNCH+A/RMNCH+A_Strategy.pdf

Narain JP (2019) Health of tribal populations in India: how long can we afford to neglect? Indian J Med Res 149(3):313. https://doi.org/10.4103/IJMR.IJMR_2079_18

Negi NS, Sekher TV, Ganguly S (2010) Antenatal care among Tribals: a study of Chhattisgarh and Jharkhand. Stud Tribes Tribals 8(2):77–86. https://doi.org/10.1080/0972639X.2010.11886621

Nongdhar J, Vyas N, Rao P, Narayanan P, Pala S (2018) Factors influencing utilization of reproductive health services among mothers in Meghalaya, India. J Family Med Prim Care 7(3):557. https://doi.org/10.4103/jfmpc.jfmpc_242_17

Nwosu CO, Ataguba JE (2019) Socioeconomic inequalities in maternal health service utilisation: A case of antenatal care in Nigeria using a decomposition approach. BMC Public Health 19(1):1493. https://doi.org/10.1186/s12889-019-7840-8

Office of the Registrar General & Census Commissioner (2011) Census of India

Ogbo FA, Dhami MV, Ude EM, Senanayake P, Osuagwu UL, Awosemo AO, Ogeleka P, Akombi BJ, Ezeh OK, Agho KE (2019) Enablers and barriers to the utilization of antenatal care services in India. Int J Environ Res Public Health 16(17):3152. https://doi.org/10.3390/ijerph16173152

Paudel YR, Jha T, Mehata S (2017) Timing of first antenatal care (ANC) and inequalities in early initiation of ANC in Nepal. Front Public Health 5:242. https://doi.org/10.3389/FPUBH.2017.00242/BIBTEX

Paul P, Chouhan P (2020) Socio-demographic factors influencing utilization of maternal health care services in India. Clin Epidemiol Glob Health 8(3):666–670. https://doi.org/10.1016/j.cegh.2019.12.023

Peña-Rosas JP, Viteri FE (2006) Effects of routine oral iron supplementation with or without folic acid for women during pregnancy. Cochrane Database Syst Rev 3:CD004736. https://doi.org/10.1002/14651858.cd004736.pub2

Rasbash J, Steele F, Browne WJ, Goldstein H (2012) A User's guide to MLwiN. In: Centre for multilevel modelling. University of Bristol, Bristol. http://www.bris.ac.uk/media-library/sites/cmm/migrated/documents/manual-web.pdf

Reddy BV (2019) Maathru Samman Pants: An initiative towards "Respectful Maternity Care". J Family Med Prim Care 8(6):1821. https://doi.org/10.4103/JFMPC.JFMPC_326_19

Register General of India (2020) Special Bulletin On Maternal Mortality In India 2016–18. https://censusindia.gov.in/vital_statistics/SRS_Bulletins/MMRBulletin 2016–18.pdf

Roy MP (2017) Underutilization of antenatal services among tribal women. Indian J Med Res 145:569–570. https://doi.org/10.4103/ijmr.IJMR_1794_16

Sanneving L, Trygg N, Saxena D, Mavalankar D, Thomsen S (2013) Inequity in India: the case of maternal and reproductive health. Glob Health Action 6(1):19145. https://doi.org/10.3402/gha.v6i0.19145

Sathiya Susuman A (2012) Correlates of antenatal and postnatal care among tribal women in India. Stud Ethno-Med 6(1):55–62. https://doi.org/10.1080/09735070.2012.11886421

Sharma S, Mohanty PS, Omar R, Viramgami AP, Sharma N (2020) Determinants and utilization of maternal health Care Services in Urban Slums of an Industrialized City, in Western India. J Family Reprod Health 14:95–101. https://doi.org/10.18502/JFRH.V14I2.4351

Singh PK, Rai RK, Alagarajan M, Singh L (2012) Determinants of maternity care services utilization among married adolescents in rural India. PLoS One 7(2):e31666. https://doi.org/10.1371/JOURNAL.PONE.0031666

Singh A, Kumar A, Pranjali P (2014) Utilization of maternal healthcare among adolescent mothers in urban India: evidence from DLHS-3. PeerJ 2014(1):e592. https://doi.org/10.7717/peerj.592

Singh A, Chakrabarty M, Chowdhury S, Singh S (2022) Exclusive use of hygienic absorbents among rural adolescent women in India: a geospatial analysis. Clin Epidemiol Glob Health 17:101116. https://doi.org/10.1016/J.CEGH.2022.101116

Sinha P, Gunagi PR, Viveki RG, Kamble M, Halki S (2019) Utilization of antenatal services under Pradhan Mantri Surakshit Matritva Abhiyan in rural area of North Karnataka: a cross-sectional study. Nat J Res Commun Med 8(2):184–188. http://journal.njrcmindia.com/index.php/njrcm/article/view/29

Sri B, Sarojini N, Khanna R (2012) An investigation of maternal deaths following public protests in a tribal district of Madhya Pradesh, Central India. Reprod Health Matters 20(39):11–20. https://doi.org/10.1016/S0968-8080(12)39599-2

Srivastava VK (2018) The National Committee Report on tribal people. Social Change 48(1):120–130. https://doi.org/10.1177/0049085717743843

Thaddeus S, Maine D (1994) Too far to walk: maternal mortality in context. Soc Sci Med 38(8):1091–1110. https://doi.org/10.1016/0277-9536(94)90226-7

Tikmani SS, Ali SA, Saleem S, Bann CM, Mwenechanya M, Carlo WA, Figueroa L, Garces AL, Krebs NF, Patel A, Hibberd PL, Goudar SS, Derman RJ, Aziz A, Marete I, Tenge C, Esamai F, Liechty E, Bucher S, Goldenberg RL (2019) Trends of antenatal care during pregnancy in low-and middle-income countries: findings from the global network maternal and newborn health registry. Semin Perinatol 43(5):297–307. https://doi.org/10.1053/j.semperi.2019.03.020

Tribal Cultural Heritage in India Foundation (2017) "Who are Scheduled Tribes?": Clarifications by the National Commission for Scheduled Tribes. https://indiantribalheritage.org/?p = 21438

Usman M, Anand E, Siddiqui L, Unisa S (2021) Continuum of maternal health care services and its impact on child immunization in India: an application of the propensity score matching approach. J Biosoc Sci 53(5):643–662. https://doi.org/10.1017/S0021932020000450

Varma GR, Kusuma YS, Babu BV (2011) Antenatal care service utilization in tribal and rural areas in a south Indian district. J Egypt Public Health Assoc 86(1&2):11–15. https://doi.org/10.1097/01.EPX.0000395395.17777.be

Verma R, Khanna P, Dhankar M (2016) Vaccination during pregnancy: today's need in India. Hum Vaccin Immunother 12(3):668. https://doi.org/10.1080/21645515.2015.1093265

Chapter 17
Utilization of Maternal Healthcare Services Among Women in Urban Slums of Prayagraj City, India

Namrata Ahirwar, Vikesh Kumar, and Kunal Keshri

Abstract Maternal healthcare is vital for the well-being of both a mother and her child. Regular maternal healthcare service (MHCS) utilization can reduce maternal deaths. This chapter, therefore, aims to study the utilization of maternal healthcare services in selected slums in Prayagraj city and examine the factors responsible for the same. We utilized primary data, which were collected by using qualitative and quantitative methods. The primary data were collected through face-to-face interviews. The study sample comprised women aged 15–49 years in the urban slums of Prayagraj city. This study found that maternal healthcare services were not utilized properly in most of the slums of Prayagraj city. The majority of the respondents registered their pregnancy in their second trimester and went for only one or two antenatal (ANC) visits. Only 18.2% of women went for three or more ANC visits. About 34% of respondents received two shots of tetanus toxoid (TT) injection, and 57% of respondents did not receive a TT injections during their pregnancy. Only 43% of respondents said that they chose an institutional delivery. Among all pregnant women, 86% of respondents had a vaginal delivery and 14% of women a caesarean delivery. This study shows that the majority of the women in the sample were unaware of maternal healthcare services. That's why more than half of the population (54%) is not utilizing healthcare facilities. Increasing awareness of and improving access to the utilization of maternal healthcare services are needed for the slum population.

Keywords Slums · Maternal health · Antenatal care · Delivery care · Postnatal care

N. Ahirwar
G B Pant Social Science Institute, A Constituent Institute of University of Allahabad, Prayagraj, Uttar Pradesh, India

V. Kumar · K. Keshri (✉)
Department of Migration and Urban Studies, International Institute for Population Sciences, Mumbai, Maharashtra, India

© The Author(s), under exclusive license to Springer Nature Singapore Pte Ltd. 2024
P. Chouhan et al. (eds.), *Sexual and Reproductive Health of Women*, https://doi.org/10.1007/978-981-97-8418-9_17

17.1 Introduction

The World Health Organization defines *maternal health* as "the health of women during pregnancy, childbirth, and after delivery" (WHO, 2020). *Maternal mortality* is defined as "the death of a woman directly related to complications of pregnancy or within 42 days of the termination of pregnancy" (Orwh 2020). The high rate of maternal mortality is a major global problem. However, India has shown a great reduction in maternal mortality in recent years. That the maternal mortality ratio in India has declined over the years to 97 in 2018–2020 from 103 in 2017–2019 and 130 in 2014–2016 is heartening, but at a regional level, high differences in India between regions remain: Southern India has an MMR of only 49 (per 100,000 live births), whereas EAG states and Assam have an MMR of 137 (per 100,000 live births), much higher than the national average, at 97 (per 100,000 live births) (SRS 2019). Also, a large rural–urban gap in the utilization of maternal healthcare services (MHCSs) persists. The utilization of MHCSs is higher among urban women than rural ones (Chauhan and Kumar 2016), but women in the slums have a lower utilization of maternal healthcare services than other urban women (Sharma et al. 2020).

The important reasons for the high maternal mortality are pregnancy at a premature age, the poor health of the mother, and home delivery unattended by trained *dais* or nurses. Pregnancy-related causes of death include a large number of disorders, such as unsafe abortion; infection; anemia; bleeding during pregnancy; fetal malposition, leading to the death of a mother; and several other causes (Mishra and Newhouse, 2007). Antenatal birth and postnatal treatment are all considered to be maternal healthcare services. Maternal healthcare services are vital for the wellbeing of both a mother and her child. Regular maternal healthcare service utilization can reduce maternal deaths. Several socioeconomic and cultural factors influence how frequently women receive healthcare during pregnancy, during childbirth, and after delivery (Fatema and Lariscy 2020).

With close to 20 million migrants moving from rural to urban areas every year, combined with intrinsic population growth inside urban areas, India's urban population growth is expected to continue. The urban share of India's population was around 31%, according to the 2011 census, and is expected to cross 40% by 2030 (United Nations, 2018). According to Census 2011, India had 454 million migrants in 2011. This had risen by 139 million from 315 million in 2001 and 220 million in 1991, a doubling from 1991–2011 (Report of the Working Group on Migration 2017). Massive issues with India's inadequate public health facilities are now plaguing the country's slums and are likely to get worse over time. Maternal healthcare service access and use are significantly impacted by migration. People living in slums have been shown to have poor health, especially women and children, who are the most vulnerable members of society (Kaviarasu and Gladston 2015). Women frequently get trapped in a cycle of bad health that becomes worse due to childbearing and severe physical labor; in particular, those who live in poor conditions have low levels of education and lack accessibility. The situation is quite dire in South

Asia due to inadequate access to healthcare services and poor utilization (Chandwani and Padhiyar 2013). The education of couples, their financial situation, and prenatal checkups seemed to have favorable effects on increasing maternal healthcare service utilization overall. The usage of services, however, was generally adversely impacted by conventional beliefs and practices, the poor status of women, distance to facilities, a lack of health knowledge, and women's employment. Maternal age, marital status, faith, traditional views, family structure, mother's education, spouse's education, and women's status are some examples of sociocultural variables. Economic accessibility includes factors like the socioeconomic standing of the household, the jobs of parents, the family's revenue, the price of institutional delivery, transit, and lost productivity due to travel time. The necessity for institutional birth might be seen differently by different women, depending on a variety of circumstances, including their awareness of pregnancy and health concerns, the significance placed on pregnancy, prior institutional use, antenatal visits, and pregnancy problems. Physical accessibility takes into account a person's place of residence, travel time to the medical institution, and choices for transportation.

Women's health, especially their reproductive health, is getting worse. Living in unhygienic, unsanitary conditions in slums with poor educational backgrounds and the low social status that accompanies slum living negatively affects their health, especially the problems that they face with their reproductive systems. This leads to lower treatment rates and, as a result, a heavier burden of illness on women than on men (Sanneving et al. 2013).

The utilization of maternal health services is impacted by a variety of factors that work at every level: individual, family, and community (Zhang et al. 2016); Garg et al. 2007). The appropriate requirements vary depending on the use of maternal healthcare. Generally speaking, women in higher socioeconomic categories have a tendency to use maternal healthcare more frequently than those in lower socioeconomic groups (Abor et al. 2011). A mother's education is a significant social factor that influences the use of services for maternity and child health in a favorable way (Barman et al. 2020). Other socioeconomic characteristics that are frequently deemed significant include domicile, religion, and household level of living (Mochache et al. 2020). The usage of prenatal care and delivery services is also influenced by the household's financial situation. Caste has a high correlation with the use or lack thereof of maternal care services (Chimankar and Sahoo 2011).

17.2 Data Source and Methods

In this chapter, the mixed-methods research design was used to determine the utilization of maternal healthcare services during the antenatal, delivery, and postnatal periods among pregnant and recently delivered women in the slums of Prayagraj city. This research further investigated the socioeconomic and demographic factors affecting the utilization of maternal healthcare services among pregnant and recently delivered women in the slums of Prayagraj city. We utilized primary data and both qualitative and quantitative methods. Primary data were collected through face-to-face interviews.

A structured schedule and semistructured qualitative interview guidelines were used as study tools in the mixed technique to gather quantitative and qualitative data, respectively. The study aimed to survey 200 respondents. In total, 16 in-depth interviews (IDIs) and seven focus group discussions (FGDs) were conducted with women who were pregnant at the time of listing and women who gave birth in the past 1 year (recently delivered women), chosen from each slum. The interview approach is useful for gathering both extensive and in-depth information. In-depth interviews covering all personal and mother–child healthcare behaviors were also carried out in the slum. Detailed interviews with pregnant mothers, new mothers (recently delivered women), traditional birth attendants (TBAs), accredited social health activists (ASHAs), and auxiliary nurse midwives (ANMs) were conducted via a conversation with the respondent. To achieve the best results, the focus group discussions were held with mothers and pregnant women in the study population. Health professionals attended the focus group discussions. The FGDs helped to collect full details on the health of women and their unborn children. It also offered broad details on mothers' experiences and perceptions of prenatal, delivery, and postpartum treatment. For data collection, four slums were selected: (1) Purapadain near Shastri Bridge, (2) Dharkar Basti, Kydganj, (3) Takiya Alopibagh, and (4) Parade Ground Jhopad Patti and Alopibagh. The study sample comprised women aged 15–49 years in the urban slums of Prayagraj city because this age bracket represents the reproductive years of women as defined by the World Health Organization (WHO 2006). First, we selected from the registered slums and nonregistered slums lists given by the municipal corporation of Prayagraj. The non-registered slums selected for the study were Takiya Alopibagh, Parade Ground Jhopad Patti (Alopibagh) and the registered slums selected were Purapadain near Shastri Bridge, Dharkar Basti, and Kydganj. Before selecting the slums, the relevant documents and reports of the municipal corporation of Prayagraj were systematically reviewed. The participants of the study included all women who were pregnant at the time of listing and women who gave birth in the past 1 year (recently delivered women), chosen from each slum. The interviews were held with government health workers, auxiliary nurse midwives (ANMs), accredited social health activists (ASHAs), and anganwadi workers (AWWs). Purposive sampling was used for this study. We selected 200 respondents for our study. Respondents were selected with the help of accredited social health activists (ASHAs), auxiliary nurse midwives (ANMs), and anganwadi workers (AWWs). Data are collected from pregnant and recently delivered women because they represent the most suitable subjects for study and for data collection. Among the 200 participants, 100 pregnant women were selected from the following areas: Purapadain near Shastri Bridge (25), Dharkar Basti, Kydganj (31), Takiya Alopibagh (24), Parade Ground Jhopad Patti, and Alopibagh (20).

Similarly, 100 recently delivered women were selected from the following areas: Purapadain near Shastri Bridge (26), Dharkar Basti, Kydganj (32), Takiya Alopibagh (19), Parade Ground Jhopad Patti (Alopibagh) (23).

17.2.1 First Step

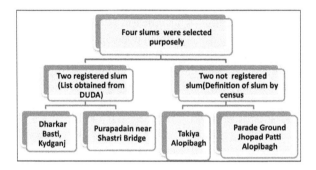

17.2.2 Second Step

See Fig. 17.1

A closed and open-ended questionnaire was used to collect the qualitative and quantitative data via the face-to-face interview technique. Section I contained the questions that were designed to collect the data on the socioeconomic background of the respondents and their utilization of maternal healthcare services. Questions on women's perceptions and experiences (problems during pregnancy, causes of home delivery, whether they received prenatal care) were used. The SPSS software package was used for the analysis in this chapter. Descriptive statistics were carried out to provide details on the study participants.

Fig. 17.1 Sampling framework

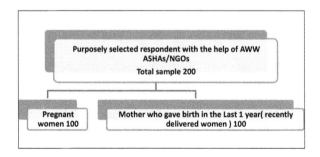

17.2.3 Selection of Study Area

17.2.3.1 Prayagraj City (Erstwhile Allahabad)

The level of urbanization has been increasing rapidly in Uttar Pradesh, specifically in Ghaziabad, Lucknow, Kanpur Nagar, Agra, Meerut, Varanasi, and Prayagraj. The percentage of the population living in urban areas is highest in Ghaziabad, followed by Lucknow, Kanpur Nagar, Agra, Varanasi, and Prayagraj. The urban percentage of Prayagraj is low compared to other the million-plus cities in Uttar Pradesh, and Prayagraj is the only million-plus city that has a low urban population according to the national average. The city with the highest slum population is Meerut, followed by Ghaziabad, Kanpur Nagar, Varanasi, Prayagraj, Agra, and Lucknow. Most of the migrants to these cities are rural-to-urban migrants. The Prayagraj district is one of the major and largest districts in Uttar Pradesh. Prayagraj has the largest rural population. Here, 75.6% of the population is in rural areas, and 24.2% in urban areas. One of the biggest cities in northern India is Prayagraj, which serves as the administrative center for Uttar Pradesh's most populated district (Prayagraj). According to the 2011 registrar general of India, the Prayagraj urban agglomeration/metropolitan area has 1,212,395 residents overall. According to the 2001 Indian Census, migrants constitute around 15% of the overall population of Prayagraj's urban agglomeration. Of the 1.5 lakh people who moved into the city in 2015, 33% moved from rural regions. The district with the highest urban population is Ghaziabad (68%) and that with the lowest is Prayagraj (25%). But the percentage of mothers who received antenatal care is highest in Lucknow (52%) and lowest in Prayagraj (30%) (Fig. 17.2).

17.3 Results

17.3.1 Socioeconomic and Demographic Characteristics

This section describes the various socioeconomic and demographic characteristics of the respondents. Supporting tables and figures and comparative information from the primary survey are provided. Using descriptive statistics, this section also presents the respondents' socioeconomic and demographic background, migration duration, age, birth order, education, caste, religion, and family type (nuclear or non-nuclear).

All 100 pregnant female respondents were interviewed during the primary survey. About 35% of the women in this category are below 20 years old, 49% are between 20 and 34 years, and 16% are between 35 and 49 years. Regarding educational status, 54% of women had no formal education, 34% had only completed primary school, and 12% had completed upper primary school. The sample respondents' primary occupations were as rag pickers, *kabaad* (junk) shop employees,

17 Utilization of Maternal Healthcare Services Among Women in Urban Slums...

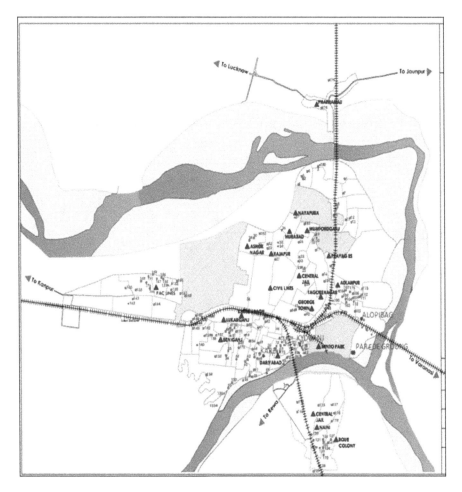

Fig. 17.2 Map showing the location of slums in Prayagraj. (*Source*: Slums in Prayagraj (Municipal Corporation Allahabad 2011))

basket makers, and sweepers. The sample respondents are divided into three groups on the basis of their monthly income, which includes their spouse's salary and other family income: those with monthly incomes of less than INR 3000, between INR 3000 and INR 5000, and between INR 5000 and 10,000. About one-fifth of the respondents (or 19%) have monthly incomes of less than INR 3000, 69% have incomes of INR 3000 to INR 5000, and 12% have incomes of INR 5000 to INR 10,000. Most participants' families earned between INR 3000 and INR 5000 per month. Of the sample respondents, 70% are from Scheduled Castes and 23% from other social groups. Of the sample respondents, 72% are Hindu and 28% Muslim. Out of the total of 100 individuals who participated in the survey, 74% are from nuclear families and 25% from joint families. Moreover, 30% of the respondents had lived in a slum for less than 5 years, 39% had lived there for 5–10 years, and 28% had lived there for more than 10 years (Table 17.1).

Interviews were conducted with 100 selected women who had given birth within last one year, among which 41% were below the age of 20 years, 43% were between the age group of 20 to 34 years, and 16% were between the ages group of 35 to

Table 17.1 Socioeconomic and demographic background characteristics of the pregnant women ($n = 100$)

Backgrounds Characteristics		Percentage
Age		
	Below 20 years	35
	20–34 years	49
	35–49 years	16
Birth order		
	1	4
	2–3	62
	4+	34
Education		
	No formal education	54
	Primary education	34
	Upper primary education	12
Type of family		
	Nuclear family	74
	Joint family	25
Religion		
	Hindu	72
	Muslim	28
Caste		
	Scheduled Caste	70
	Other	30
Occupation		
	No work	27
	Rag picking	47
	Working at a *kabaad* (junk) shop	19
	Basket making	1
	Sweeping	6
Family income per month (in INR)		
	Below 3000	19
	3000–5000	69
	5000–10,000	12
Migration duration		
	Below 5 years	33
	5–10 years	39
	Above 10 years	28

Source: Author's fieldwork, 2018–2019

49 years. Regarding educational qualification, 64% did not have any formal education, 25% had completed primary school, and 11% had completed upper primary schooling. The sample respondents' primary occupations were rag pickers, *kabaad* (junk) shop employees, basket makers, and sweepers. On the basis of monthly income of the respondent they are categorized into three categories, which includes their spouse's salary and other family income. First, 53% respondent had monthly incomes less than INR 3000, second, 43% had incomes between INR 3000 to INR 5000, and third, 4% had monthly incomes between INR 5000 to INR 10,000. Among the caste categories (social groups), 66% were from Scheduled Castes and 34% from other groups. Regrading religious groups, 30% were Muslims and 70% Hindus. In terms of family size, 74% were in nuclear families and 25% in joint families. If we look at the migration duration of respondent, 29% had been living in a slum for less than 5 years, 39% respondents were living from 5–10 years, and 32% respondents were living more than 10 years (Table 17.2).

17.3.2 Utilization of Antenatal Care Services

We carried out a primary survey for the collection of data by using structured questions. The study aimed to survey 100 pregnant respondents during fieldwork, and data on the socioeconomic and demographic characteristics of the respondents were collected.

Table 17.3 shows that 66% of the pregnant respondents were registered during their pregnancy. Of the respondents, 66.7% registered their pregnancy during their second trimester, 22.7% during their first trimester, and 10.6% during their third trimester. Only 33% of the respondents never registered their pregnancy. The majority of respondents received only one or two ANC checkups. Only 18.2% went for three or more ANC visits. Of the respondents, 34% received two TT injections, 9% received one TT injection, and 57% did not receive any TT injections during their pregnancy (Table 17.4).

17.3.3 Utilization of Delivery and Postnatal Care Services

In this section, we carried out a primary survey for data collection, asking closed questions. For this survey, we asked 100 recently delivered women a series of questions, after which, percentage analyses were performed.

The results show that the majority of women received advice from a health worker within the past 3 months of pregnancy. More than 70% of women received a health checkup during pregnancy. Among the respondents, 57% chose home delivery and 43% selected institutional delivery. Most of the women had a vaginal delivery (86%), and 14% had a caesarean delivery. The majority of women who gave birth at a hospital used a government ambulance. More than 50% of

Table 17.2 Socioeconomic and demographic backgrounds characteristics of women who gave birth in the last 1 year and recently delivered (*n* = 100)

Backgrounds Characteristics		Percentage
Age		
	Below 20 years	41
	20–34 years	43
	35–49 years	16
Birth order		
	1	24
	2–3	50
	≥ 4	26
Education		
	No formal education	64
	Primary education	25
	Upper primary education	11
Type of family (in INR) type of Family		
	Nuclear family	66
	Joint family	34
Religion		
	Hindu	70
	Muslim	30
Caste		
	Scheduled Caste	66
	Other	34
Occupation		
	No work	12
	Rag picking	49
	Working at a *kabaad* shop	7
	Basket making	25
	Sweeping	5
	Beedi rolling	2
Family income		
	Below 3000	53
	3000–5000	43
	5000–10,000	4
Migration duration		
	Below 5 years	29
	5–10 years	39
	Above 10 years	32

Source: Author's fieldwork, 2018–2019

transportations for delivery were arranged by anganwadi workers. Most of the women incurred expenses during delivery in hospital, in amounts ranging from INR 5000 to INR 10,000. Of those women who went for a health checkup after childbirth, most had a checkup at a government hospital or anganwadi center (Table 17.4).

Table 17.3 Percentage distribution of pregnant women according to their utilization of ANC services (n = 100)

Variable		Percentage
Month when pregnancy was discovered		
	1 month	36.0
	2 months	34.0
	Does not remember	30.0
Pregnancy registration		
	Yes	66.0
	No	34.0
Registration during pregnancy		
	First trimester	22.7
	Second trimester	66.7
	Third trimester	10.6
Reason for not going to antenatal checkups		
	Not necessary/ cost too much	38.2
	Too far/No transportation	23.5
	Family did not allow	17.6
	Lack of knowledge	20.6
Health problems during pregnancy		
	Swelling on head and feet	45.0
	Eyesight problem	22.0
	Heavy bleeding	15.0
	Weak ovary	7.0
	Swelling on head and feet & Eyesight problem	10.0
	Swelling on head and feet, Eyesight problem & Heavy bleeding	1.0
Type of health facility visited during pregnancy		
	None	21.0
	Govt. Clinic/Hospital	38.0
	Private Clinic/Hospital	23.0
	Traditional Birth attendant	18.0
Reason for not going to health facility		
	Service not satisfactory	4.8
	Long waiting time	6.5
	Unavailability of doctor	9.7
	Unavailability of Medicines	3.2
	Long distance	75.8
Mode of transportation to health facility		
	NA	52.0
	Walking	26.0

(continued)

Table 17.3 (continued)

Variable		Percentage
	Public Transport	22.0
Registration performed by		
	ANM	28.8
	ASHA	25.8
	AWW	36.4
	Doctor	9.1
No. of ANC visits		
	1 visit	40.9
	2 visit	40.9
	3 or more visits	18.2
ANC received		
	Weight, BP Check, Iron & Folic Acid tablet	6.1
	Weight, Hemoglobin test, Advice on food & rest	16.7
	Weight, Hemoglobin test, Iron & Folic Acid tablet	9.1
	Weight, Advice on food & rest, Iron & Folic Acid tablet	10.6
	Weight, Height, Advice on food & rest, Iron & Folic Acid tablet	12.1
	Weight, BP Check, Advice on food & rest, Iron & Iron–folic acid (IFA) tablet	25.8
	Weight, Urine & Stomach test, Hemoglobin test, Iron & Folic Acid tablet	10.6
	BP Check, Iron & Folic Acid tablet, Blood test, Ultrasound	9.1
Regular consumption of IFA tablets		
	Yes, taken	37.0
	No, not taken	56.0
	NA	7.0
Mother and child protection card received after registration		
	Yes	81.8
	No	18.2
Consultation for pregnancy care		
	Yes	82.0
	No	18.0
Consultant for pregnancy care		
	Doctor	16.0
	ANM/nurse/midwife/LHV	7.0
	DAI/traditional	14.0
	Anganwadi/ICDS Worker	4.0

(continued)

Table 17.3 (continued)

Variable		Percentage
	ASHA	14.0
	Doctor/ANM/nurse/midwife/LHV	7.0
	DAI/traditional & ASHA	11.0
	Anganwadi/ICDS worker & ASHA	9.0
	NA	18.0
No. of TT injections received during pregnancy		
	1	9.0
	2	34.0
	Does not know	57.0
Received supplementary food during pregnancy		
	Yes	34.0
	No	66.0
IFA tablets received during pregnancy		
	Yes	61.0
	No	39.0

Source: Author's fieldwork, 2018–2019

Table 17.4 Percentage distribution of recently delivered women according to their use of delivery and postnatal care services ($n = 100$)

Percentage		Variable
Consultancy of health worker within past 3 months of pregnancy		
	Yes	70.0
	No	30.0
Advice received on		
	Importance of institutional delivery	18.0
	Cord care	9.0
	Family planning or delay or avoid other pregnancy	43.0
	NA	30.0
Health checkup during pregnancy		
	Yes	72.0
	No	28.0
Place of delivery		
	Home	57.0
	Hospital	43.0
Heavy bleeding during delivery		
	Yes	20.0
	No	42.0
	Don't Know	38.0

(continued)

Table 17.4 (continued)

Percentage		Variable
Type of delivery		
	Vaginal	86.0
	Caesarean	14.0
Assistant during delivery		
	Doctor	12.0
	ANM/Nurse/Midwife/LHV	2.0
	DAI/TBA	8.0
	Mother/mother-in-law	30.0
	Other relative	19.0
	Doctor/nurse	29.0
Type of transportation to place of delivery		
	Govt. ambulance	53.5
	Other ambulance	2.3
	Jeep/car	7.0
	Motorcycle/scooter	2.3
	Tempo/auto/tractor	34.9
Expenses during delivery in hospital		
	Below INR 5000	30.2
	INR 5000–10,000	46.3
	Above INR 10,000	23.3
Who arranged transportation to place of delivery		
	ANM	2.3
	Anganwadi worker	58.1
	ASHA	2.3
	Spouse/other relatives	37.2
No. of days spent in health services after delivery		
	1	20.9
	2	20.9
	4	14.0
	5	20.9
	6	2.3
	7	20.9
Time of checkup after birth		
	HRS after Birth	9.0
	DAYS after Birth	30.0
	WKS after Birth	24.0
	Don't know	33.0
	Not done	4.0
Place of checkup after birth		
	Home	20.0

(continued)

Table 17.4 (continued)

Percentage		Variable
	Govt. hospital	37.0
	Private hospital/clinic	5.0
	Anganwadi	33.0
	Other	5.0
Checkups performed by		
	Doctor	42.0
	ANM/nurse/midwife/LHV	9.0
	Anganwadi worker	8.0
	DAI/TBA	10.0
	ASHA	26.0
	NA	5.0
Checkups performed within 2 months after discharge		
	Yes	74.0
	No	26.0
Reason for no checkups		
	High cost	61.5
	No transportation/too far	7.7
	No information to spouse/family	11.5
	Not important	19.2
Clean blade used to cut umbilical cord		
	Yes	91.0
	No	2.0
	Don't know	7.0
Problems within first 2 months after delivery		
	Heavy bleeding	46.0
	High fever	18.0
	Other	36.0
Time when baby feeding started		
	Within 2 h after birth	65.0
	After 2 h on same day after birth	25.0
	After 3 days	7.0
	Don't know	3.0
Any food given to baby apart from mother's milk in first week?		
	Yes	18.0
	No	82.0
Are you feeding mother's milk to baby at present?		
	Yes	89.0
	No	11.0

Source: Author's fieldwork, 2018–2019

17.3.4 Qualitative Findings

This section is based on qualitative field research using an open-ended questionnaire. The qualitative approach was adopted to determine which factors affect maternal healthcare service utilization. This chapter aims to understand women's experiences, feelings, and perspectives on the utilization of maternal healthcare services and explore the factors associated with the utilization of maternal healthcare services. In total, 16 in-depth interviews (IDIs) and seven focus group discussions (FGDs) were conducted with women who were pregnant at the time of listing and women who gave birth in the past year (2017) (recently delivered women). Women were chosen from each slum. IDIs with ANMs, ASHAs, and AWWs in their area were conducted to gather information on the nearest government health facility. For the in-depth interviews, we asked questions related to the utilization of maternal healthcare services (antenatal care, delivery service, and postnatal care), choosing a place of delivery and the nature of the delivery (reason for preference for homebirth or hospital delivery), and knowledge and awareness of MHCSs. During the focus group discussions, the questions were asked related to respondents' family support and their spouse's involvement in antenatal, delivery, and postnatal services; the behavior of maternal healthcare providers toward pregnant women and recently delivered women; the distance to the health facility; and exposure to social media (how social media influences women's attitudes, knowledge, and behavior when they are utilizing MHCSs).

The results from the above themes are discussed in this chapter. Most women registered for ANC after the first trimester of pregnancy. We tried to determine the reasons for this. Women opt for ANC only if they experience a complication during pregnancy. Otherwise, they do not consider going to be necessary.

As one pregnant respondent said,

> Main Anganwadi Kendra kuchmahine bad gayi, kyokimeriamma [mother] ne kahathakikuchmahine bad hi jana, aurtabhijana jab koi dikkatho, kyoki agar bastikemaherian [women] ko teen mahina se pahlepatachaljayega to tumharebalbacchako koi na koi dikkathojayegi (IDI with a 23-year-old pregnant woman).

Translation: "I went to the anganwadi center a few months later because my mother told me to go only after a few months and only if there was a problem, because if the women of the settlement get to know before three months, then your child will have some trouble."

As another pregnant respondent stated,

> Madam ji, aapko batayen ki meri padosan hain unke sabhi bacche ghar par hi huyehai, wo kabhi kahi nahi gayi, koi goli bhi nahi khayi. Wo kahti bhi hai ki jab tak sab theek hai kahi jane ke jarurt nahi hai. Isliye ham tab gaye the jab khoon bah rahaa tha, ruk hi naahi raha tha (IDI with a 27-year-old pregnant woman).

Translation: "Madam, I want to tell you that my all neighbor's children have been delivered at home; she never went anywhere and did not even take any pills. She also said that as long as everything is fine, there is no need to go anywhere. That is why we went when the bleeding was not stopping."

In this study, most women reported that frequent visits were unnecessary as justification for their delaying registration or avoiding registration for full antenatal care services. Some women said, the cost was too high. Some women told the family member that they did not give permission. Some women informed us that they did not have time to go, and some were unaware.

As one pregnant respondent from a Purapadain slum said,

Ghar par bahut kam hota hai. Hamarladkabitiya [children] ghar par akelanahi rah payega. Main kai bar checkupkeliyenahijasakti. Hamara admi bhi kam par chala jata hai. ham usko bina btaye bhi nahi ja sakte. Itne bar Jane ko bhi nahi kah sakte, kyoki kam rukega to ghar kais echalega, chulha naa jale to bacche kaisejiyenge. Ham khhayengekya, sath hi hamarii tnikamayinahihai (IDI with a 25-year-old pregnant woman).

Translation: "There is much work at home. Our children will not be able to live alone at home. I can only go for a checkup a few times. My husband also goes to work; we cannot even go without informing him. You cannot even ask them to go so often because if the work stops, how will the house run? If the stove is not on, how will the children live? What will we eat when we only have a little income?"

As another recently delivered respondent from a Takiya slum said,

Didi bar-bar jane ki jarurat nahi hai. Jab lagega ki ab bachenge nahi to jayenge. Kyoki ham sune hai ham bar bar jayenege to, Asha Didi Logan ko hamare jane se paisa milta hai. Hame kaha mana to samay kharab hota hai. Apne mard ki gali khhao so alag (IDI with a 23-year-old recently delivered woman).

Translaton: Most women living in a slum do not know medications like iron tablets and calcium tablets. "They know iron/calcium tablets by [names like] 'lalgoli' or 'khoon badhane wali goli,' 'saved goli,' 'bacche ki haddi majboot karne wali goli.'"

Only one out of the four selected slums had a proper anganwadi center. Women gave many reasons for not taking iron tablets; they said that they received them from anganwadi centers or Asha Didi but had yet to eat.

As a 28-year-old pregnant woman from Parade Ground Jhopad Patti, Alopibaghslum, said,

I start vomiting as soon as I eat an iron tablet; it smells awful, and after eating, it starts burning in the stomach, so I threw it after eating only 1–2 tablets.

A 29-year-old recently delivered woman shared her experience: "She said, I knew iron tablets should be taken during pregnancy, so I had brought them from anganwadi centers, but my mother-in-law threw them out. In addition, madam is asking for increasing your blood so that when your baby will born, she will ask you to go to the hospital for delivery and take out the amount of blood from your body and then she will sell it. I had eight children, but I have never needed a pill like this."

Some women have to make decisions according to their mother-in-law and other women in the family. As one 26-year-old pregnant woman said in an IDI, "Asha Didi told me to take iron tablets at night. However, I always forget because I get tired after working all day. I cannot remember to take pills every day."

Due to distance and a lack of transportation, going to the hospital for delivery was deemed unnecessary: "We did not have money to go to the hospital." The educational status of women and their spouses, household economic status, and visits to ANC were the significant factors that influenced them.

An AWW shared her views: "AWW said that some women's husbands are unemployed, and I also found that some women's husbands do not work. In addition, she said that someone's condition is so bad that someday food is not even available. That is why, even after our persuasion, they do not go to the hospital for delivery, even if there is a problem. They need the money to go to them, as the hospital is also far away. That is why most women give birth to children at home. If any woman is sick, she will tell her husband or family members; if her husband is not allowed to go, then such women will not have access to healthcare services."

A 33-year-old recently delivered woman from a Purapadain slum shared her experience: "We were getting treatment in a government hospital. So, everyone there said that an average child would be born here. Everything will go well; there is no need to be afraid. We did not know anyone in the slum. My husband and I were at my house, so we went to the hospital. The nurse took me inside the room and gave birth to the baby through the operation; it would have been expected if we had not gone to the hospital. She also said that when I told some women of the Basti, they said that this would have been what happened in the hospital; if you had talked to us, the operation would not have occurred, and the child would have been born quickly. Now I have many problems. A lot of money was also spent. So now I am afraid to go to the hospital."

These qualitative findings reveal that women who delivered in a hospital and those who went for more than three ANC visits had received postnatal care. On the other hand, women who gave birth at home did not receive postnatal care.

Key issues that influenced postnatal care utilization were identified from the IDIs with women/AWW/ASHAs.

> Women come to the anganwadi centers for postnatal care services when there is difficulty during delivery and if the child has any problem. Most of the time, we tell women how to breastfeed, keep the number of children low, cleanliness, we talk about why it is important, nutrition, hygiene, and advice about safe sex (a 27-year-old AWW).

> I have given birth to all my children at home, so I never needed any treatment. I never went to the hospital. We usually go to the health facility to get the child vaccinated, but there are some women in the Basti whose child was born in the hospital. They have been seen going to the hospital sometimes (IDI with 27-year-old recently delivered woman).

Most women believed that if a woman gave birth at home and everything went well with the delivery, then she did not need to go to a health facility unless she faced a serious problem.

The use of postnatal care services for women and their newborns depends on the mother's health status and that of her newborn. Women who experienced complications during delivery and who had a caesarean section went to the hospital a few days later.

Most women are unaware of the warning signs and difficulties that might occur throughout pregnancy, delivery, and the postnatal period. A lack of awareness, believing that home delivery is easier, and feeling ashamed to go to the hospital for delivery are some of the factors that influence women's utilization of maternal healthcare services in the study area. During an FGD, we found that most migrant women had heard about maternal healthcare services from other women in their families. Most women were unaware of what services to get during pregnancy at the time of delivery and as part of postnatal care.

Due to their lack of awareness, women take a long time to decide whether they should seek maternal healthcare services and to decide when to visit a health facility. Some FDG participants reported that by the time that they had decided to go to the hospital, they were too late. As a 30-year-old recently delivered woman said,

Ye hi karan meri badi bahniya [elder sister] ke jan gayi thi. Babua ko paida huye kucch ghante huye the ki achanak se unki tabiyat kharab ho gayi, peeli ho gayi thi, basti ke kucch logo ke kaha ki asptal le jao lekin tab tak bhut der ho gayi thi.

Translation: This is the reason why my elder sister died. A few hours after Babua (son) was born, suddenly his health deteriorated; he turned yellow, and some people in the settlement had to take him to the hospital, but by then, it was too late.

The study found that most of the women were late for ANC registration. Apart from this, anganwadi workers go door to door in Basti, but women do not go to the centers even after being called repeatedly. According to them, they have no need for it. The research found that the low intake of iron and calcium tablets among respondents resulted from the respondents' lacking information on their importance.

As a recently delivered woman said in an in-depth Parade Ground Jhopad Patti interview, "Didi, if we go to the hospital, they will give us so many medicines. I will provide injections by thinking of which tears would come out. I don't know how many times we have to go to the hospital and what will happen in the end that she (Dr.) will say that the child will born only through the operation. They give the medicine, so that child is taken only after the procedure. Also, we fear the hospital because they want to make their money. Because to go there means to cause trouble. Everything is quickly done at home with the help of relatives; there is no unnecessary drama" (IDI with a 37-year-old recently delivered woman).

A 35-year-old recently delivered woman shared her experience: "We have been living in this slum for 6 years, and we have four children. There are six members in our family. Our family income is less than 3,000 INR per month. My two children were born in our village at home, and two were born here in a slum. My husband works as a rag picker, and I do not work; their work does not fulfill our needs, so I do not even think of giving birth to a child in a hospital. Even if I die giving birth to a child at home. I don't want to cause of tension for my husband. I know that when we go to the hospital for healthcare, some things are also accessible in the government hospital. But we have to buy medicines and such things are very expensive. When I was pregnant for the fourth time, I had lots of complications. I wanted to go to the hospital, but we did not have money, so we didn't go to the hospital. At this time, it was fifth time when I got pregnant. In the 8th months pregnancy, my baby was not moving, and there was light bleeding, so it was essential to go to the hospital, but at that time, we didn't even have the money to reach the hospital. We had arranged the money from relatives living in the neighborhood. But at the end we to lose out child, it was still birth."

During pregnancy, at the time of delivery, and after delivery, the support of the spouse and family members is very crucial; along with this, many problems must be faced due to excessive family involvement. Women are not able to make decisions related to themselves . Most of the women said that during pregnancy and delivery, only the spouse or other family members decide: "We cannot go to the hospital or anganwadi centers without asking the spouse." The spouse or elders of the household also arrange funding for ANC visits and delivery. Some women say that their spouses are alcoholics, so they also keep some money with them. And sometimes, without informing the family, they even go to the hospital for treatment. The spouse also arranges the place for delivery (home delivery/hospital delivery). The slum spouses or others arrange transportation for the delivery.

A 24-year-old recently delivered woman shared her experience:

> She told me that the child was not born when I had labor pain for 2 days. Then Asha Didi said that you should go to the hospital. We went to the hospital. The doctor told me my child would be born from the operation there. Hearing this, the family members brought me back to the slum. I could not do anything but want my baby to be born in the hospital. The child died a day after birth.

As a 31-year-old pregnant woman from Dharkar Basti said, "We have four members in our family. My husband leaves for work at 8 in the morning. I cannot go out of the house, leaving my children alone at home. Then, no matter how important it is, I never go to the hospital or anganwadi centers like in two previous births without taking any medicine, it will happen the same way. Once, I thought of going to an anganwadi center because some women of the Basti were going. That day, the husband was at home, but I did not dare to ask him because he also did not like me to leave my house, leaving the children alone. After all, there is no need for it unless there is any problem. And I don't have any problem."

Some of the women shared their experiences during the focus group discussion. When they go to the hospital for treatment and meet with the reception staff or the doctor, their expertise has not been good. The majority expressed terrible experiences. "In FGD, four respondents mutually said nurses often scolded them during labor. Sometimes, they are abusive and rude. We never got the correct information. They only asked me to move from one room to another."

Previous experiences of services received during pregnancy and delivery affect the use of MHCSs. "FGD participants reported that nurses and doctors mistreat us in the hospital. When we reached the hospital, seeing our dirty clothes, they talked severely to us and told my husband to go to the market first and get some clothes; only then we will touch him. From then onwards, we have decided that no matter how many problems there are, we will not go to the hospital."

A 26-year-old pregnant woman shared her experience: "When we went to the government hospital for delivery, I had an expected delivery; my baby girl was born.

We both had no health problems for some time; we were OK. Then, all of a sudden, my daughter started having problems. So, she gave some medicine to my daughter. After a few hours, my daughter was dead. They didn't tell us how it happened. On the contrary, they told that it was our fault, we did not care, so the baby died. We were sure that our daughter was not in this world because of their carelessness. When we told docter, he abused us badly and slapped my husband. We had a daughter, so be quiet; if we had a son, we would have gone to the police, even if we had to borrow money from someone for this. We have two daughters and wanted a son, but we didn't need a daughter. Two daughters were born quickly at home, so we will not go to the hospital this time, and if we have to go, I will go to a private hospital. We have heard that even though money may be spent there, the mother and child do not have to face any problems."

Asha, who works in Basti, told me about an incident with a woman we took to a government hospital for delivery. "Where she died a few hours after delivery. There was no negligence. Everything had happened well. There was a [vaginal] delivery. Both mother and child were fine, but the woman was already weak. We brought her home. Suddenly, her health started deteriorating, and then we came and took her to the nearest nursing home. She was not admitted due to his serious condition. Much time has passed in this process. When we reached the government hospital again, his pulse had stopped. There can be many reasons for sudden deteriorating health, but her family blamed us. Allegations were made against the hospital staff. Since then, we clearly said that if we come to take healthcare and those registered during pregnancy, we will take them to the hospital for delivery. Otherwise, we will not go."

The duration of migration also affects whether women use maternal healthcare services. Women who had lived in the city for a longer period utilized maternal health services more often than those who had lived there for a shorter period.

As a 28-year-old pregnant woman who recently migrated said during an FGD,

Abhi do sal hi shahar mai aaye hyuye hai, 2–4 sal to sahi se kam hi nahi milta, hmarae pas rupya hi nahihota fir doctor dawai ka chakkar kheka. Hmare bacchan ka khana naseeb ho jata ye bhibadi bat hai.

Translation: "The main reason for this is that it's been 2 years since we came to this city, we have not gotten proper work for 2–4 years, due to which we do not have money to go to the hospital, our children and we get food, this is the big thing."

As another 22-year-old pregnant woman said,

Jo aourte pahle se basti mai rah rahi hai unhe koi dikkat nahi hai. Unke liye to sabhi ka sahara hai. Anganwadi wali didi bhi unhi ki bat sunti. Aur unhone unse ye bhi kaha ki koi bhi jaruraat hogi ham sath denge chahe paise ko leke ho ya koi aur jarurt. Lekin wo hmse yesa kuchh nahi kahi. Ham yhan naye hai isliye wo hamse jyada bat nahi karti ham bhi nahi karte. Ham kisi par viswas bhi nahi karte meri mummy ne bola hai ki aram se ghar par hi sab ho jayega.

Translation: "Those who are already living in the settlement have no problem. For them, everyone has support. Anganwadi Asha didi also listened to them. And he also told them that we will support any need, whether it is about money or any other condition. But he didn't say anything like that to us. We are new here, so she only talks to us a little; we also do not. We don't trust anyone; my mother said everything will be done comfortably at home."

According to women's own testimony, they rarely care of themselves; their family and spouse are their priorities, and they lack access to any formal source of knowledge, such as radio, television, or medical personnel, that could raise their awareness of complications during the antenatal period.

In an FGD in Dharkar Basti, a 29-year-old pregnant woman talked about how she gets information from mobile TV: "She says that her husband is educated; he keeps watching on mobile and shows her how she should care for herself at such a time. Checkups are also necessary during pregnancy; the mobile has received this information."

As a 34-year-old recently delivered woman said in an FGD,

Jab mera Lalla (baby boy) hone wala tha ham bacchahoobaykhatirasptalgaye the kyokishaadike 3 saal bad pet se huyithi. Hamari sass ne kah rakha thi ki 1 sal aur kucch nahi hoga to bhaga dengi aur apne Lalla (son) ka dusar vayah karegi. ja khhhtir ham aur hamarr pati dhyan dete the jhan se janakri mil jaye lete rahte the. Us time hamne kam paisa mai aik purana phone bhi kharida tha jisse hame janakari milti rahe.

Translation: "When my lalla [baby boy] was about to be born, we went to the hospital for delivery because I got pregnant after 3 years of marriage. Our mother-in-law said that if nothing happens for 1 more year, she will kick me out and marry off her lalla [son] again. My husband and I used to pay attention to it, where we got information. At that time, we bought an old phone for less money to get information."

17.4 Discussion and Conclusion

Maternal health is an important factor in the development of any country. India has implemented many policies and programs to improve maternal health, such as Janani Suraksha Yojana (JSY), Pradhan Mantri Surakshit Matritva Abhiyan (PMSMA), comprehensive abortion care (CAC), and the Labour Room Quality Improvement Initiative (LaQshya), among others, to improve maternal healthcare and childcare. Because of these policies and programs, India has shown good improvement in reducing maternal death, but a large regional gap between the southern and northern states of India persists. On the other hand, a large rural–urban gap persists in the utilization of maternal healthcare. Such use is higher among urban women than rural ones (Chauhan and Kumar 2016), but women in the slums have a lower utilization of maternal health than other urban women do (Sharma et al. 2020).

This study found that only 43% of pregnant women were able to utilize maternal healthcare in the slums of Prayagraj, Uttar Pradesh. The educational and occupational status of mothers and the distance and time taken to reach a health facility are consistently strong predictors of the use of all the maternal health services considered in this study (Sharma et al. 2020) (Barman et al. 2020). At the individual, most of the women (64%) hadn't undergone any type of formal education, and most of the women (about 75%) worked in rag picking and basket making. Also, a strong relationship exists between poverty and the use of maternal care (Kumar 2010). About 70% of women have to spend more than INR 5000 during delivery, and more than 90% of a woman's family's income was no more than INR 5000 per month.

Many studies have suggested that women with high-quality relations with their family members are more likely to use maternal care (Allendorf 2010) (Zhang et al. 2016). Along with family relations, cultural and gender norms also affect the utilization of maternal health (Mochache et al. 2020) (Wai et al. 2015). This study found a misconception in taking iron pills and regular ANC checkups; found that most of the currently pregnant women had to perform home care; and found that their behavior was influenced by their in-laws and neighbors (Upadhyay et al. 2014).

Migration status has both positive and negative effects on the utilization of maternal healthcare in urban areas, depending on the geographic distance and availability of transportation to health facilities, especially in rural areas. Many studies have shown that migration to urban areas leads to a higher utilization of maternal healthcare (Lindstrom and Muñoz-Franco 2006) (Ali et al. 2018). However, this study found that migrants in slums have to face some problems because of their lack of a support network and their low trust in their neighbors.

Most of the time, the behavior of healthcare professionals is not cooperative with slum women. Many women shared their bad experiences during delivery. The negative attitude and behaviors of healthcare providers was found to erect a barrier that impedes increasing the utilization of maternal healthcare (Mannava et al. 2015; Agarwal et al. 2019).

The results of this study demonstrated that the use of maternal healthcare services depended on a woman's prior pregnancies and deliveries. Women were more likely to use maternal health services if their prior pregnancies or deliveries were problematic. Women who had a good prior pregnancy and delivery experience where everything went smoothly did not consider maternal healthcare service utilization as necessary. Women who had unsatisfactory past experiences with maternal healthcare services were found to have used such services less frequently. Women who were aware of the benefits of these services used maternity healthcare services more often (Choudhury and Ahmed 2011).

Declaration

Availability of Data and Materials The data analyzed in this study are available from the corresponding author upon reasonable request. The corresponding author takes responsibility for the integrity and accuracy of the data analysis.

Ethics Approval and Consent to Participate Verbal consent was needed from all adult study participants, and we obtained verbal consent from adult participants (parents and key informants) and women ages below 18 years who are considered emancipated minors in this context.

Competing Interests The authors declare that they have no competing interests.

Funding This research received no specific grant from public, commercial, or not-for-profit funding agencies.

References

Abor PA, Abekah-Nkrumah G, Sakyi K, Adjasi CKD, Abor J (2011) The socio-economic determinants of maternal health care utilization in Ghana. Int J Soc Econ 38(7):628–648. https://doi.org/10.1108/03068291111139258

Agarwal S, Curtis SL, Angeles G, Speizer IS, Singh K, Thomas JC (2019) The impact of India's accredited social health activist (ASHA) program on the utilization of maternity services: a nationally representative longitudinal modelling study. Hum Resour Health 17(1):68. https://doi.org/10.1186/s12960-019-0402-4

Ali I, Jaleel CPA, Maheshwari N, Rahman H (2018) Migration and maternal health care services utilisation in Uttar Pradesh, India. Social Science Spectrum 4(3):136–146

Allendorf K (2010) The quality of family relationships and use of maternal health-care Services in India. Family Planning 41(4):263. https://about.jstor.org/terms

Barman B, Saha J, Chouhan P (2020) Impact of education on the utilization of maternal health care services: an investigation from National Family Health Survey (2015–16) in India. Child Youth Serv Rev 108:104642. https://doi.org/10.1016/j.childyouth.2019.104642

Chandwani H, Padhiyar N (2013) Utilization of maternal health Care Services in an Urban slum of Gujarat, India. Electronic Physician 5:672

Chauhan BG, Kumar A (2016) Rural-urban differential in utilization of maternal healthcare Services in India: a decomposition analysis. Soc Sci Spect 2(1):49

Chimankar DA, Sahoo H (2011) Factors influencing the utilization of maternal health care services in Uttarakhand. Stud Ethno Med 5(3):209. https://doi.org/10.1080/09735070.2011.11886411

Choudhury N, Ahmed SM (2011) Maternal care practices among the ultra-poor households in rural Bangladesh: a qualitative exploratory study. BMC Pregnancy Childbirth 11:1. https://doi.org/10.1186/1471-2393-11-15

Fatema K, Lariscy JT (2020) Mass media exposure and maternal healthcare utilization in South Asia. SSM—Population Health 11:100614. https://doi.org/10.1016/j.ssmph.2020.100614

Garg S, Agarwal P, Singh M (2007) Maternal health-care utilization among women in an urban slum in Delhi. Indian J Community Med 32(3):203. https://doi.org/10.4103/0970-0218.36829

Kaviarasu SJ, Gladston GX (2015) Status of Women's health in urban sub-standard settlements of Chennai, Tamil Nadu state, India. Eur Acad Res 2(11):14473

Kumar S (2010) Reducing maternal mortality in India: policy, equity, and quality issues. Indian J Public Health 54(2):57–64. https://doi.org/10.4103/0019-557X.73271

Lindstrom DP, Muñoz-Franco E (2006) Migration and maternal health services utilization in rural Guatemala. Soc Sci Med 63(3):706–721. https://doi.org/10.1016/j.socscimed.2006.02.007

Mannava P, Durrant K, Fisher J, Chersich M, Luchters S (2015) Attitudes and behaviours of maternal health care providers in interactions with clients: a systematic review. Glob Health 11(1):36. https://doi.org/10.1186/s12992-015-0117-9

Mochache V, Wanje G, Nyagah L, Lakhani A, El-Busaidy H, Temmerman M, Gichangi P (2020) Religious, socio-cultural norms and gender stereotypes influence uptake and utilization of maternal health services among the Digo community in Kwale, Kenya: a qualitative study. Reprod Health 17(1):71. https://doi.org/10.1186/s12978-020-00919-6

Orwh (2020) Maternal morbidity and mortality: what do we know? how are we addressing it? www.nih.gov/women/maternalhealth

Report of the Working Group on Migration (2017)

Sanneving L, Trygg N, Saxena D, Mavalankar D, Thomsen S (2013) Inequity in India: the case of maternal and reproductive health. Glob Health Action 6(1):19145. https://doi.org/10.3402/gha.v6i0.19145

Sharma S, SarathiMohanty P, Omar R, Viramgami AP, Sharma N (2020) Determinants and utilization of maternal health Care Services in Urban Slums of an Industrialized City, in Western India. J Family Reprod Health. 10.18502/jfrh.v14i2.4351 14:95

SRS (2019) SRS_MMR_Bulletin_2018_2020

Upadhyay P, Liabsuetrakul T, Shrestha AB, Pradhan N (2014) Influence of family members on utilization of maternal health care services among teen and adult pregnant women in Kathmandu, Nepal: a cross-sectional study. Reprod Health 11(1):1. https://doi.org/10.1186/1742-4755-11-92

Wai KM, Shibanuma A, Oo NN, Fillman TJ, Saw YM, Jimba M (2015) Are husbands involving in their spouses' utilization of maternal care services?: a cross-sectional study in Yangon, Myanmar. PLoS One 10(12):e0144135. https://doi.org/10.1371/journal.pone.0144135

Zhang L, Xue C, Wang Y, Zhang L, Liang Y (2016) Family characteristics and the use of maternal health services: a population-based survey in eastern China. Asia Pac Fam Med 15(1):1–8. https://doi.org/10.1186/s12930-016-0030-2

Chapter 18
Inadequate Iron–Folic Acid Consumption Among Pregnant Mothers in India: A Spatial Analysis

Aditya Singh ⓘ, Mahashweta Chakrabarty ⓘ, Sourav Chowdhury ⓘ, Shivani Singh ⓘ, and Rakesh Chandra ⓘ

Abstract Despite guidelines recommending that every expectant mother take 100 iron–folic acid (IFA) tablets or an equivalent amount of syrup for 100 days, over 70% of Indian mothers do not adhere to this recommendation. Understanding the geographical distribution of insufficient IFA intake and the factors influencing it is crucial for developing targeted prevention and intervention strategies. However, prior to this chapter, research exploring the geographic disparities in IFA consumption and its determinants in India has been limited. Therefore, this chapter aims to address this research gap by examining the spatial patterns of inadequate IFA consumption at the district level and identifying the factors explaining these district-level spatial patterns. This chapter analyzed data from 141,875 married women aged 15–49, using the fourth round of the NFHSs (2019–2021). The dependent variable, inadequate IFA, was defined as consuming fewer than the recommended 100 IFA tablets or equivalent syrup. A district-level prevalence map was prepared to assess the spatial pattern of inadequate IFA consumption. Further, spatial clustering in IFA consumption was evaluated by using Moran's I statistic and bivariate local indicators for spatial association (BiLISA) maps. Finally, the correlates of inadequate IFA consumption were examined by using ordinary least squares, spatial lag,

---

A. Singh (✉)
Banaras Hindu University, Varanasi, Uttar Pradesh, India
e-mail: adityasingh@bhu.ac.in

M. Chakrabarty
Department of Geography, Banaras Hindu University, Varanasi, Uttar Pradesh, India

S. Chowdhury
Department of Geography, Raiganj University, Raiganj, West Bengal, India
Department of Geography, Shishuram Das College, Bhusna, West Bengal, India

S. Singh
Independent Researcher, Lucknow, Uttar Pradesh, India

R. Chandra
School of Health System Studies, Tata Institute of Social Sciences, Mumbai, Maharashtra, India

© The Author(s), under exclusive license to Springer Nature Singapore Pte Ltd. 2024
P. Chouhan et al. (eds.), *Sexual and Reproductive Health of Women*,
https://doi.org/10.1007/978-981-97-8418-9_18

and spatial error models. The overall prevalence of inadequate IFA consumption in India was 70%, with substantial spatial heterogeneity across different regions, districts, and even socioeconomic groups. The statistically significant spatial autocorrelation value for inadequate IFA consumption indicated the existence of clustering in the distribution of inadequate IFA consumption across the districts of India. Further analysis revealed that several clusters of high values of inadequate IFA were concentrated primarily in the districts of empowered action group (EAG) states—i.e., Bihar, Uttar Pradesh, Madhya Pradesh, Jharkhand, and Rajasthan. BiLISA analysis revealed that the districts with high rates of inadequate IFA consumption also had high rates of poverty and illiteracy, a higher number of Scheduled Caste (SC) and Scheduled Tribe (ST) mothers, high rates of early marriage, the inadequate coverage of antenatal care (ANC), and low levels of mass-media exposure. Among the three regression models applied, the spatial error model was the best. The results of the model suggested that inadequate IFA consumption at the district level was positively associated with ANC visits and negatively associated with a respondent's education. Considerable spatial heterogeneity exists at the district level in the consumption of inadequate IFA among expectant mothers in India. Redirecting resources to vulnerable subgroups and geographical areas that were identified as lagging in this study would be critical to ensuring equitable progress in reducing IFA deficiency-related anemia among expectant mothers across the country. In addition, appropriate interventions need to be introduced to increase the average number of ANC visits in districts where IFA consumption is substantially low.

Keywords IFA · Iron–folic acid · Spatial analysis · Spatial error model · NFHS · India

18.1 Introduction

India lost an opportunity to meet the fourth and fifth United Nations' *Millennium Development Goals* (MoSPI and G.O.I 2015). Worldwide, 0.28 million maternal deaths occurred in 2015, and India accounted for one-quarter of those deaths (Kassebaum et al. 2016). Despite a half-fold drop in maternal mortality in India (from 482.1 to 248 deaths per 100,000 live births) between 1990 and 2015, the country has a long way to go before achieving the third Sustainable Development Goal by 2030 (from 248 maternal deaths in 2015) (Kassebaum et al. 2016).

Over 20% of all maternal deaths in India are caused by anemia, directly or indirectly (Ministry of Health and Family Welfare 2013b). Iron deficiency anemia during pregnancy is particularly concerning (Lynch 2011; Noronha et al. 2012), with almost half of all pregnant mothers affected according to the report from the fourth round of the National Family Health Surveys (NFHS-4) (International Institute for Population Sciences (IIPS) and ICF 2017; WHO 2011). This condition, resulting from folate and iron deficiencies, has been linked to adverse birth outcomes like preterm labor, low birth weight, and poor child health (Abu-Ouf and Jan 2015; Allen 2000; Di Renzo et al. 2015; Lynch 2011; Wiegersma et al. 2019). To mitigate these risks, iron–folic acid (IFA) supplementation is crucial during pregnancy, administered in tablet or syrup form to boost hemoglobin levels and reduce the likelihood of anemia (Sanghvi et al. 2010).

Under the Reproductive, Maternal, Newborn, Child plus Adolescent Health (RMNCH+A) program, pregnant women receive 100 IFA tablets or an equivalent amount in syrup to support their health during pregnancy (Ministry of Health and Family Welfare 2013a). In 2013, the government of India launched the National Iron+ Initiative as a comprehensive strategy to combat anemia caused by iron deficiency (MoHFW 2013). Despite these efforts, the coverage of adequate IFA among pregnant women remains dismally low, with over 70% not meeting the recommended intake, as per the latest available data (International Institute for Population Sciences (IIPS) and ICF 2017).

Marked geographical inequalities in health and healthcare are common in a country like India, which has continental dimensions. Previous studies have noted significant regional and state-level variation in IFA consumption. However, none of the studies on IFA consumption has assessed the spatial heterogeneity in inadequate IFA consumption among pregnant mothers and associated predictive factors at the district level in India, even though it is needed to inform policy and identify specific programming interventions to achieve greater coverage and rectify geographical inequality in coverage (Banerjee et al. 2020; Mishra et al. 2021; Yeneneh et al. 2018; Chourasia et al. 2017).

Geographical variation in the prevalence of inadequate IFA consumption among mothers may not be observable in an individual-level data analysis (Anselin 1995). Therefore, in this research, district-level spatial data are reorganized by aggregating individual-level data to determine whether any spatial clustering is present in the inadequate IFA consumption among mothers at the district level. If any clustering is present, this research aims to determine whether those clusters are of high or low values and where they are in the country. In addition, spatial regression is conducted to evaluate the factors associated with inadequate IFA consumption across Indian districts.

18.2 Data and Methods

18.2.1 Data Source

The data for this chapter were sourced from NFHS-4, conducted between 2015 and 2016 (International Institute for Population Sciences (IIPS) and ICF 2017). The NFHS is a nationally representative cross-sectional survey that gathers data on diverse demographic, socioeconomic, and health-related topics. Employing a two-stage stratified random sampling approach, NFHS-4 surveyed 699,686 mothers aged 15 to 49 from 601,509 households, achieving a response rate of 97%. The sample for this chapter comprises only mothers who had at least one child in the

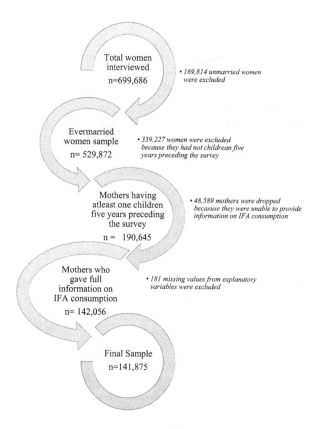

Fig. 18.1 Process of sample selection for this study

5 years preceding the survey and for whom IFA consumption data were available in the NFHS-4 dataset ($n = 141{,}875$). Figure 18.1 illustrates the process of sample selection for this chapter. The data are accessible on the DHS website at www.measuredhs.com.

18.2.2 Outcome Variable

In this chapter, the dependent variable is inadequate IFA consumption, meaning mothers do not consume the 100 IFA tablets or equivalent amount in syrup for 100 days, as recommended by the National Iron+ Initiative (MoHFW 2013). The mothers were asked the following question in the NFHS-4 survey: "During the whole pregnancy, for how many days did you take the tablet or syrup?" The dependent variable was recoded into a binary variable with two categories: (1) inadequate (<100 IFA tablets/equivalent syrup), coded as 1, and (2) adequate (≥100 IFA tablets/equivalent syrup), coded as 0.

18.2.3 Predictor Variables

After conducting an extensive review of the prior research in this area, a wide variety of prospective explanatory variables were chosen for this study (Chourasia et al. 2017; Ogundipe et al. 2012; Roy et al. 2013; Varghese et al. 2019; Wendt et al. 2015). These included the mother's household wealth index, education, social group, religion, year at marriage, mass-media exposure, pregnancy registration, number of ANC visits, and place of residence.

18.2.4 Statistical Analysis

The chapter's main aim is to explore district-level spatial patterns of inadequate IFA consumption and explain them. We employed relevant geospatial techniques, such as Moran-I statistics, univariate LISA, and bivariate LISA, to identify clustering in the distribution and used a set of spatial regression to investigate the relevant correlates of the inadequate IFA consumption at the district level.

In examining spatial patterns, the objective generally is to determine whether spatial features (in our case, districts) with similar values of a variable (e.g., inadequate IFA) are clustered, randomly distributed, or dispersed. Spatial clustering is usually taken as an indication that something of interest is in the spatial distribution that calls for further investigation to understand the reasons behind the observed spatial variation. Although clusters of similar values can be discerned simply by looking at a choropleth map of the variable of interest, such discernment is not always straightforward. Also, a qualitative description of clustering is not always sufficient. Therefore, we quantify the degree to which districts with similar values cluster and where such clustering occurs on the map.

In scientific parlance, the degree to which observations (values) at one spatial location (district) are similar to those of the surrounding locations is referred to as spatial autocorrelation or spatial dependence. A positive spatial autocorrelation occurs when adjacent districts have similar observations. Conversely, negative spatial autocorrelation occurs when neighboring districts tend to have contrasting observations. The presence of spatial autocorrelation in a dataset means that the observations are not independent, which violates a fundamental assumption of statistics, namely the independence of observations. The presence of dependence in observations invalidates most statistical tests. Therefore, checking for the presence of clustering or spatial autocorrelation in spatial datasets is critical for correct statistical inference. Several ways to test for spatial autocorrelation are available, but one of the most popular is Moran's I.

We employed two forms of Moran's I, namely univariate and bivariate Moran's I, to measure spatial autocorrelation at the global scale (Anselin 1995; Anselin et al. 2009). Univariate Moran's I measures the spatial autocorrelation of neighborhood values around a certain geographical position, whereas bivariate Moran's I analyses the correlation between a variable and the weighted average of another variable in the neighborhood.

Local measures of spatial association (LISA) are sued to identify local clusters (observations nearby have similar attribute values) or spatial outliers (observations nearby have different attribute values), unlike global measures that summarize the overall spatial autocorrelation of the study area in one single value. In other words, local measures allow users to identify local "pockets" of spatial autocorrelation that may not be recognized when using global measures. Univariate LISA and bivariate LISA maps were utilized in this chapter to trace the spatial clusters and spatial outliers.

Later in this chapter, a group of regression models was employed to find out the significant correlates of the prevalence of inadequate IFA consumption at the district level in India. To determine the level of autocorrelation in the error term, a spatial ordinary least squares (OLS) regression model was employed. We estimated the spatial lag model (SLM) and the spatial error model (SEM) after the OLS revealed spatial autocorrelation in its error term for the dependent variable (Anselin 1995; Yandell and Anselin 1990). We used ArcGIS 10.5, GeoDa, GeoDaSpace, and Stata 13.1 to analyze our data.

18.3 Results

Table 18.1 presents the socioeconomic background of the mothers who were included in the sample used for analysis in this chapter. More than one-third of mothers were poor, about one-fifth were uneducated, nearly one-third belonged to the Scheduled Caste (SC) and Scheduled Tribe (ST) categories. Most of them were Hindus, about one-third of mothers were married before the age of 18 years (child marriage), and about one-fifth did not have any mass-media exposure. About one-tenth of mothers did not register their pregnancy, and around two-fifth of all mothers did not have four ANC visits, as recommended by the World Health Organization, or WHO (WHO and UNICEF 2003).

Figure 18.2 shows the prevalence of inadequate IFA consumption among pregnant mothers across the districts of India. The color pattern depicts the differences in prevalence throughout the districts. The dark-red color indicates the districts with higher prevalence values for inadequate IFA consumption, whereas the dark-blue color indicates the districts with lower prevalence values for inadequate IFA consumption. More than 75% of the prevalence (higher prevalence) of inadequate IFA consumption is found in the districts of Uttar Pradesh, Bihar, Arunachal Pradesh, Nagaland, and Tripura. Similarly, the central districts of West Bengal and Rajasthan, western districts of Jharkhand, and northern districts of Madhya Pradesh also had higher prevalence values (>75%) for inadequate IFA consumption. We also found that almost all the districts of northern, central, eastern, western, and northeastern regions of India had prevalence values of 50–75% (comparatively high prevalence) for inadequate IFA consumption.

Table 18.1 Background characteristics of the study population, India, 2015–2016

Background characteristics	Weighted % (n = 141,875)
Consumption of IFA	
Adequate (≥100 tablet)	30.00
Inadequate (<100 tablets)	70.00
Wealth quintiles	
Nonpoor	60.40
Poor	39.60
Mother's education	
Educated	77.88
Uneducated	22.12
Social classes	
Non-SC/ST	68.37
SC/ST	31.63
Religion	
Non-Muslim	85.24
Muslim	14.76
Child marriage	
No	65.09
Yes	34.91
Media exposure	
Yes	80.55
No	19.45
Pregnancy registration	
Yes	90.62
No	9.38
ANC visits	
>4 times	59.24
<4 times	40.76
Place of residence	
Urban	32.08
Rural	67.92

n sample

Table 18.2 shows that the Moran's I value of spatial autocorrelation for inadequate IFA consumption is 0.66, indicating the clustering distribution of inadequate IFA consumption across the districts of India. Among the explanatory variables, the highest Moran's I value comes from mothers who had fewer than four ANC visits (0.76), followed by mothers who had a child marriage (0.72), those from the poor wealth quintile (0.71), those with no education (0.71) and those who had no mass-media exposure (0.70). The spatial autocorrelation of mothers who had inadequate IFA consumption and who had fewer than four ANC visits was 0.62 and that of mothers who had inadequate IFA consumption and who had no mass-media exposure was 0.52. Additionally, the spatial autocorrelation of mothers who had inadequate IFA consumption and mothers from the poor wealth quintile was 0.48, and

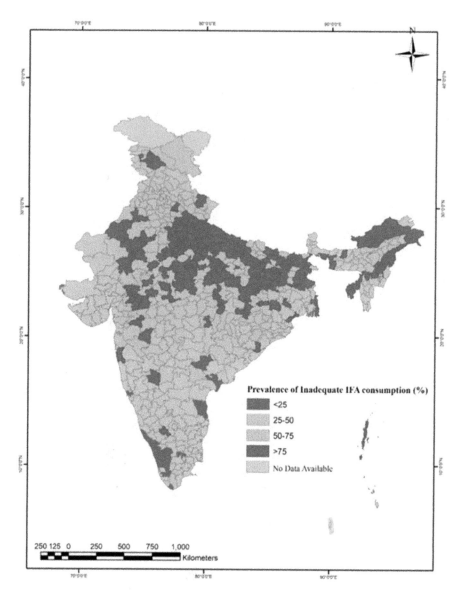

Fig. 18.2 Prevalence of inadequate IFA consumption among pregnant mothers in India, 2015–2016

that of mothers who had inadequate IFA consumption and who had no education was 0.48.

Figure 18.3 depicts the univariate LISA maps for the dependent and independent variables across Indian districts. A significant high-high clustering (hot spots) of inadequate IFA consumption was discovered in the districts of Uttar Pradesh, Bihar, Arunachal Pradesh, West Bengal, Jharkhand, and Madhya Pradesh, which is similar

Table 18.2 Univariate and bivariate Moran's I values for outcomes and predictors in India, 2015–16

Variables	Univariate Moran's I (p-value)	Bivariate Moran's I (p-value)
Inadequate IFA consumption	0.66 (<0.001)	
Poor	0.71 (<0.001)	0.48 (<0.001)
No education	0.71 (<0.001)	0.48 (<0.001)
SC/ST	0.58 (<0.001)	0.06 (0.003)
Muslim	0.69 (<0.001)	0.03 (0.048)
Child marriage	0.72 (<0.001)	0.44 (<0.001)
No mass-media exposure	0.70 (<0.001)	0.52 (<0.001)
No pregnancy registration	0.53 (<0.001)	0.34 (<0.001)
<4 ANC visits	0.76 (<0.001)	0.62 (<0.001)
Rural	0.30 (<0.001)	0.29 (<0.001)

to the hot spots of poor mothers, noneducated mothers, mothers married as children, those with no mass-media exposure, those who went to fewer than four ANC visits, and rural mothers. The districts of Arunachal Pradesh, Nagaland, Meghalaya, Mizoram, Manipur, Jharkhand, Odisha, and Gujarat had SC/ST hotspots. Higher concentrations of Muslim mothers were seen in the areas of West Bengal, Arunachal Pradesh, Jammu & Kashmir, Kerala, and a few districts in western Uttar Pradesh.

The bivariate LISA cluster maps (Fig. 18.4) reveal considerable high-high clustering in both the dependent and independent variables. In the districts of Uttar Pradesh, Madhya Pradesh, Bihar, Jharkhand, West Bengal, Arunachal Pradesh, and Nagaland, high inadequate IFA consumption was clustered with higher proportions of poor mothers, mothers with no education, mothers belonging to the SC/ST social classes, mothers who went to fewer than four ANC visits, mothers with no exposure to mass media, and mothers who married as children.

Table 18.3 presents the spatial regression estimates for the prevalence of inadequate IFA consumption and associated predictors for 640 districts in India. The OLS model revealed that poor mothers (β: 0.115, p: 007), uneducated mothers (β: 0.154, p: 0.002), Muslim mothers (β: 0.115, p: 0.000), mothers who married as children (β: 0.105, p: 0.034), mothers with no mass-media exposure (β: −205, p: 0.003), mothers who went to fewer than four ANC visits (β: 0.526, p: 0.000), and rural mothers (β: 0.075, p: 0.019) were significant ($p < 0.05$) spatial predictors of inadequate IFA consumption in India.

The lag coefficient (Rho) in the SLM was 0.40 (p: 0.000), indicating that a change in inadequate IFA consumption in a particular district may statistically lag behind the prevalence of inadequate IFA consumption in neighboring districts by 40%. In the spatial lag model, uneducated mothers (β: 0.093, p: 0.036), Muslim mothers (β: 0.126, p: 0.000), mothers with no media exposure (β: −0.137, p: 0.024), mothers who went to fewer than four ANC visits (β: 0.362, p: 0.000), and rural mothers (β: 0.086, p: 0.003) were all significantly associated with the prevalence of inadequate IFA consumption in India.

The model with the lowest Akaike information criterion (AIC) and highest R-square value is considered the best model. In our case, SEM had the lowest AIC

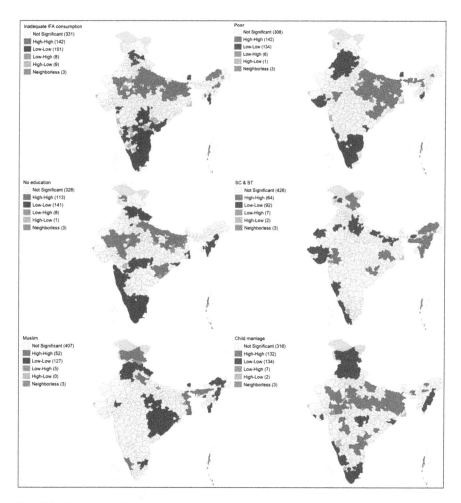

Fig. 18.3 Univariate LISA (cluster) maps for dependent and explanatory variables for districts of India, 2015–2016. *Note*: High-High: districts with higher prevalence share boundaries with districts with the same prevalence; Low-Low: districts with lower prevalence share boundaries with districts with the same prevalence; Low-High: districts with lower prevalence surrounded by higher-prevalence districts; and High-Low: districts that have higher prevalence are bordered by lower-prevalence districts

and the highest adjusted R-square value, making it the best model out of the three. The AIC value for the spatial error model was −958.5, and the adjusted R-square value was 0.72. The Lambda value (spatial autoregressive coefficient)/error lag was 0.55 ($p < 0.001$), indicating that a spatial influence on the prevalence of inadequate IFA consumption from the omitted variables was not present in the SEM.

According to the model, if the proportion of mothers with no education increased by 10% in a district, the prevalence of inadequate IFA consumption would rise by 1.3%. Similarly, if the proportion of Muslim mothers in a district rose by 10%, the

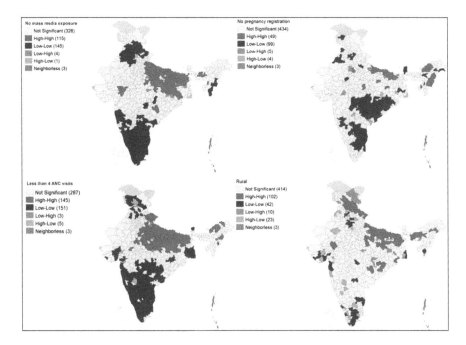

Fig. 18.3 (continued)

prevalence of inadequate IFA consumption would rise by 1%. If a 10% increase in the proportion of mothers who did not follow the WHO guideline of four ANC visits (fewer than four ANC visits) in a district took place, inadequate IFA consumption would increase by 4.6%, and if the proportion of mothers from rural areas increased 10%, the prevalence of inadequate IFA consumption would increase by 1%. These results simply imply that districts with a higher percentage of mothers who went to than four ANC visits and who had no education have a higher likelihood for the prevalence of inadequate IFA consumption.

18.4 Discussion

This chapter examined the spatial variation in inadequate IFA consumption among India mothers during pregnancy. A positive Moran's I indicates the presence of high spatial autocorrelation—i.e., the clustering distribution of inadequate IFA consumption across the districts of India. Inadequate IFA consumption was very high, over 70%, in many districts in Uttar Pradesh, Bihar, Arunachal Pradesh, Nagaland, and Tripura. In the end, mothers with no education, Muslim mothers, mothers who went to fewer than four ANC visits, and mothers from rural areas were observed to be positively associated with inadequate IFA consumption at the district level in India.

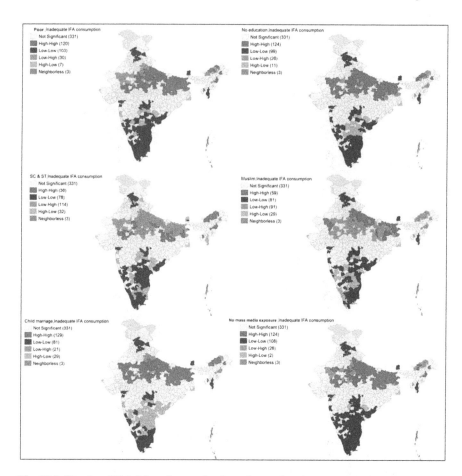

Fig. 18.4 Bivariate LISA (cluster) maps for dependent and explanatory variables for districts of India, 2015–2016. *Note*: High-High: districts with higher prevalence share boundaries with districts with the same prevalence; Low-Low: districts with lower prevalence share boundaries with districts with the same prevalence; Low-High: districts with lower prevalence surrounded by higher-prevalence districts; and High-Low: districts that have higher prevalence are bordered by lower-prevalence districts

This study revealed that inadequate IFA consumption is concentrated among illiterate mothers in empowered action group (EAG) states (Arokiasamy and Gautam 2008). Mothers who are illiterate do not have adequate opportunities to learn about pregnancy and childbirth (Anya et al. 2008). Thus, they are less informed about good healthcare practices and medications during pregnancy, which results in inadequate IFA consumption. Other research has found similar outcomes (Chourasia et al. 2017).

In India, mothers from Bihar, Uttar Pradesh, and Madhya Pradesh, where about 89%, 78%, and 72% of the entire population, respectively, resides in rural regions, are more susceptible to inadequate IFA consumption (Office of the Registrar

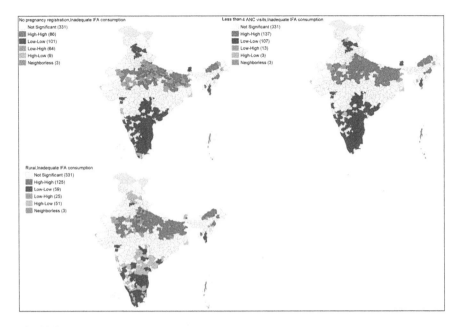

Fig. 18.4 (continued)

Table 18.3 Spatial regression estimates showing factors associated with inadequate IFA consumption in India, 2015–2016

Variables	OLS (p-value)	SLM (p-value)	SEM (p-value)
Poor	0.115 (0.007)	0.060 (0.116)	0.062 (0.206)
No education	0.154 (0.002)	0.093 (0.036)	0.127 (0.031)
SC/ST	0.025 (0.304)	0.038 (0.083)	0.015 (0.588)
Muslim	0.155 (0.000)	0.126 (0.000)	0.108 (0.008)
Child marriage	0.105 (0.034)	0.064 (0.148)	0.102 (0.082)
No mass-media exposure	−0.205 (0.003)	−0.137 (0.024)	−0.095 (0.178)
No pregnancy registration	0.086 (0.111)	0.024 (0.615)	0.011 (0.853)
< 4 ANC visits	0.526 (0.000)	0.362 (0.000)	0.455 (0.000)
Rural	0.075 (0.019)	0.086 (0.003)	0.086 (0.006)
Rho		0.40 (0.000)	
Lambda			0.55 (0.000)
AIC	−855.9	−955.3	−958.5
Adjusted R	0.64	0.71	0.72

AIC Akaike information criterion, *OLS* ordinary least squares, *SLM* spatial lag model, *SEM* spatial error model

General and Census Commissioner 2011). Previous research has indicated that geographical access to health facilities has a heavy impact on healthcare services utilization, especially in rural areas with low availability of services (Kesterton et al. 2010; Singh et al. 2012; Tanou et al. 2021; Weisgrau 1995). Apart from accessibility, deep-rooted traditional perceptions—"lay health culture"—about childbirth among rural mothers might be another factor contributing to their inadequate IFA consumption (Mattson 2010). Childbirth is still considered a natural state of being rather than a medical condition for mothers in rural India, and mothers rarely seek preventive and curative medical services to safeguard their own health and well-being (Kumar and Singh 2016).

Inadequate IFA consumption is higher among Muslim mothers, indicating that the utilization of maternal healthcare services was lower among Muslim mothers than non-Muslim mothers, similar to the findings in previous research (Barman et al. 2020; Gogoi et al. 2014; Navaneetham and Dharmalingam 2002; Singh et al. 2014a. The Sachar Committee, which was formed to perform a comprehensive assessment of the Muslim community's social, economic, and educational status, concluded that Muslims "exhibit deficits and deprivation in practically all dimensions of development" and that "the deficits are particularly salient in the areas of female schooling and economic status" (Haneefa 2020). Apart from poverty and illiteracy, religious and societal limitations like the burka/niqab, the physical separation of girls/women from boys/men, and the obligation for mothers to cover and hide their bodies seem to adversely affect mothers' healthcare behaviors (Singh et al. 2014b). Muslim mothers' lack of autonomy restricts their contact with men outside of their own household. Therefore, the presence of male doctors in hospitals may be a barrier to the utilization of healthcare services given that Muslim mothers often avoid male physicians for prenatal care and delivery support (Singh et al. 2014a).

One of the major findings of our study is that mothers who went to fewer than four ANC visits had inadequate IFA consumption, especially in the districts of Uttar Pradesh, Bihar, Madhya Pradesh, Rajasthan, and Arunachal Pradesh. Full ANC (four or more ANC visits) is effective in improving the health of mothers and birth outcomes. According to the WHO, every pregnant mother should go to at least four antenatal visits, with the first one preferably in the first trimester (WHO and UNICEF 2003). A skilled ANC provider usually provides IFA tablets/equivalent amounts of syrup for only 1 month at a single ANC visit (Kumar et al. 2019). This indicates that if a mother has fewer ANC visits, she is more likely to consume an inadequate number of IFA tablets.

Despite the government's Anemia Mukt Bharat (AMB) strategy, launched in 2018, which included preventive iron–folic acid supplementation in target groups of mothers, children, and adolescents in all Indian states, IFA consumption is not evenly distributed. The districts in Uttar Pradesh, Bihar, Jharkhand, and Madhya Pradesh exhibited the largest clustering of inadequate IFA consumption across all explanatory factors. During policy intervention, greater attention should be paid to the districts of these states to minimize inadequate IFA consumption. In short-term interventions, the number of ANC visits should be increased for all the high-high clustering districts of India. Simultaneously, the focus should be on mass awareness campaigns and door-to-door visitation programs. Frontline health workers like accredited social health activists (ASHA) can play important roles in disseminating crucial information about the benefits of adequate IFA consumption during pregnancy, particularly in the rural areas of high-high clustering districts that were identified in this chapter. Girls' education should be prioritized in long-term interventions, particularly in the states of Uttar Pradesh, Bihar, and Madhya Pradesh. In addition, religious beliefs that obstruct the utilization of proper healthcare services, including adequate IFA consumption, particularly for Muslim mothers, should be eliminated.

This chapter has certain limitations that the reader should be aware of. First, the number of IFA tablets consumed by mothers during pregnancy in the NFHS-4 is based on self-reporting. Even though the NFHS-4 has made several attempts to address the issue of data falsification, we cannot assume that the data are always 100% accurate, due to the inability to recall. As a result, while applying the findings and interpretations presented in this work, readers and users must keep this in mind. Second, because the data come from a cross-sectional survey, the association between dependent and independent factors in this chapter cannot be regarded as causality. Hence, the result must always be regarded with caution. Third, because this chapter included only those variables that were available in the NFHS-4 data, omitted variable bias may be present.

18.5 Conclusion

In India, around 70% of pregnant mothers do not consume the recommended 100 IFA tablets during pregnancy. No doubt, the reproductive and child health (RCH) initiative and the National Iron+ Initiative in India have reduced inadequate IFA consumption among pregnant mothers, yet a substantial geographic heterogeneity persists in IFA consumption. Inadequate IFA consumption was highly concentrated in the EAG states. Being illiterate, rural, and Muslim and going to fewer than four ANC visits were some of the factors explaining the district-level heterogeneity in inadequate IFA consumption among mothers. Districts where vulnerable groups of women are concentrated should be targeted with appropriate policy measures and programmatic interventions to increase the consumption of IFA.Declaration

Availability of Data and Material Data and materials for this chapter are sourced from publicly available secondary sources and accessible at https://dhsprogram.com/methodology/survey/survey-display-541.cfm. Interested individuals can register at the provided link to freely download the necessary data.

Ethics Approval and Consent to Participate This chapter is based on secondary data, which are available in the public domain. Therefore, ethical approval is not required to conduct this study.

Competing Interests The authors declare that they have no competing interests.

Funding This chapter did not receive any specific grant from funding agencies in the public, commercial, or not-for-profit sectors.

References

Abu-Ouf NM, Jan MM (2015) The impact of maternal iron deficiency and iron deficiency anemia on child's health. Saudi Med J 36(2):146. https://doi.org/10.15537/SMJ.2015.2.10289

Allen LH (2000) Anemia and iron deficiency: effects on pregnancy outcome. Am J Clin Nutr 71(5):1280S–1284S. https://doi.org/10.1093/AJCN/71.5.1280S

Anselin L (1995) Local indicators of spatial association—LISA. Geogr Anal 27(2):93–115. https://doi.org/10.1111/j.1538-4632.1995.tb00338.x

Anselin L, Syabri I, Kho Y (2009) GeoDa: an introduction to spatial data analysis. In: Handbook of applied spatial analysis, pp 73–89. https://doi.org/10.1007/978-3-642-03647-7_5

Anya SE, Hydara A, Jaiteh LE (2008) Antenatal care in The Gambia: missed opportunity for information, education and communication. BMC Pregnancy Childbirth 8(1):1–7. https://doi.org/10.1186/1471-2393-8-9

Arokiasamy P, Gautam A (2008) Neonatal mortality in the empowered action group states of India: trends and determinants. J Biosoc Sci 40(2):183–201. https://doi.org/10.1017/S0021932007002623

Banerjee A, Singh AK, Chaurasia H (2020) An exploratory spatial analysis of low birth weight and its determinants in India. Clin Epidemiol Global Health 8(3):702–711. https://doi.org/10.1016/j.cegh.2020.01.006

Barman B, Saha J, Chouhan P (2020) Impact of education on the utilization of maternal health care services: an investigation from National Family Health Survey (2015–16) in India. Child Youth Serv Rev 108:104642. https://doi.org/10.1016/J.CHILDYOUTH.2019.104642

Chourasia A, Pandey CM, Awasthi A (2017) Factors influencing the consumption of iron and folic acid supplementations in high focus states of India. Clin Epidemiol Global Health 5(4):180–184. https://doi.org/10.1016/j.cegh.2017.04.004

Di Renzo GC, Spano F, Giardina I, Brillo E, Clerici G, Roura LC (2015) Iron deficiency anemia in pregnancy. Womens Health 11(6):891–900. https://doi.org/10.2217/WHE.15.35

Gogoi M, Unisa S, Prusty RK (2014) Utilization of maternal health care services and reproductive health complications in Assam, India. J Public Health 22(4):351–359. https://doi.org/10.1007/S10389-014-0614-Y

Haneefa M (2020) The educational status of Indian Muslims a decade after the Sachar Committee report. SSRN Electron J. https://doi.org/10.2139/SSRN.3647513

International Institute for Population Sciences (IIPS) and ICF (2017) National Family Health Survey (NFHS-4), 2015–16: India. IIPS, Mumbai

Kassebaum NJ, Barber RM, Dandona L, Hay SI, Larson HJ, Lim SS, Lopez AD, Mokdad AH, Naghavi M, Pinho C, Steiner C, Vos T, Wang H, Achoki T, Anderson GM, Arora M, Biryukov S, Blore JD, Carter A et al (2016) Global, regional, and national levels of maternal mortality, 1990–2015: a systematic analysis for the global burden of disease study 2015. Lancet 388(10053):1775–1812. https://doi.org/10.1016/S0140-6736(16)31470-2

Kesterton AJ, Cleland J, Sloggett A, Ronsmans C (2010) Institutional delivery in rural India: the relative importance of accessibility and economic status. BMC Pregnancy Childbirth 10(1):1–9. https://doi.org/10.1186/1471-2393-10-30

Kumar A, Singh A (2016) Explaining the gap in the use of maternal healthcare services between social groups in India. J Public Health 38(4):771–781. https://doi.org/10.1093/pubmed/fdv142

Kumar G, Choudhary TS, Srivastava A, Upadhyay RP, Taneja S, Bahl R, Martines J, Bhan MK, Bhandari N, Mazumder S (2019) Utilisation, equity and determinants of full antenatal care in India: analysis from the National Family Health Survey 4. BMC Pregnancy Childbirth 19(1):1–9. https://doi.org/10.1186/S12884-019-2473-6

Lynch SR (2011) Why nutritional iron deficiency persists as a worldwide problem. J Nutr 141(4):763S–768S. https://doi.org/10.3945/JN.110.130609

Mattson J (2010) Transportation, distance, and health care utilization for older adults in rural and small urban areas. Transp Res Rec 2265(1):192–199. https://doi.org/10.3141/2265-22

Ministry of Health and Family Welfare (2013a) A strategic approach to reproductive, maternal, newborn, child and adolescent health (RMNCH+A) in India. https://nhm.gov.in/images/pdf/RMNCH+A/RMNCH+A_Strategy.pdf

Ministry of Health and Family Welfare (2013b) Guidelines for control of iron deficiency anaemia. National Rural Health Mission, p 54

Mishra PS, Kumar P, Srivastava S (2021) Regional inequality in the Janani Suraksha Yojana coverage in India: a geo-spatial analysis. Int J Equity Health 20(1):1–14. https://doi.org/10.1186/S12939-020-01366-2

MoHFW (2013) National Iron+ Initiative: guidelines for control of iron deficiency anaemia. https://www.nhm.gov.in/images/pdf/programmes/child-health/guidelines/Control-of-Iron-Deficiency-Anaemia.pdf

MoSPI & G.O.I (2015) Millennium Development Goals: India Country Report 2015. http://mospi.nic.in/sites/default/files/publication_reports/mdg_2july15_1.pdf

Navaneetham K, Dharmalingam A (2002) Utilization of maternal health care services in southern India. Soc Sci Med 55(10):1849–1869. https://doi.org/10.1016/S0277-9536(01)00313-6

Noronha JA, Al Khasawneh E, Seshan V, Ramasubramaniam S, Raman S (2012) Anemia in pregnancy—consequences and challenges: a review of literature. J South Asian Fed Obstetr Gynaecol 4(1):64–70. https://doi.org/10.5005/jp-journals-10006-1177

Office of the Registrar General & Census Commissioner (2011) Census of India, Ministry of Home Affairs, Government of India. http://censusindia.gov.in/

Ogundipe O, Hoyo C, Østbye T, Oneko O, Manongi R, Lie RT, Daltveit AK (2012) Factors associated with prenatal folic acid and iron supplementation among 21,889 pregnant women in northern Tanzania: a cross-sectional hospital-based study. BMC Public Health 12(1):1–10

Roy MP, Mohan U, Kumar Singh S, Kumar Singh V, Kumar Srivastava A, Pratim Roy M (2013) Socio-economic determinants of adherence to iron and folic acid tablets among rural ante-natal mothers in Lucknow, India. Natl J Commun Med 4(3):386–391. www.njcmindia.org

Sanghvi TG, Harvey PWJ, Wainwright E (2010) Maternal iron–folic acid supplementation programs: evidence of impact and implementation. Food Nutr Bull 31(2 Suppl):S100. https://doi.org/10.1177/15648265100312S202

Singh PK, Rai RK, Alagarajan M, Singh L (2012) Determinants of maternity care services utilization among married adolescents in rural India. PLoS One 7(2):e31666. https://doi.org/10.1371/JOURNAL.PONE.0031666

Singh A, Kumar A, Pranjali P (2014a) Utilization of maternal healthcare among adolescent mothers in urban India: evidence from DLHS-3. PeerJ 2014(1):e592. https://doi.org/10.7717/peerj.592

Singh PK, Kumar C, Rai RK, Singh L (2014b) Factors associated with maternal healthcare services utilization in nine high focus states in India: a multilevel analysis based on 14 385 communities in 292 districts. Health Policy Plan 29(5):542–559. https://doi.org/10.1093/HEAPOL/CZT039

Tanou M, Kishida T, Kamiya Y (2021) The effects of geographical accessibility to health facilities on antenatal care and delivery services utilization in Benin: a cross-sectional study. Reprod Health 18(1):1–11. https://doi.org/10.1186/S12978-021-01249-X

Varghese JS, Swaminathan S, Kurpad AV, Thomas T (2019) Demand and supply factors of iron–folic acid supplementation and its association with anaemia in north Indian pregnant women. PLoS One 14(1):e0210634

Weisgrau S (1995) Issues in rural health: access, hospitals, and reform. Health Care Financ Rev 17(1):1

Wendt A, Stephenson R, Young M, Webb-Girard A, Hogue C, Ramakrishnan U, Martorell R (2015) Individual and facility-level determinants of iron and folic acid receipt and adequate consumption among pregnant women in rural Bihar, India. PLoS One 10(3):e0120404. https://doi.org/10.1371/JOURNAL.PONE.0120404

WHO (2011) The global prevalence of anaemia in 2011. https://apps.who.int/iris/bitstream/handle/10665/177094/9789241564960_eng.pdf

WHO & UNICEF (2003) Antenatal care in developing countries: promises, achievements, and missed opportunities: an analysis of trends, levels, and differentials. World Health Organization, Geneva

Wiegersma AM, Dalman C, Lee BK, Karlsson H, Gardner RM (2019) Association of prenatal maternal anemia with neurodevelopmental disorders. JAMA Psychiatry 76(12):1294. https://doi.org/10.1001/JAMAPSYCHIATRY.2019.2309

Yandell BS, Anselin L (1990) Spatial econometrics: methods and models. J Am Stat Assoc 85:905. https://doi.org/10.2307/2290042

Yeneneh A, Alemu K, Dadi AF, Alamirrew A (2018) Spatial distribution of antenatal care utilization and associated factors in Ethiopia: evidence from Ethiopian demographic health surveys. BMC Pregnancy Childbirth 18(1):1–12. https://doi.org/10.1186/S12884-018-1874-2

Chapter 19
Maternal and Child Healthcare Utilization and Corresponding Expenditure in India

Rupa Dutta

Abstract This chapter provides a comprehensive contextualization of maternal and child healthcare utilization and associated expenditure in India, drawing insights from National Sample Survey data and employing descriptive statistics. The findings highlight commendable immunization coverage in the country, with minimal socioeconomic disparities, yet they reveal a slight discrepancy in expenditure based on the place of residence. Despite a significant increase in pre- and postnatal care services, substantial variation persists across social and economic groups and among states. This chapter emphasizes a consistent rise in expenditure on pre- and postnatal care in India, accompanied by discernible socioeconomic and residential differences. Institutional deliveries in government hospitals have notably increased, with some states leading in the accessibility of private facilities. The utilization expenditure for maternal healthcare, particularly in private facilities, has seen a gradual rise. Given these findings, policy recommendations are crucial to further improve healthcare outcomes. Targeted strategies for equitable immunization funding should be implemented, addressing residence-based expenditure disparities. Tailoring healthcare outreach programs to diverse socioeconomic groups and regions can enhance the utilization of pre- and postnatal care services. Policymakers should focus on making maternal healthcare more affordable and accessible, with investments in infrastructure and training to bridge gaps in access to private facilities. These policy measures aim to build on existing achievements and ensure that maternal and child healthcare services are accessible and equitable across the socioeconomic spectrum and geographical locations in India.

Keywords Maternal and child healthcare · Healthcare expenditure · Healthcare inequality · India

R. Dutta (✉)
Department of Promotion of Industry and Internal Trade (DPIIT), Ministry of Commerce and Industry, New Delhi, India

19.1 Introduction

Maternal and child healthcare (MCH) utilization has been positively correlated with maternal and child survival and well-being (Roy et al. 2021). Recognizing the pivotal role of maternal health in addressing broader economic, social, and developmental challenges, the World Health Organization (WHO) advocates for a comprehensive approach known as the maternal continuum of care (CoC). The maternal CoC, endorsed by the WHO, emphasizes key components essential for ensuring the health and well-being of mothers and newborns. This continuum comprises four crucial elements: eight or more antenatal care visits, skilled birth attendant delivery, and postnatal care within 48 h (Rahaman et al. 2024b). This structured approach serves as instrumental support, promoting maternal and newborn well-being through routine antenatal health screenings, safe delivery practices, and postnatal care support. Over time, the government of India (GoI) has undertaken various maternal and child health programs to align itself with global initiatives and achieve a United Nations' Sustainable Development Goal (SDG), which focuses on ensuring healthy lives and promoting well-being for all (Rana and Goli 2021). These initiatives aim to enhance healthcare accessibility, particularly for maternal and child health, contributing to the broader agenda of achieving sustainable and inclusive development.

In particular, the government of India (GoI), through its National Health Mission (NHM), has implemented a comprehensive range of maternal and child health programs aimed at enhancing the safety of maternity experiences by improving both the coverage and quality of healthcare services (Ghosh and Ghosh 2020). A noteworthy initiative under this mission is the Janani Suraksha Yojana (JSY), introduced in 2005 as a call promotion scheme. JSY focuses on reducing maternal and infant mortality rates and operates as a conditional cash transfer program for pregnant women who opt for institutional deliveries. In addition to JSY, the Janani Shishu Suraksha Karyakram (JSSK), launched in 2011, strives to eliminate out-of-pocket expenses (OOPEs) for pregnant women, newborns, and infants by covering costs related to drugs, diet, diagnostics, user charges, referral transport, and more (Ajmer et al. 2023). JSSK ensures that all pregnant women delivering in public health institutions receive free and comprehensive care, including caesarean sections. Further fortifying the maternal health landscape is the Pradhan Mantri Surakshit Matritva Abhiyan (PMSMA), launched in 2016 by the Ministry of Health & Family Welfare. This initiative aims to provide assured, high-quality antenatal care at no cost to all pregnant women. Simultaneously, the DAKSHATA scheme, also implemented by the government of India, strengthens intrapartum and immediate postpartum care by enhancing the competency of healthcare providers on the basis of evidence-based practices and established labor room protocols.

India has made commendable progress in reducing maternal deaths over the past two decades. In 1990, the maternal mortality ratio (MMR) was alarmingly high at 600 deaths per hundred thousand live births. However, due to concerted efforts and the implementation of various programs, the MMR declined significantly. It dropped from 301 per hundred thousand live births in 2001–2003 to 97 in 2018–2020 (Meh et al. 2022). Similarly, the neonatal mortality rate (NNMR) decreased from 43 per thousand live births in 2011 to 25 per thousand live births in 2021. This remarkable improvement underscores the effectiveness of India's maternal and child health initiatives in enhancing the well-being of mothers and infants (Ajmer et al. 2023). Despite significant strides in maternal and child healthcare utilization and well-being in India, substantial geographical and socioeconomic disparities persist (Roy et al. 2021). Existing studies have underscored the lower levels of maternal and child healthcare utilization, particularly in economically weaker states, known as empowered action group (EAG) states, and among socioeconomically vulnerable groups (Rana et al. 2019). The discourse on regional and social inequalities in maternal healthcare utilization and overall well-being points to both structural and socioeconomic factors. Structural factors play a pivotal role, with healthcare infrastructure varying significantly across the country. For instance, the level of healthcare services in Tamil Nadu are notably higher than are those in Bihar, due to limited access to quality healthcare options in Bihar (Roy et al. 2021). Moreover, sociocultural indicators such as female education levels, women's autonomy, and the formal workforce participation rate are lower in EAG states compared to non-EAG states (Roy et al. 2023). These factors are positively associated with a lack of awareness regarding maternal healthcare, insufficient knowledge about modern healthcare sources, and a preference for traditional maternity practices, collectively leading to reduced maternal healthcare utilization in EAG states. In addition to structural and sociocultural drivers, the high OOPEs associated with maternal and child healthcare emerges as a significant barrier to service utilization (Balla et al. 2022). Recent studies have highlighted that despite the government's promotion of free comprehensive maternal and child health services in public health facilities, the imbalance between demand and capacity forces socioeconomically disadvantaged individuals to seek services from profit-making healthcare facilities (Roy et al. 2021). Consequently, a substantial number of households in India face financial distress daily while attempting to access maternal and child health services (Kumar and Anil Kumar 2021). Beyond the public health service demand and supply debate, certain maternal services, medications, and routine travel costs to maternal health and well-being centers are not included in public maternal health schemes (Leone et al. 2013). This omission significantly contributes to OOPEs. Furthermore, the low coverage of health insurance among Indians is another contributing factor to issues related to OOPEs in India. The narrative highlights the persisting disparities in maternal and child healthcare, shedding light on the multifaceted challenges that need attention to achieve more-equitable healthcare outcomes in the country. Given the existing disparities in maternal and child health and well-being across various social and administrative strata in India (Roy et al. 2021; Yadav and Jena 2022), this chapter seeks to explore the variations in maternal and child healthcare utilization levels. The focus extends to understanding these variations across different social groups, wealth quintiles, and state boundaries. A critical aspect of this examination involves addressing the question of whether the gaps in maternal and child healthcare utilization across these factors have diminished or remained constant over time.

Through these analyses, this chapter aims to provide valuable insights into identifying segments of the population that may have been neglected in the progress toward improved maternal and child health outcomes.

19.2 Data and Methodology

This research relies primarily on unit-record data extracted from the most recent three rounds of the National Sample Survey (NSS) focusing on healthcare: the 60th round (January–June 2004), the 71st round (January–June 2014), and the 75th round (2017–2018). These rounds employed a multistage stratified sampling approach to gather extensive information on morbidity, healthcare usage, and healthcare expenses, among other pertinent parameters. The NSS data utilized in this investigation span a wide array of details, encompassing personal characteristics, household features, education, health status, housing amenities, access to facilities, household possessions, and living conditions. The surveys conducted during these specific rounds comprehensively addressed healthcare services, contributing to a holistic assessment of health outcomes. The unit-record data from the NSS rounds play a pivotal role in this study, providing intricate insights into health-related aspects, healthcare expenditure, and various sociodemographic and economic dimensions. By concentrating on NSS data, the study ensures a nuanced examination of healthcare dynamics and their intersections with different socioeconomic factors. The robust multistage stratified sampling methodology applied in NSS rounds enhances the representativeness and reliability of the gathered data, thereby reinforcing the analytical foundation of the study. In essence, this research taps into the wealth of NSS data to shed light on patterns and trends in health outcomes, healthcare expenditure, and sociodemographic and economic characteristics. This approach not only highlights the significance of NSS as a valuable data source but also underscores the depth and comprehensiveness of the study's exploration into the complexities of healthcare dynamics and their broader implications. Descriptive statistics, specifically employing percentage distribution and proportions, were utilized to present the findings in each chapter. The expenditures of maternal and child healthcare utilization are presented in this chapter by adjusting for inflation while considering the NSS 75th round expenditure as the baseline.

19.3 Results

19.3.1 Coverage and Expenditure Related to Child Immunization

Figure 19.1 clearly shows the substantial changes in immunization levels over time, irrespective of an individual's place of residence. The percentage of children receiving vaccines has increased from 89% in 2004 to 97% in 2018 in rural areas. In urban areas, it has increased from 94% to 98% during the same period.

Figure 19.2 displays the levels of average immunization expenditure according to Indians' place of residence during 2004 to 2018. The average immunization expenditure was higher in urban areas (INR 251) than in rural ones (INR 36) during 2018. A similar rural–urban gap in average immunization expenditure (INR 20 in rural and INR 113 in urban) was also observed in 2004. The average spending on immunization in both rural and urban areas doubled between 2004 and 2018.

A significant difference appeared in average expenditure on immunization according to gender in India, irrespective of an individual's place of residence (Fig. 19.3). In 2004, the average expenditure was INR 22 for boys and INR 17 for girls in rural areas. However, the expenditure increased to INR 42 for boys and INR 29 for girls in 2018 in rural areas. In urban areas, the average expenditure was INR 109 for boys and INR 118 for girls in 2004, which increased to INR 243 for boys and INR 260 for girls in 2018. In addition, the average immunization expenditure gap was lower in urban settings than in their rural counterparts (Fig. 19.3).

No significant difference was found in immunization coverage based on social group throughout the NSS rounds. A small difference in immunization coverage was observed between the first wealth quintile (94.2%) and fifth wealth quintile (97.8%) groups in 2018 (Table 19.1). The level of receiving immunization increased slightly from 2004 to 2018 across the social and wealth quintile groups (Table 19.1).

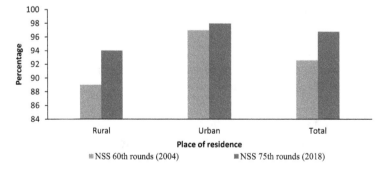

Fig. 19.1 Children receiving any vaccine according to place of residence, India, NSS, 2004 and 2018. (*Source*: Author's estimation from NSS 60th and 75th rounds)

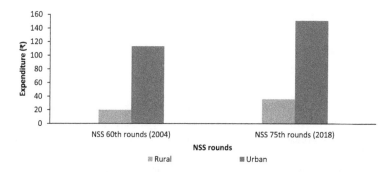

Fig. 19.2 Average immunization expenditure in India according to place of residence, 2004 and 2018. (*Source*: Author's estimation from NSS 60th and 75th rounds. All results are inflation adjusted)

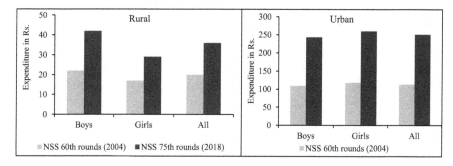

Fig. 19.3 Average immunization expenditure in India according to gender and place of residence, 2004 and 2018. (*Source*: Author's estimation from NSS 60th and 75th rounds. All results are inflation adjusted)

The average expenditure has increased manifold between 2004 and 2017, about twofold for the bottom-most income quintile and about threefold for the richest income quintile (Table 19.2).

19.3.2 Coverage and Expenditure Related to Pre- and Postnatal Care

Figure 19.4 clearly shows remarkably high coverage for pre- and postnatal care, where prenatal care even in rural areas has risen from 69.8% to 97% over a 20-year period, whereas that for urban areas has risen from 83.6% to 98%. For postnatal care, the concomitant increase has been from 62.6% to 87% in rural areas and from 72.9% to 90% in urban areas.

Table 19.1 Number of children receiving any immunization according to their social group and household wealth quintile in NSS 60th and 75th rounds

	NSS 60th rounds (2004)	NSS 75th rounds (2018)
Social group		
ST	91.6	96.2
SC	92.6	96.2
OBC	92.0	97.1
General	93.9	97.0
Wealth quintile		
1st quintile	92.9	94.2
2nd quintile	92.4	97.1
3rd quintile	92.0	95.9
4th quintile	92.7	97.4
5th quintile	93.2	97.8

Source: Author's estimation from NSS 60th and 75th rounds

Table 19.2 Average expenditure on immunization according to social group and household wealth quintile in NSS 60th and 75th rounds

	NSS 60th round (2004)	NSS 75th round (2018)
Social group		
ST	22	29
SC	38	39
OBC	46	84
General	51	187
Total	43	91
Wealth quintile		
1st quintile	22	41
2nd quintile	27	23
3rd quintile	32	34
4th quintile	51	64
5th quintile	73	235

Source: Author's estimation from NSS 60th and 75th rounds. All results are inflation adjusted

The average expenditure on antenatal care has almost doubled between 2004 and 2018 in both rural and urban areas. However, the change in postnatal care expenditure was comparatively lower than that in prenatal care expenditure (Fig. 19.5).

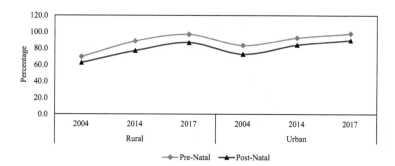

Fig. 19.4 Women's availing themselves of antenatal and postnatal care across NSS rounds, India, 2004–2017 (%). (*Source*: Author's estimation from NSS 60th, 71st, and 75th rounds)

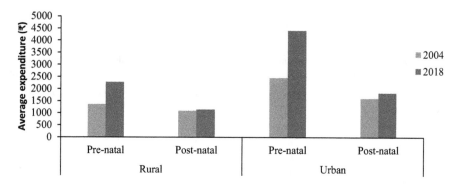

Fig. 19.5 Average expenditure on pre- and postnatal care according to place of residence across NSS 60th and 75th rounds, India, 2004–2018. (*Source*: Author's estimation from NSS 60th and 75th rounds. All results are inflation adjusted)

19.3.3 Coverage and Expenditure Related to Institutional Delivery Care

Another relevant process input is the levels of institutional delivery. A comparative picture over the rounds indicates that the percentage distribution of institutional delivery, including private and public sector, has improved. The percentage of home delivery has reduced from 34.5% in 2004 to 8.2% in India in 2018 (Table 19.3).

As a result, the increase at all levels in India from 64% to 69.2% between the 71st and 75th rounds reveals a higher share of public/government hospitals, with states like Assam, Bihar, Chhattisgarh, Uttar Pradesh, and Uttaranchal showing the greatest number of government hospitals (Figs. 19.6 and 19.7). Under the NHM, these were the target states. The share of government hospitals for delivery continues to rise over rounds, as well (Figs. 19.6 and 19.7).

The government of India has been promoting institutional delivery in government hospitals, but in 2018, private sector childbirth remained high in states such as

19 Maternal and Child Healthcare Utilization and Corresponding Expenditure in India

Table 19.3 Breakdown of births according to place of residence across NSS rounds, India, 2004–2018 (%)

NSS rounds	India			Rural			Urban		
	Public	Private	At home	Public	Private	At home	Public	Private	At home
NSS 60th round (2004)	26.5	39.0	34.5	23.7	34.5	41.8	33.9	51.2	14.9
NSS 71st round (2014)	60.6	36.0	3.3	65.9	30.0	3.8	45.4	52.9	1.7
NSS 75th round (2018)	64.1	27.9	8.2	68.0	22.4	9.5	50.6	45.5	3.9

Source: Author's estimation from NSS 60th, 71st, and 75th rounds

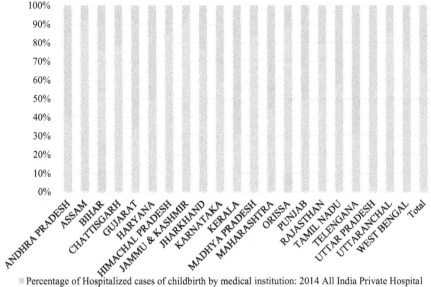

■ Percentage of Hospitalized cases of childbirth by medical institution: 2014 All India Private Hospital

■ Percentage of Hospitalized cases of childbirth by medical institution: 2014 All India Govt/Public Hospital

Fig. 19.6 State-wise distribution of births according to hospital type (%) in NSS 71st round, 2014, India. (*Source*: Author's estimation from NSS 71st round)

Kerala (68.8%), Andhra Pradesh (49.5%), Gujarat (48%), Karnataka (45.2%), and Punjab (46.9%) (Fig. 19.7).

Figure 19.8 illustrates the average expenditure per childbirth during the 75th round in India. The data reveal a significant discrepancy in expenditure. For normal deliveries in rural India, the average expenditure was ten times higher in private hospitals than in government hospitals. Likewise in rural areas, caesarean deliveries cost five times more in private hospitals than in government hospitals. This disparity

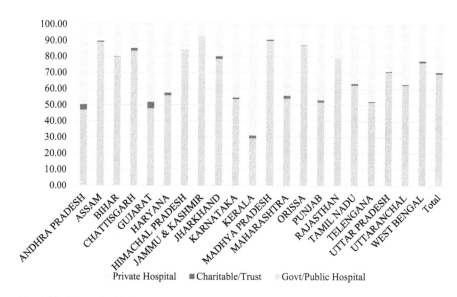

Fig. 19.7 State-wise births according to place of delivery (%) in NSS 75th round, 2018, India. (*Source*: Author's estimation from NSS 75th round)

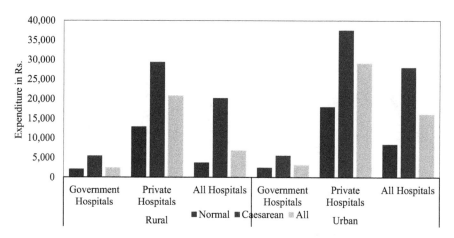

Fig. 19.8 Average expenditure per childbirth according to type of delivery and place of residence in NSS 75th round, India. (*Source*: Author's estimation from NSS 75th round)

in delivery expenditures between government and private hospitals is also evident in urban areas, as depicted in Fig. 19.6.

Across socioeconomic classes and wealth quintiles in 2017–2018, the average medical, total, and OOPE varied significantly (Table 19.4). The expenditure levels are high among the General category and topmost household wealth quintiles.

The percentage distribution in cases of childbirth across social groups and income quintiles is progressive in nature and increases for the General category and

Table 19.4 Average medical expenditure, overall expenditure, and OOPE per childbirth in 75th round, 2018, India

	Medical expenditure	Total expenditure	OOPE
Social group			
ST	6872	8292	6560
SC	5395	6641	5301
OBC	8993	10,514	8712
General	14,080	15,795	13,038
Total	9223	10,721	8800
Wealth quintile			
1st quintile	3706	4741	3625
2nd quintile	4436	5588	4274
3rd quintile	6111	7432	6025
4th quintile	9329	10,968	9140
5th quintile	16,318	18,215	15,184

Source: Author's estimation from NSS 75th round

Table 19.5 Breakdown of hospitalizations for childbirth according to ward, NSS 71st round, 2014, India (%)

	India			Rural			Urban		
	Free	Paying general	Paying special	Free	Paying general	Paying special	Free	Paying general	Paying special
Social group									
ST	79.0	16.7	4.3	82.9	15.3	1.8	47.4	28.1	24.6
SC	71.8	24.0	4.3	74.9	22.4	2.7	60.5	29.5	10.0
OBC	57.6	31.5	11.0	62.2	29.8	8.0	45.1	35.8	19.1
GEN	47.2	39.3	13.6	52.5	38.4	9.2	37.7	40.9	21.4
Wealth quintile									
1st quintile	80.7	17.6	1.7	79.0	19.2	1.8	65.7	30.6	3.8
2nd quintile	72.8	24.1	3.1	71.5	24.1	4.4	55.6	31.7	12.7
3rd quintile	66.9	27.2	5.9	67.9	26.4	5.7	42.7	39.3	18.0
4th quintile	61.4	30.4	8.2	58.8	33.6	7.6	37.5	37.7	24.8
5th quintile	48.0	36.5	15.5	54.5	35.2	10.3	31.0	39.7	29.3

Source: Author's estimation from NSS 71st round

higher-income quintiles. For the year 2018, the percentage of the people using free wards decreased from 82.8% to 47.5% at all levels in India for the lowest income quintile to the highest income quintile, as well as across income quintiles and socio-economic groupings, this figure has declined from 84.2% for STs to 53.7% for the General category (Tables 19.5 and 19.6).

Table 19.6 Hospitalizations for childbirth according to ward type, NSS 75th round, 2018, India (%)

	India			Rural			Urban		
	Free	Paying general	Paying special	Free	Paying general	Paying special	Free	Paying general	Paying special
Social group									
ST	84.2	13.3	2.5	85.9	12.4	1.8	68.4	22.1	9.6
SC	77.9	19.1	3.0	81.6	16.2	2.2	62.5	31.3	6.3
OBC	64.0	28.3	7.8	69.7	24.7	5.6	48.2	38.1	13.8
GEN	53.7	37.6	8.7	63.3	31.3	5.4	38.9	47.3	13.7
Wealth quintile									
1st quintile	82.8	15.1	2.1	83.0	16.0	1.0	65.0	29.0	6.0
2nd quintile	79.6	17.6	2.9	79.0	19.0	2.0	59.0	34.0	7.0
3rd quintile	72.3	24.5	3.2	76.0	21.0	3.0	46.0	43.0	11.0
4th quintile	66.3	27.2	6.5	69.0	25.0	6.0	33.0	49.0	17.0
5th quintile	47.5	39.6	12.9	57.0	33.0	11.0	19.0	54.0	27.0

Source: Author's estimation from NSS 75th round

19.3.4 Average Healthcare Expenditure by Medical Institutions

Table 19.7 reveals an upward trend in maternal healthcare expenditure in India during 2004–2018, regardless of the healthcare facility used. The average total expenditure for maternal healthcare has increased from INR 19,591 in 2004 to INR 22,046 in 2018. In private hospitals, this expenditure has seen a similar trend, increasing from INR 25,465 in 2004 to INR 33,249 in 2018. The results also reveal that OOPE for maternal healthcare utilization has been on the rise over time, especially in private hospitals (Table 19.7).

Table 19.8 shows that the average medical expenditure, overall health expenditure, and OOPE (in INR) for care during hospital stays per case of hospitalization in the past 365 days increased across the NSS rounds, irrespective of social group. Medical expenditure has nearly tripled from 2004 to 2018, regardless of social group, and a similar positive trend has been observed in nonmedical health expenditure and OOPE during this period.

A look across social groups indicates a fourfold increase in total expenditure, with OOPE forming 80% of all expenditure, but the proportion of OOPE in total health expenditure has not shown a marked increase across social groups. State-wise details indicate a remarkably high degree of OOPE as a proportion of total heath expenditure for states like Bihar, UP, Chhattisgarh, and Jharkhand, as

Table 19.7 Maternal healthcare expenditure according to type of facility across NSS rounds, 2004–2018, India (in INR)

		Type of hospital		
	Place of hospital	Public	Private	Total
NSS 60th round (2004)				
Medical expenditure	Rural	8980	20,078	15,429
	Urban	10,118	31,707	23,453
	Total	9316	23,873	17,944
Nonmedical expenditure	Rural	1343	1519	1587
	Urban	1211	1592	1647
	Total	894	1750	1825
Total expenditure	Rural	10,324	21,595	17,016
	Urban	11,012	33,457	25,278
	Total	10,527	25,465	19,591
OOPE	Rural	7366	17,882	13,408
	Urban	8853	25,127	19,355
	Total	7840	20,691	15,550
NSS 71st round (2014)				
Medical expenditure	Rural	6584	25,956	17,841
	Urban	9070	38,678	29,193
	Total	7311	30,883	21,824
Nonmedical expenditure	Rural	2084	2722	2493
	Urban	2010	2753	2511
	Total	1833	2814	2547
Total expenditure	Rural	8667	28,677	20,336
	Urban	10,903	41,491	31,740
	Total	9321	33,635	24,336
OOPE	Rural	6414	25,129	17,291
	Urban	8590	34,597	26,265
	Total	7050	28,795	20,439
NSS 75th round (2018)				
Medical expenditure	Rural	5351	26,137	16,407
	Urban	6464	37,522	26,132
	Total	5678	30,588	19,818
Nonmedical expenditure	Rural	1668	2833	2297
	Urban	1633	2661	2228
	Total	1551	2394	2099
Total expenditure	Rural	7019	28,970	18,705
	Urban	8014	39,915	28,231
	Total	7311	33,249	22,046
OOPE	Rural	5130	24,971	15,685
	Urban	5856	31,005	21,803
	Total	5343	27,330	17,830

Source: Author's estimation from NSS 60th, 71st, and 75th rounds. Note: All results are inflation adjusted expenditures where NSS 75th round expenditure taken as constant

Table 19.8 Average medical expenditure, overall health expenditure, and OOPE (in INR) for care broken down according to social group during hospital stays per case of hospitalization in the past 365 days, India, 2004–2018

	NSS 60th round (2004)			NSS 71st round (2014)			NSS 75th round (2017–2018)		
	Rural	Urban	Total	Rural	Urban	Total	Rural	Urban	Total
Medical expenditure									
ST	9281	18,789	10,665	10,378	35,904	14,087	10,950	18,268	12,020
SC	11,488	16,566	12,829	13,736	16,557	14,501	14,510	19,261	15,798
OBC	15,634	18,938	16,566	18,255	25,798	20,906	15,946	21,519	17,838
General	18,868	29,823	23,250	22,893	37,570	29,396	20,332	33,909	26,488
Non-ST	15,824	23,558	18,315	18,520	29,013	22,347	16,870	26,332	20,310
All	15,429	23,453	17,944	17,841	29,193	21,824	16,407	26,132	19,818
Health expenditure									
ST	10,524	21,693	12,138	12,596	38,122	16,330	13,334	20,332	14,357
SC	12,772	17,977	14,123	15,919	18,515	16,622	16,721	21,126	17,915
OBC	17,246	20,395	18,129	20,822	28,254	23,431	18,182	23,579	20,014
General	20,674	31,976	25,189	25,584	40,472	32,179	22,777	36,136	28,834
Non-ST	17,427	25,362	19,967	21,032	31,570	24,872	19,160	28,432	22,531
All	17,016	25,278	19,591	20,336	31,740	24,336	18,705	28,231	22,046
OOPE									
ST	8401	16,691	9831	9261	32,519	12,640	10,559	12,349	10,821
SC	9029	14,835	10,532	13,422	15,390	13,955	13,668	17,437	14,690
OBC	14,394	18,232	15,621	18,059	24,453	20,306	15,458	19,112	16,698
General	15,791	21,741	18,743	21,713	32,131	26,328	19,213	26,766	22,638
Non-ST	13,682	19,407	15,789	18,019	26,097	20,966	16,119	22,043	18,273
All	13,408	19,355	15,550	17,291	26,265	20,439	15,685	21,803	17,830

Source: Author's estimation from NSS 60th, 71st, and 75th rounds. Note: All results are inflation adjusted expenditures where NSS 75th round expenditure taken as constant

indicated in Fig. 19.9. Bihar, Uttar Pradesh, Chhattisgarh, and Jharkhand are all characterized as socioeconomically poor states.

Table 19.9 indicates the state-wise major source of finance for hospitalization expenditure, for the year 2017–2018. Table 19.9 reflects that Andhra Pradesh has a higher percentage of insurance coverage, household income, or savings funds, covering 80% of hospitalization expenditure. Table 19.9 also indicates similar data for rural and urban areas.

19.4 Discussion

This chapter aims to investigate disparities in maternal and child healthcare utilization across social and administrative strata in India (Roy et al. 2021; Yadav and Jena 2022). The analysis focuses on variations in healthcare utilization among different

19 Maternal and Child Healthcare Utilization and Corresponding Expenditure in India 349

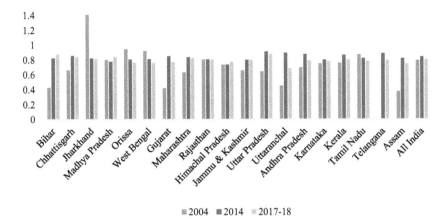

Fig. 19.9 State-wise OOPE as proportion of total health expenditure, India, NSS, 2004–2018. (*Source*: Author's estimation from NSS 60th, 71st, and 75th rounds and RBI)

social groups, wealth quintiles, and states, with an emphasis on assessing whether these gaps have changed over time. By exploring these variations, this chapter seeks to identify segments of the population that may still face challenges in achieving improved maternal and child health outcomes.

This chapter begins by highlighting the positive impact of increasing immunization levels on the reduction in the infant mortality rate (IMR) and child mortality rate (CMR) over time (Ajmer et al. 2023; Rana et al. 2019). The government of India's provision of a free and complete immunization package has positively influenced immunization coverage, although socioeconomic and spatial heterogeneity persists (Srivastava et al. 2020; International Institute for Population Sciences and ICF 2021). Studies have indicated that factors such as a mother's low education level and lack of awareness contribute to the undercoverage of immunization, particularly in rural areas (Khan et al. 2019). Urban areas show higher average immunization expenditure, potentially attributed to a considerable number of individuals' opting for immunization from private facilities, thereby increasing the average cost of immunization (Sarveswaran et al. 2019; Mathur et al. 2020). Gender disparity in immunization expenditure is minimal in urban areas but significantly pronounced in rural regions, indicating a preference for male children and a presence of gender-biased childcare and cost allocation in rural India (Rawat et al. 2021; Khan and Saggurti 2020). This chapter emphasizes the need for further qualitative research to uncover the reasons behind lower immunization spending for girls than boys in rural settings, aligning with previous studies (Rawat et al. 2021; Khan and Saggurti 2020). In summary, this chapter delves into the evolving landscape of maternal and child healthcare utilization, shedding light on disparities and advocating for a nuanced understanding of these dynamics for targeted interventions.

Aligned with previous research (Rana et al. 2019), our study emphasizes the remarkable progress in the utilization of pre- and postnatal care in India, contributing to a reduction in both the infant mortality rate (IMR) and the child mortality rate

Table 19.9 Distribution of the sources of health expenditure in NSS 75th round, India, 2018 (%)

States	Household income/ savings	Borrowings	Sale of physical assets	Contribution from friends and relatives	Other sources	All sources
Andhra Pradesh	56.3	21.7	0.2	9.1	12.7	100
Assam	94.2	3.4	0.2	0.5	1.7	100
Bihar	87.9	9.1	0.1	1.7	1.3	100
Chhattisgarh	87.1	5.0	0.4	2.2	5.2	100
Gujarat	93.0	4.0	0.0	2.6	0.4	100
Haryana	87.5	9.3	0.1	2.3	1.0	100
Himachal Pradesh	93.2	3.7	0.1	2.0	1.0	100
Jharkhand	82.9	6.4	0.2	2.8	7.7	100
Karnataka	79.6	15.6	0.2	3.0	1.7	100
Kerala	77.9	10.4	0.6	6.2	4.9	100
Madhya Pradesh	82.1	7.1	0.3	1.1	9.4	100
Maharashtra	88.8	5.6	0.2	3.0	2.5	100
Odisha	87.0	9.8	0.5	1.5	1.1	100
Punjab	85.8	7.6	0.2	5.4	1.1	100
Rajasthan	84.9	13.1	0.1	1.8	0.2	100
Tamil Nadu	78.0	16.7	0.4	4.2	0.8	100
Telangana	79.4	12.3	0.3	1.4	6.6	100
Uttar Pradesh	83.2	9.3	0.3	2.4	4.7	100
Uttaranchal	91.4	5.0	0.5	2.3	0.8	100
West Bengal	83.5	5.8	0.3	3.8	6.6	100
Total	83.1	9.5	0.3	3.1	3.9	100

Source: Author's estimation from NSS 75th round

(CMR) (Ajmer et al. 2023). However, a noteworthy increase in expenditure on pre- and postnatal care over time raises public health concerns (Balla et al. 2022). Socioeconomic and residential disparities in average expenditure on pre- and postnatal care are also worrisome for the nation (Kumar and Anil Kumar 2021). This chapter reveals a heartening fourfold reduction in home deliveries from 2004 to 2018, a key indicator for reducing the MMR and IMR (Ajmer et al. 2023; Meh et al. 2022). Despite India's significant contribution to the global burden of communicable, maternal, perinatal, and nutritional deficiency (CMPND) conditions, the increasing trend in maternal healthcare utilization is aiding in the decline of these fatalities (Yadav and Singh 2020). Promoting institutional deliveries, awareness campaigns, community involvement, and social mobilization are essential to decreasing maternal and child health vulnerability. The imperative is to enhance public health facilities, making them cost-efficient and accessible. Nationwide, the utilization of private healthcare facilities for child delivery has nearly tripled, with a similar trend observed in rural India, reflecting the positive impact of ongoing maternal and child health programs like JSY schemes and the National Health Mission (Dutta 2019; Sen et al. 2020). Although a considerable proportion of childbirths occur in private hospitals in urban areas, enhancing public healthcare facilities through population-based targeting and socioeconomic equity-focused approaches is crucial (Mishra and Mohanty 2019). The increasing number of institutional deliveries in government hospitals across Indian states underscores the positive impact of initiatives like Janani Suraksha Yojana, highlighting remarkable progress in promoting institutional delivery (Sen et al. 2020). The vital role of accredited social health activist (ASHA) workers in enhancing the acceptance of institutional delivery, particularly in rural areas, has been highlighted by previous literature (Paul and Pandey 2020). Despite the government's promotion of institutional delivery in government hospitals, the high prevalence of private sector childbirth in states like Kerala, Andhra Pradesh, Gujarat, Karnataka, and Punjab raises concerns. While private sector involvement in maternity care is acceptable with controlled costs and regulated profits, the extensive reliance on private healthcare for maternal care in a country with low health insurance coverage and a significant impoverished population poses challenges related to distress financing (Mishra and Mohanty 2019; Goli et al. 2018).

The current study also found a notable disparity in delivery expenditures between government and private hospitals, particularly in urban areas. Previous studies have reported similar findings (Joudyian et al. 2021) and emphasized that the high-cost deliveries in private healthcare facilities pose a significant concern for OOPE in India (Mishra and Mohanty 2019). Therefore, a pressing need to place greater emphasis on regulating costs for treatments and child deliveries in private healthcare facilities has arisen. Concurrently, the expenditure levels are high among the General category and topmost household wealth quintiles in the present study. The high expenditures, especially for OOPEs, are undoubtedly concerning (Mishra and Mohanty 2019). Thus, the equitableness in preventive healthcare services in terms of childcare is a matter of grave concern. The access might have improved due to focused attention and the implementation of various government programs, but availability, quality, and cost remain causes of concern (Dutta 2019). A further study can help answer how these numbers have changed over time and what the respective roles of the public and private sectors are in the process. The current chapter also highlights that the average total expenditure for maternal healthcare has increased from INR 19,591 in 2004 to INR 22,046 in 2018. In private hospitals, this expenditure has seen a similar trend, increasing from INR 25,465 in 2004 to INR 33,249 in 2018. Comparable trends have been observed in government hospitals, although the degree of change is lower than that in private hospitals. Comparable results from previous studies (Balla et al. 2022; Mohanty et al. 2019) have suggested the need to control the rapid increase in maternal healthcare expenditure in India. Expenditure in private hospitals has consistently been higher than in government hospitals across the NSS rounds, emphasizing the necessity to address private maternal healthcare expenses in India. Simultaneously, the infrastructure and the quality of government hospitals need to be enhanced to encourage the public to access government facilities for maternal healthcare. Past studies have highlighted the poor infrastructure and quality issues in government hospitals, which deter people from choosing government hospitals for maternal services, especially during critical situations (Ali et al. 2020; Roy et al. 2021). Significant spatial heterogeneity in the infrastructure and quality of government hospitals exists in India (Khan et al. 2019; Rahaman et al. 2024a). Therefore, infrastructural development in underperforming regions in India needs to be focused on.

The current study results also reveal that OOPE for maternal healthcare utilization has been on the rise over time in India, especially in private hospitals. Previous studies have also underscored the significant issue of OOPE for maternal healthcare, often resulting in distress financing (Balla et al. 2022; Kumar and Anil Kumar 2021). Hence, the government should prioritize the expansion of maternal healthcare insurance coverage in India. Such a step can help alleviate the burden of OOPE so that maternal healthcare can become accessible and affordable for all. The current study also found that medical expenditure has nearly tripled from 2004 to 2018, regardless of social group. A similar positive trend was observed in nonmedical health expenditure and OOPE during this period (Kumar and Anil Kumar 2021). However, the increase in maternal healthcare expenditure among socioeconomically disadvantaged groups, such as the Other Backward Classes (OBC), Scheduled Tribes (ST), and Scheduled Castes (SC), is a concern for India (Issac et al. 2016). When these marginalized groups bear the burden of maternal healthcare expenses, it often leads to distress financing (Mishra and Mohanty 2019). Existing studies have suggested that the problem of OOPE related to maternal healthcare utilization among socioeconomically disadvantaged groups is strongly associated with resorting to credit from unorganized sources and paying high interest rates. This, in turn, pushes them further into chronic poverty (Issac et al. 2016; Mishra and Mohanty 2019). Therefore, the present study suggests that public insurance and healthcare facilities in India need to be strengthened, particularly in these socioeconomically deprived states.

19.4.1 Limitations

The current chapter's findings, derived from descriptive statistics, have not revealed a significant level of variation. Consequently, a potential for bias exists in the results. To enhance reliability, a further study employing robust statistical analyses should be conducted. Additionally, because this study relies on cross-sectional data, it does not establish causal relationships. To address this limitation, conducting a subsequent study that explores the research issues of using data from multiple sources would be advisable. This approach would contribute to a more comprehensive and nuanced understanding of the factors influencing the outcomes under investigation. Although this chapter has several limitations, it contributes to the literature by providing comprehensive insights into maternal and child healthcare utilization and corresponding expenditure in India. The findings of this chapter are helpful to understand the temporal, spatial, sociodemographic, and economic variation in maternal and child health in Indian settings.

19.5 Conclusion

In conclusion, India has made commendable progress in immunization coverage, but addressing disparities in immunization expenditure on the basis of one's place of residence remains an area for improvement. While significant strides have been achieved in pre- and postnatal care utilization, notable disparities persist across socioeconomic groups and administrative units. The increasing expenditure on pre- and postnatal care highlights the urgent need to bridge socioeconomic and residential gaps in this crucial aspect of healthcare. Institutional deliveries in government hospitals have increased, but access to private facilities remains uneven. This chapter revealed that approximately 70% of one of the highest global OOPEs is for health, posing a significant risk to those near or below the poverty line. To build on achievements and address persistent disparities, policymakers should consider the following suggestions:

(a) Implement strategies for equitable funding in immunization programs, reducing expenditure gaps between urban and rural areas.
(b) Tailor healthcare outreach programs to meet the specific needs of diverse socioeconomic groups and regions, promoting wider pre- and postnatal care utilization.
(c) Focus on policies that make maternal healthcare more affordable and accessible in both public and private healthcare settings.
(d) Invest in infrastructure and training in regions with limited access to private healthcare facilities, ensuring broader accessibility.

Incorporating these recommendations into healthcare policies will strengthen India's healthcare system, making immunization, pre- and postnatal care, and maternal healthcare accessible to all, irrespective of socioeconomic background or place of residence.Declaration

Availability of Data and Material This chapter used secondary data, which are publicly available.

Ethics Approval and Consent to Participate None.

Competing Interests The author declare that no competing interests.

Funding None.

References

Ajmer S, Rahaman M, Rana MJ, Sheikh I (2023) Contextualising under-five deaths in Bihar, India: insights from primary and secondary data. Child Youth Serv Rev 144:106718. https://doi.org/10.1016/j.childyouth.2022.106718

Ali B, Dhillon P, Mohanty SK (2020) Inequalities in the utilization of maternal health care in the pre- and post-National Health Mission periods in India. J Biosoc Sci 52(2):198–212. https://doi.org/10.1017/S0021932019000385

Balla S, Sk MIK, Ambade M, Hossain B (2022) Distress financing in coping with out-of-pocket expenditure for maternity care in India. BMC Health Serv Res 22(1):1–14. https://doi.org/10.1186/s12913-022-07656-5

Dutta S (2019) Access to maternal health care services and socioeconomic disparities in pre- and post nrhm period in India: evidence from national sample survey. AJMR 8(4):294–308. https://doi.org/10.5958/2278-4853.2019.00161.7

Ghosh A, Ghosh R (2020) Maternal health care in India: a reflection of 10 years of National Health Mission on the Indian maternal health scenario. Sex Reprod Healthc 25:100530. https://doi.org/10.1016/j.srhc.2020.100530

Goli S, Nawal D, Rammohan A, Sekher TV, Singh D (2018) Decomposing the socioeconomic inequality in utilization of maternal health care services in selected countries of South Asia and sub-Saharan Africa. J Biosoc Sci 50(6):749–769. https://doi.org/10.1017/S0021932017000530

International Institute for Population Sciences & ICF (2021) National Family Health Survey, 2019–21. 2021. Retrived from: https://iipsindia.ac.in/content/national-family-health-survey-nfhs-5-india-report (Accessed on 1st January, 2024).

Issac A, Chatterjee S, Srivastava A, Bhattacharyya S (2016) Out of pocket expenditure to deliver at public health facilities in India: a cross sectional analysis. Reprod Health 13(1):1–9. https://doi.org/10.1186/s12978-016-0221-1

Joudyian N, Doshmangir L, Mahdavi M, Tabrizi JS, Gordeev VS (2021) Public-private partnerships in primary health care: a scoping review. BMC Health Serv Res 21(1):1–18. https://doi.org/10.1186/s12913-020-05979-9

Khan N, Saggurti N (2020) Socioeconomic inequality trends in childhood vaccination coverage in India: findings from multiple rounds of National Family Health Survey. Vaccine 38(25):4088–4103. https://doi.org/10.1016/j.vaccine.2020.04.023

Khan J, Shil A, Mohanty SK (2019) Hepatitis B vaccination coverage across India: exploring the spatial heterogeneity and contextual determinants. BMC Public Health 19(1):1–14. https://doi.org/10.1186/s12889-019-7534-2

Kumar S, Anil Kumar K (2021) Out-of-pocket expenditure and catastrophic health spending on maternity care for hospital-based delivery care in empowered action group (EAG) states of India. Glob Soc Welf 8:231–241. https://doi.org/10.1007/s40609-020-00192-2

Leone T, James KS, Padmadas SS (2013) The burden of maternal health care expenditure in India: multilevel analysis of national data. Matern Child Health J 17:1622–1630. https://doi.org/10.1007/s10995-012-1174-9

Mathur M, Mathur N, Khan N, Kumar D, Verma A (2020) Predictors of 'out-of-pocket Expenditure' on routine immunization of under-five children: a regression analysis. Cureus 12(12):e11859. https://doi.org/10.7759/cureus.11859

Meh C, Sharma A, Ram U, Fadel S, Correa N, Snelgrove JW et al (2022) Trends in maternal mortality in India over two decades in nationally representative surveys. BJOG 129(4):550–561. https://doi.org/10.1111/1471-0528.16888

Mishra S, Mohanty SK (2019) Out-of-pocket expenditure and distress financing on institutional delivery in India. International journal for equity in health, 18:1–15. https://doi.org/10.1186/s12939-019-1001-7.

Mohanty SK, Panda BK, Khan PK, Behera P (2019) Out-of-pocket expenditure and correlates of caesarean births in public and private health centres in India. Soc Sci Med 224:45–57. https://doi.org/10.1016/j.socscimed.2019.01.048

Paul PL, Pandey S (2020) Factors influencing institutional delivery and the role of accredited social health activist (ASHA): a secondary analysis of India human development survey 2012. BMC Pregnancy Childbirth 20(1):1–9. https://doi.org/10.1186/s12884-020-03127-z

Rahaman M, Roy A, Chouhan P, Malik NI, Bashir S, Ahmed F, Tang K (2024a) Contextualizing the standard maternal continuum of care in Pakistan: an application of revised recommendation of the World Health Organization. Front Public Health 11:1261790. https://doi.org/10.3389/fpubh.2023.1261790

Rahaman M, Roy A, Kapasia N, Chouhan P, Muhammad T (2024b) Factors associated with public and private healthcare utilization for outpatient care among older adults in India: a Wagstaff's decomposition of Anderson's behavioural model. Int J Health Plann Manage 2024:1–25. https://doi.org/10.1002/hpm.3771

Rana MJ, Goli S (2021) The road from ICPD to SDGs: health returns of reducing the unmet need for family planning in India. Midwifery 103:103107. https://doi.org/10.1016/j.midw.2021.103107

Rana MJ, Gautam A, Goli S, Reja T, Nanda P, Datta N, Verma R (2019) Planning of births and maternal, child health, and nutritional outcomes: recent evidence from India. Public Health 169:14–25. https://doi.org/10.1016/j.puhe.2018.11.019

Rawat S, Yadav A, Bhate K (2021) Gender determination and gender gap: a cross sectional comparative study of mothers attending under five immunisation clinics in urban and rural areas. J Family Med Prim Care 10(9):3470. https://doi.org/10.4103/jfmpc.jfmpc_1726_20

Roy A, Paul P, Chouhan P, Rahaman M, Kapasia N (2021) Geographical variability and factors associated with caesarean section delivery in India: a comparative assessment of Bihar and Tamil Nadu. BMC Public Health 21:1–15. https://doi.org/10.1186/s12889-021-11750-4

Roy A, Rahaman M, Bannerji R, Adhikary M, Kapasia N, Chouhan P, Das KC (2023) Spatial clustering and drivers of open defecation practice in India: findings from the fifth round of National Family Health Survey (2019-21). Global Transit 5:55–63. https://doi.org/10.1016/j.glt.2023.05.002

Sarveswaran G, Krishnamoorthy Y, Sakthivel M, Vijayakumar K, Priyan S, Thekkur P, Chinnakali P (2019) Preference for private sector for vaccination of under-five children in India and its associated factors: findings from a nationally representative sample. J Trop Pediatr 65(5):427–438. https://doi.org/10.1093/tropej/fmy071

Sen S, Chatterjee S, Khan PK, Mohanty SK (2020) Unintended effects of Janani Suraksha Yojana on maternal care in India. SSM Popul Health 11:100619. https://doi.org/10.1016/j.ssmph.2020.100619

Srivastava S, Fledderjohann J, Upadhyay AK (2020) Explaining socioeconomic inequalities in immunisation coverage in India: new insights from the fourth National Family Health Survey (2015–16). BMC Pediatr 20(1):1–12. https://doi.org/10.1186/s12887-020-02196-5

Yadav AK, Jena PK (2022) Explaining changing patterns and inequalities in maternal healthcare services utilization in India. J Public Aff 22(3):e2570. https://doi.org/10.1002/pa.2570

Yadav AK, Singh A (2020) Age-and sex-specific burden of morbidity and disability in India: a current scenario. Eval Health Serv 1:11–13

Part VI
Societal Perspective of Women's Sexual and Reproductive Health

Chapter 20
Addressing Menstrual Stigma in South Asia: A Holistic Approach Toward Gender Equality and Public Health

Raka Sarkar, Puja Das, and Mahua Chatterjee

Abstract Menstruation is a natural and human biological function of women of reproductive age, yet it is treated as a taboo in many communities across the world. Such taboos may have positive or negative effects, but in all cases, they affect the health of individuals and women's communities as a whole. This article aims to describe how both men and women express stigmatizing attitudes toward menstruation and how menstruating women have to bear physical pain and psychological stress during those days. Undoubtedly, long-standing gender stereotyping and social structuring keep menstrual taboos alive and well in the contemporary world. This chapter is descriptive, using secondary data. It concludes that improving female education, adequate policy measures, and social respect for women could reduce the stigma around menstruation.

Keywords Reproductive age · Taboo · Stress · Contemporary world · Social respect

20.1 Introduction

Menstruation, a physiological process inherent to women's reproductive biology, has been imbued with cultural significance and stigma throughout history. The etymology of the term, derived from the Latin word *menses* meaning "moon," underscores its cyclical nature, typically spanning 28 days and involving intricate

---

R. Sarkar (✉)
Center for the Study of Regional Development (CSRD), Jawaharlal Nehru University, New Delhi, India
e-mail: rakasa22_ssf@jnu.ac.in

P. Das
Department of Geography, University of Gour Banga, Malda, West Bengal, India

M. Chatterjee
Lady Brabourne College, Kolkata, India

© The Author(s), under exclusive license to Springer Nature Singapore Pte Ltd. 2024
P. Chouhan et al. (eds.), *Sexual and Reproductive Health of Women*, https://doi.org/10.1007/978-981-97-8418-9_20

hormonal changes within the female body (Majeed et al. 2022; ACOG 2015). However, since ancient Vedic times, menstruation has been laden with guilt and taboo, interpretations suggesting a symbolic connection to the monthly flow of a Brahmana's blood as a form of expiation (Chawla 1994). Despite its biological importance, menstruation remains a largely taboo subject, particularly in low- and middle-income countries like India, where discussions surrounding menarche and menstruation are rare even among girls and women within families (Singh 2006).

This stigma surrounding menstruation is especially pronounced in South Asia, where it is deeply entrenched in cultural, religious, and socioeconomic factors (Johnston-Robledo and Chrisler 2020). In many communities, menstruation is perceived as a simultaneous rite of passage and a source of impurity and pollution, perpetuating mixed messages and conflicting emotions for young girls (Patkar 2020). The age-old taboos and rituals centering on menstruation exclude women and girls from performing certain activities during their menstruation period. Menstruating Hindu girls are usually restricted from offering puja and touching holy books. Before the 2019 Supreme Court verdict, women under the age of 50 were not allowed into the Sabarimala temple of Kerala, in the southwestern state of India, though nearly 50 million devotees each year make the pilgrimage to Sabarimala temple. India is a land of mixing culture. In one state, a prohibition against bleeding women in Hindu temples is undergirded by considering them as "impure"; in another state, in the northeast, period blood is considered a matter of optimal respect. In Manipur, a girl's first bloodied cloth is kept by her mother and gifted back to her once she has married because it is believed to protect the girl and her family against poor health. Some people believe that a woman's energy goes downward during menstruation and that, in contrast, energy moves upward in the Hindu temple. According to this believe, a menstruating woman might experience severe pain just because of this conflict in energy movement. In Jharkhand, many people fear that period blood might be used for black magic and that women who do not discretely destroy their cloths are witches. This superstition has caused nearly 400 women to die every year in the state. In some cases, menstruating women are not allowed to enter a kitchen to cook food for others. Women themselves do not want to see their own blood because it is considered unclean or dirty and feel embarrassed and ashamed if their menstrual status were to become known. Women sometimes become reluctant to take part in sexual intercourse during these days from their culturally imbued concern that their partners might feel dirty or smell bad. At the community level, menstrual stigma reinforces harmful norms that portray menstruation as dirty or shameful, further marginalizing women and excluding them from certain activities or roles (Patkar 2020). Despite some efforts to address menstrual stigma through initiatives like menstrual hygiene management programs, these interventions often fall short due to insufficient community involvement and their failure to challenge deeply ingrained cultural norms (Johnston-Robledo and Chrisler 2020).

Addressing menstrual stigma requires taking a multifaceted approach that encompasses improving female education, implementing effective policy measures, and fostering social respect for women (Johnston-Robledo and Chrisler 2020). By challenging existing taboos and promoting inclusivity and understanding, societies can work toward accepting menstruation without shame or discrimination (Singh 2006). Through a thorough examination of historical, cultural, and social contexts, coupled with a review of the existing literature and data, this chapter aims to provide a comprehensive understanding of menstrual stigma and contribute to the advancement of policies and practices that promote gender equality and women's health on a global scale. The objectives of this review are twofold: first, to delve into the various manifestations of menstrual taboos and stigma across different societies and cultures, with a particular focus on understanding the deeply entrenched attitudes toward menstruation in South Asia, and second, to analyze the multifaceted impact of menstrual stigma on the physical and psychological health of menstruating individuals by exploring the role of gender stereotypes and social constructs in perpetuating this stigma and discussing potential strategies to mitigate its effects and promote menstrual health and dignity, especially within the South Asian context.

20.2 Understanding Menstruation Stigma

The phenomenon of social exclusion surrounding menstruation, often referred to as menstruation stigma, is a complex issue deeply ingrained in sociocultural norms and beliefs. Goffman's definition of *stigma* as a distinguishing mark that sets individuals or groups apart applies aptly here, as menstruation is often viewed as dirty, embarrassing, and something to be hidden. This stigma manifests in various ways, from religious taboos such as restrictions on temple entry or participation in certain rituals to cultural practices like the fear of menstrual blood being used for black magic (Goffman 1969; Barrington et al. 2021). Menstruation stigma refers to the negative perception of menstruation and those who menstruate. It characterizes the menstruating body as abnormal and abject, leading to a sense of shame, embarrassment, or hesitation to talk about periods (Johnston-Robledo and Chrisler 2020). This stigma is not just an individual problem but a societal one in that it influences norms and behaviors at various levels, from personal to institutional (UNICEF 2022). In South Asia, where cultural and religious beliefs heavily influence perceptions of menstruation, stigma can have profound effects on girls' education, mental health, and overall well-being. The taboo surrounding menstruation perpetuates gender inequality, reinforcing notions of women's impurity and inferiority (McCammon et al. 2020). The impact of menstruation stigma on individuals can be profound. It can lead to discrimination, isolation, and violence, which can result in mental health issues, including depression and anxiety (van Lonkhuijzen 2022). The stigma also affects access to education in that many girls are forced to drop out of school during their periods due to a lack of sanitary facilities and a fear of ridicule (Girls Not Brides 2020).

At the community level, menstruation stigma can perpetuate gender inequality. It reinforces the notion that menstruation is a "dirty" process, undermining the dignity and worth of women (McCammon et al. 2020). This can lead to societal norms that exclude menstruating women from certain activities or roles, further marginalizing them in society (McCammon et al. 2020). Addressing menstruation stigma requires taking a multifaceted approach. While initiatives like menstrual hygiene management programs in schools have been implemented, they have often fallen short of addressing deeply entrenched cultural and societal norms. Structural inequalities, such as inadequate sanitation facilities and limited access to menstrual hygiene products, further perpetuate stigma and marginalization. Therefore, effective interventions must not only address the physical aspects of menstruation but also challenge the underlying gender stereotypes, cultural beliefs, and systemic inequalities that sustain stigma (Johnston-Robledo and Chrisler 2020; UNICEF 2022). In essence, menstruation stigma is a product of historical practices, gender inequalities, and societal views that frame menstruation as impure or shameful. Overcoming this stigma necessitates comprehensive interventions that tackle both the structural barriers and the deeply ingrained attitudes and beliefs surrounding menstruation. Only through such efforts can we create a society where menstruation is viewed with dignity and respect rather than shame and discrimination.

In many cultures, menstruation is surrounded by a web of beliefs and practices that contribute to the stigmatization of menstruating individuals. Menstruation, a natural biological process, is often encased in cultural and religious frameworks that contribute to its stigmatization. Cultural beliefs and practices vary widely, but many cultures view menstruation through a lens of impurity, leading to seclusion and restrictions on women's participation in social and religious activities during menstruation (Olson et al. 2022; Johnston-Robledo and Chrisler 2020; Gottlieb 2020). Similarly, religious taboos characterize menstruation as unclean or defiling, resulting in prohibitions on women's engagement in religious rituals or entry into sacred spaces during their periods (Mukherjee et al. 2020; Johnston-Robledo and Chrisler 2020). These cultural and religious norms not only reinforce the stigma surrounding menstruation but also affect women's spiritual connection and sense of equality within their communities. In some cultures and religions, menstruating women are considered impure or unclean. This can lead to social exclusion and restrictions on their activities during their menstrual cycle. For instance, in some religious practices, menstruating women are banned from attending religious ceremonies, adding another layer of stigma and exclusion (Anand and Garg 2015; Chaturvedi et al. 2021). The psychological impact of the cultural and religious stigma surrounding menstruation cannot be understated. Women may experience shame, embarrassment, and isolation, leading to feelings of inadequacy and low self-esteem. Being excluded from religious or social activities during menstruation can exacerbate these effects, contributing to a sense of marginalization and emotional distress (Johnston-Robledo and Chrisler 2020).

Socioeconomic factors significantly influence menstrual stigma, contributing to its perpetuation in various societies. Rossouw and Ross (2021) highlight that in many communities, menstruation remains a taboo subject, steeped in secrecy and shame due to entrenched social norms and cultural beliefs. This stigma is particularly pronounced in low-income households, where inadequate resources and knowledge about menstruation exacerbate the challenges faced by menstruating individuals (Rossouw and Ross 2021). In rural communities, menstruation is often subjected to various kinds of social stigmata. Young girls or women dealing with menstrual stigma often face challenges due to their socioeconomic background (Thapa et al. 2019). Studies by Dhingra et al. (2009) and Guterman et al. (2007) underscore the profound impact of socioeconomic status on menstrual practices. Affluent families can often afford sanitary napkins, whereas girls from urban slums resort to cloth due to financial constraints (Garg et al. 2012). Economic disparities thus manifest in differential menstrual hygiene practices, highlighting the need for accessible menstrual products for marginalized communities.

Education emerges as a pivotal determinant of menstrual hygiene awareness (Majeed et al. 2022). Kumar and Srivastava (2011) emphasize the role of maternal education, with educated mothers fostering open discussions and dispelling menstruation-related taboos. Moreover, educated girls exhibit a heightened consciousness of menstrual hygiene, accentuating the importance of comprehensive menstrual education in school curricula. Education plays a pivotal role in breaking down menstrual stigma by equipping girls with accurate knowledge about menstruation, which dispels common myths and misunderstandings, while also encouraging a more informed and accepting view of this natural biological process (Sommer et al. 2015). However, socioeconomic disparities in access to education and employment opportunities can hinder efforts to effectively address menstrual stigma (Majeed et al. 2022). Furthermore, the lack of access to essential resources, such as sanitation facilities and affordable menstrual hygiene products, perpetuates menstrual stigma, particularly in marginalized communities. Economic constraints faced by women and girls in these communities exacerbate the challenges related to menstrual hygiene management, reinforcing the stigma surrounding menstruation. The intersection of socioeconomic factors with cultural and religious beliefs further complicates the issue (Hennegan et al. 2021; Rossouw and Ross 2021). In many communities, traditional practices and beliefs shape access to resources and opportunities, amplifying the stigma associated with menstruation. This complex interplay of factors underscores the need for comprehensive interventions that prioritize economic empowerment, education, and access to resources.

Menstruation, often perceived solely as a biological phenomenon, is intricately intertwined with cultural beliefs and practices across different societies. This chapter aims to explore the multifaceted dimensions of menstruation within various cultural contexts, focusing on aspects such as ritual impurity, social exclusion, taboos, and gender dynamics and their impacts on women's experiences. Around the world, cultural beliefs and practices surrounding menstruation indeed vary widely, reflecting diverse perspectives on this natural biological process. In certain cultures, menstruation is revered as a sacred time, symbolizing a woman's connection to fertility and the ability to bear children. Women may be honored and celebrated during their menstrual cycles, viewed as embodying the divine feminine and participating in rituals that mark this significant aspect of womanhood. Conversely, in other cultural contexts, menstruation is perceived through a lens of impurity or dirtiness, leading to the imposition of restrictions and social exclusion for women during their menstrual periods. These beliefs often stem from traditional religious teachings and societal norms that associate menstruation with notions of contamination or taboo. Cultural and religious beliefs significantly shape menstrual practices and perceptions. Variations in terminology, such as *periods*, *MC*, or *masik*, reflect the cultural nuances surrounding menstruation (Mahon and Fernandes 2010).

As a result, menstruating individuals may face limitations on their participation in various activities, including religious ceremonies, communal gatherings, and even everyday interactions with others. Judaism and Hinduism serve as prime examples of how cultural beliefs and practices shape attitudes toward menstruation within their respective communities. In Judaism, the concept of menstruation, known as niddah, is imbued with a sense of separation and ritual purity. The guidelines outlined in Leviticus 15 of the Hebrew Bible delineate specific rules and regulations on menstruation, emphasizing the importance of maintaining physical and spiritual cleanliness during this time (Cohen 2020; Meacham 2009). These instructions not only govern individual behavior but also dictate societal attitudes toward menstruation within Jewish communities, framing it as a period of distinct religious observance and reverence. Similarly, Hinduism prescribes codes of conduct for menstruation, found in texts like the Manu Smriti, which encapsulate deeply rooted religious teachings and traditions surrounding this biological process (Cohen 2020). Within Hindu culture, menstruation is often associated with concepts of purity and impurity, with menstruating women expected to observe certain restrictions and rituals to maintain spiritual cleanliness. These practices reflect broader cultural norms and religious beliefs that shape the understanding and management of menstruation within Hindu communities (Dunnavant and Roberts 2012).

In both Judaism and Hinduism, each of these cultural frameworks provides a comprehensive lens through which menstruation is understood and managed. They not only inform individual practices and behaviors but also contribute to the broader societal attitudes toward menstruation, influencing how menstruating individuals are perceived and treated within their respective communities. Understanding these cultural beliefs and practices is crucial for gaining insights into the diverse experiences of menstruation worldwide and for promoting greater awareness and acceptance of menstruation as a natural and integral aspect of women's lives (Cohen 2020).

20.3 Ritual Impurity and Social Exclusion

Ritual impurity and social exclusion related to menstruation stigma stem from deeply entrenched cultural norms and religious doctrines (Cohen 2020). The perceived impurity of menstruating individuals often leads to their exclusion from religious practices, communal gatherings, and even the household. This exclusion can result in a sense of isolation and shame for menstruating individuals, impacting their mental well-being and sense of belonging in their communities.

In some cultures, menstruating individuals are required to observe specific rituals and practices to cleanse themselves of impurity before being welcomed back into the community. These rituals can vary widely, including periods of seclusion or designated cleansing ceremonies. The enforcement of such practices perpetuates the notion of menstrual impurity, further ostracizing menstruating individuals and reinforcing the stigma associated with menstruation. Menstruating women are often considered impure, leading to restrictions on their participation in religious ceremonies or entry into temples (Cohen 2020; Dunnavant and Roberts 2012; Oster and Thornton 2011). Among Orthodox Jewish communities, menstrual blood is viewed as polluting, resulting in prohibitions on physical contact between menstruating women and others (Cohen 2020; Dunnavant and Roberts 2012). These practices underscore the societal stigma surrounding menstruation and its implications for social interactions within these cultural contexts.

20.4 Taboos and Restrictions

Taboos surrounding menstruation serve to perpetuate stigma and reinforce gender inequalities across cultures. These taboos often dictate restrictive behaviors and practices, shaping women's attitudes toward and perceptions of menstruation (Cohen 2020; White 2012). For example, in some cultures, menstruating women are required to isolate themselves from communal activities and refrain from food preparation (Cohen 2020; White 2012). In both Judaism and Hinduism, strict guidelines dictate various restrictions on menstruating individuals, emphasizing the perceived impurity associated with menstruation (Cohen 2020; Meacham 2009). These cultural taboos reflect broader societal norms and power structures that govern women's bodies and behaviors.

20.5 Impact on Gender Dynamics

Menstrual stigma not only impacts women's physical and mental well-being but also plays a significant role in shaping gender dynamics within societies. The taboos, restrictions, and social exclusion related to menstruation contribute to the marginalization and disempowerment of women, reinforcing existing gender inequalities (Olson et al. 2022; Xue 2023). The perception of menstruation as impure or polluting reinforces the notion of women as inherently unclean, shaping societal attitudes toward women's bodies and perpetuating gender-based discrimination (Johnston-Robledo and Chrisler 2020; Sonawane and Kannake 2020). This not only impacts the daily lives of menstruating women but also influences broader gender dynamics, contributing to the normalization of discrimination and unequal treatment based on biological functions (Johnston-Robledo and Chrisler 2020).

Moreover, the restriction on menstruating individuals from religious practices and communal activities further reinforces the subordinate position of women within these cultural and religious contexts, limiting their participation and agency. This perpetuates gender disparities and restricts women's access to spaces of power and decision-making, ultimately reinforcing existing gender hierarchies (Cohen 2020; Meacham 2009). Additionally, the societal stigma surrounding menstruation contributes to the invisibility of women's experiences and needs, further marginalizing their voices within public discourse and policymaking. This reinforces unequal power dynamics and hinders the advancement of gender equality because women's reproductive health and experiences remain undervalued and overlooked.

The cultural construction of menstruation significantly influences gender dynamics within these religious communities. In Judaism, patriarchal attitudes toward women's bodies are reflected in the laws of niddah, where men exert control over women's reproductive health and sexuality (Cohen 2020; Meacham 2009). Similarly, in Hinduism, menstrual taboos perpetuate traditional gender norms and hierarchies, where men dictate women's roles and behaviors on the basis of religious teachings (Cohen 2020; Johnston-Robledo and Chrisler 2020). Menstruation becomes a tool for regulating women's bodies and upholding male privilege within these religious traditions (Cohen 2020).

20.6 Access to Menstrual Hygiene Products

In a country like India, where female literacy is quite impressionable, 91.95% as per 2021 Census, many adolescent girls have no idea what periods are until they experience one. In the developing world, a certain mindset and conservative social structure compels many in society to believe not only that menstruation is a social taboo but also that it prevents adolescent girls from gaining proper knowledge and accessing menstrual health care, which is vital to their maintaining their physical and mental health. Particularly in rural areas, women have to use cloths or leaves instead of sanitary pads. According to the fourth round of the National Family Health Surveys (NFHS-4), conducted in 2015–2016, 42% of women in India use sanitary napkins, 62% use cloths, and 16% use locally prepared napkins. In the same survey, only 48% of rural women were found to use a hygienic method of menstrual protection, as compared to 78% of women in urban areas. Unhygienic methods cause bacterial and fungal infections in the reproductive and urinary tracts. Part of this is because of the social stigma associated with menstruation, where, in some cultures, women can not take baths or wash their hair. Women are prevented from going to work or attaining schools due to their fear of the negative mental health effects from menstruation stigma.

Ensuring access to period hygiene products is a crucial component of combating menstruation stigma. These activities aim to enhance product availability, affordability, and distribution channels, as outlined by Mahon and Fernandes (2010), Hennegan and Montgomery (2016), Kuhlmann et al. (2017, 2019). To reduce the burden of menstruation and the stigma associated with it, we can overcome obstacles like financial limits or the limited availability of menstrual hygiene products in rural areas. Education is particularly significant in confronting menstruation stigma. Empowering individuals with comprehensive and age-appropriate menstrual health education can provide them with knowledge about their bodies, menstruation, and menstrual hygiene practices. This information can dispel myths and misconceptions about menstruation, foster positive attitudes toward menstrual health, and promote open communication about periods. Raising awareness and speaking up about menstruation can uncover inequalities in several areas of life, leading to the development of comprehensive policies beyond only addressing menstrual issues (Goddard and Sommer 2020).

The limited availability of menstrual hygiene products poses substantial obstacles for many women, especially those in marginalized areas. Financial limitations frequently restrict the purchasing of menstrual hygiene products, resulting in the use of makeshift and unclean alternatives that may carry health hazards (Sommer et al. 2015). In rural and underserved areas, the scarcity of menstrual hygiene products worsens the situation, hindering individuals from adequately maintaining their menstrual health (Goddard and Sommer 2020). Cultural taboos and the shame related to menstruation can hinder access to these items. In many cultures, openly talking about or buying menstrual hygiene products might be seen as taboo, causing individuals to feel shame and humiliation when trying to obtain these necessary health products (Rossouw and Ross 2021). This maintains the concealment and obscurity of menstruation, impeding the availability of products and strengthening the negative perception linked to menstrual health. Poor sanitation facilities are major obstacles to obtaining menstrual hygiene products (Mahon and Fernandes 2010). The inadequate number of private and clean facilities for managing menstruation can hinder women's ability to use menstrual hygiene products efficiently and with dignity. A lack of clean and private facilities can hinder women's maintenance of their menstrual hygiene, which can result in health risks and pain.

Inadequate menstrual hygiene practices can lead to serious health consequences for individuals. Using unsanitary alternatives or mismanaging menstruation can heighten the likelihood of infections, like urinary tract infections and reproductive tract infections. Infections can occur due to unhygienic materials or incorrect disposal practices, leading to the proliferation and transmission of germs (Rossouw and Ross 2021).

Examining the intersection of multiple forms of discrimination and the resulting marginalization reveals that menstrual stigma is connected to gender inequality, poverty, and limited access to education and healthcare for women, creating a complex web of marginalization and discrimination (Chaturvedi et al. 2021). The overlapping issues worsen the difficulties experienced by marginalized individuals in handling their menstrual health. The interaction of menstrual stigma with other types of marginalization and discrimination has a compounding impact on women's capacity to handle their menstrual health (Stangl et al. 2019). This cumulative effect will likely lead to negative health consequences for individuals.

Moreover, the dearth of thorough research on menstrual health management impedes efforts to properly tackle these difficulties. Thorough methods must be created to address the multifaceted issues surrounding menstruation stigma, which are influenced by social, cultural, and economic factors. By acknowledging the interconnectedness of menstruation stigma with other types of marginalization and discrimination, we might be able to create more- comprehensive and more-efficient solutions. The stigma associated with menstruation has significant consequences on human rights, such as dignity, bodily autonomy and integrity, health, privacy, and freedom from discriminatory and degrading treatment (Verma et al. 2021; Johnson 2019; Loughnan et al. 2020). Menstrual stigma has wide-ranging effects on individuals' physical and mental well-being and on their access to resources and opportunities. To tackle these issues and reduce the harmful effects of menstruation stigma, a thorough and intersectional strategy must be implemented.

20.7 Challenges and Strategies

Menstrual stigma remains a serious societal challenge, especially in marginalized populations and cultural contexts where deep-rooted beliefs sustain unfavorable views of menstruation. This stigma has various consequences, including limiting individuals' access to reliable menstrual health information and worsening socioeconomic inequalities in accessing menstrual hygiene products. This analysis emphasizes the need for a comprehensive approach to tackle menstruation stigma from various angles. The current education systems' failure to provide thorough menstrual health education contributes to the persistence of myths and misunderstandings about menstruation. The absence of comprehensive menstrual health education in schools and community programs sustains cultural stigmas and hinders open discussions about menstruation. As a result, people, especially young girls, lack the essential information needed to question conventional standards and promote positive views on menstruation. Community-based interventions are essential in challenging deeply entrenched cultural attitudes, as they provide a platform for open discussions about menstruation and promote a more informed, positive perspective within local contexts. By including community leaders and stakeholders, these programs establish forums for discussion, enabling individuals to address existing taboos and promote change within their communities. The success of these interventions depends on their capacity to manage intricate sociocultural processes and guarantee inclusivity, especially for marginalized groups. Furthermore, media and lobbying activities have substantial impacts on changing cultural views on menstruation. By utilizing different media platforms, these campaigns can challenge stereotypes, debunk myths, and support policy changes to improve access to menstrual hygiene products and facilities (Wakefield et al. 2020). However, the success of media campaigns depends on their capacity to incorporate culturally relevant messages and involve various stakeholders to encourage significant discussions and bring about concrete changes. By utilizing global frameworks and successful interventions like Kerala's She- Pad initiative and community-based programs such as Goonj, South Asian countries can customize their strategies to effectively tackle the cultural intricacies of menstrual stigma (Parthasarathy 2022). Governmental policy measures are essential in reducing menstruation stigma. Policymakers can provide resources, draft legislation, and implement initiatives to address menstruation stigma by focusing on period health in public health and gender equality agendas. The effectiveness of policy interventions depends on how effectively they adhere to international frameworks and best practices and how they adapt to the specific sociocultural settings of the groups they aim to assist.

20.8 Conclusion

The issue of menstrual stigma is a complex and multifaceted problem that requires a holistic approach for effective management (Chaturvedi et al. 2021; Johnston-Robledo and Chrisler 2020). This approach should address not only the physical aspects of menstruation, such as hygiene and access to menstrual products, but also the social and cultural factors that contribute to stigma and discrimination (Chaturvedi et al. 2021). By adopting comprehensive strategies that include education, awareness campaigns, and the involvement of diverse stakeholders, we can begin to challenge the societal norms and perceptions surrounding menstruation and promote a more supportive and rights-based environment for menstruating individuals. This approach should also prioritize the integration of menstrual health into broader sexual and reproductive health agendas, recognizing the interconnectedness of these issues. Additionally, the specific needs and experiences of marginalized groups within the menstruating population, such as refugees, people with disabilities, and the LGBTQ+ community, must be considered.

By embracing examples of successful interventions from India and other neighboring countries, South Asian nations can tailor their interventions to suit the cultural, social, and economic dynamics within their own communities. Case studies from similar cultural contexts can provide valuable insights into effective strategies for addressing menstrual stigma and promoting menstrual rights, thereby serving as guiding examples for policy implementation and adaptation.

Through the convergence of national and international policy frameworks, as well as the integration of best practices, these efforts can lead to tangible and sustainable changes in challenging menstrual stigma and promoting menstrual health as an essential component of gender equality and public health agendas. To achieve these goals, diverse stakeholders, including government agencies, nongovernmental organizations (NGOs), healthcare providers, educators, community leaders, and individuals with first-hand experiences must be included. Only through collaboration and a comprehensive approach can we hope to dismantle the stigma surrounding menstruation and create a more inclusive and supportive society for menstruating individuals. Overall, this review of sources highlights the importance of addressing menstrual stigma as a complex and interconnected issue.

By integrating these policy implications and interventions, South Asian countries can take significant strides in managing, preventing, and reducing the stigma associated with menstruation. Through a comprehensive approach that incorporates the policy landscape in the region, international frameworks and guidelines, and best practices and case studies, governments and stakeholders can work toward creating an environment that upholds the dignity, rights, and well-being of menstruating individuals, ultimately fostering a more inclusive and equitable society.

Declarations

Availability of Data and Materials All the data related to this study are reported in this document.

Ethics Approval and Consent to Participate Ethical approval is not applicable.

Competing Interests The authors declare that they have no competing interests.

Funding The authors did not receive financial assistance from any funding agency.

References

ACOG (2015) Menstruation in girls and adolescents: using the menstrual cycle as a vital sign. Acog. org. https://www.acog.org/clinical/clinical-guidance/committee-opinion/articles/2015/12/menstruation-in-girls-and-adolescents-using-the-menstrual-cycle-as-a-vital-sign

Anand T, Garg S (2015) Menstruation related myths in India: strategies for combating it. J Fam Med Prim Care 4(2):184. https://doi.org/10.4103/2249-4863.154627

Barrington DJ, Robinson HJ, Wilson E, Hennegan J (2021) Experiences of menstruation in high income countries: a systematic review, qualitative evidence synthesis and comparison to low- and middle-income countries. PLoS One 16(7):e0255001. https://doi.org/10.1371/journal.pone.0255001

Chaturvedi B, Goswami S, Pal N, Singh RP, Yadav T, Gangwar S, Mishra KN, Kumudhavalli MV (2021) A brief note on menstrual stigma: social assumptions and responsibilities. Int J Curr Res Rev 13(06):60–63. https://doi.org/10.31782/ijcrr.2021.13604

Chawla J (1994) Mythic origins of menstrual taboo in Rig Veda. Econ Pol Wkly 29(43):2817–2827. https://www.jstor.org/stable/4401940

Cohen I (2020) In: Bobel C, Winkler IT, Fahs B, Hasson KA, Kissling EA, Roberts T-A (eds) Menstruation and religion: developing a critical menstrual studies approach. Palgrave Macmillan, London. https://www.ncbi.nlm.nih.gov/books/NBK565592/

Dhingra R, Kumar A, Kour M (2009) Knowledge and practices related to menstruation among tribal (Gujjar) adolescent girls. Stud EthnoMed 3(1):43–48. https://doi.org/10.1080/09735070.2009.11886336

Dunnavant NC, Roberts T-A (2012) Restriction and renewal, pollution and power, constraint and community: the paradoxes of religious women's experiences of menstruation. Sex Roles 68(1–2):121–131. https://doi.org/10.1007/s11199-012-0132-8

Garg R, Goyal S, Gupta S (2012) India moves towards menstrual hygiene: subsidized sanitary napkins for rural adolescent girls—issues and challenges. Matern Child Health J 16:767–774. https://doi.org/10.1007/s10995-011-0798-5

Girls Not Brides (2020) Girls not brides impact report 2020. https://www.girlsnotbrides.org/learning-resources/resource-centre/girls-not-brides-impact-report-2020/

Goddard SJ, Sommer M (2020) Menstrual health and hygiene management and WASH in urban slums: gaps in the evidence and recommendations. J Gender Water 7:1

Goffman E (1969) Stigma: notes on the management of spoiled identity. Postgrad Med J 45(527):642–642. https://doi.org/10.1136/pgmj.45.527.642

Gottlieb A (2020) Menstrual taboos: moving beyond the curse. In: The Palgrave handbook of critical menstruation studies, pp 143–162. https://doi.org/10.1007/978-981-15-0614-7_14

Guterman MA, Mehta P, Gibbs MS (2007) Menstrual taboos among major religions. Int J World Health Soc Polit 5:1

Hennegan J, Montgomery P (2016) Do menstrual hygiene management interventions improve education and psychosocial outcomes for women and girls in low and middle income countries? A systematic review. PLoS One 11(2):e0146985. https://doi.org/10.1371/journal.pone.0146985

Hennegan J, Winkler IT, Bobel C, Keiser D, Hampton J, Larsson G, Chandra-Mouli V, Plesons M, Mahon T (2021) Menstrual health: a definition for policy, practice, and research. Sex Reprod Health Matters 29(1):1911618. https://doi.org/10.1080/26410397.2021.1911618

Johnson ME (2019) Menstrual justice. SSRN Electron J. https://doi.org/10.2139/ssrn.3389773

Johnston-Robledo I, Chrisler JC (2020) In: Bobel C, Winkler IT, Fahs B, Hasson KA, Kissling EA, Roberts T-A (eds) The menstrual mark: menstruation as social stigma. Palgrave Macmillan, London. https://www.ncbi.nlm.nih.gov/books/NBK565611/

Kuhlmann AS, Henry K, Wall LL (2017) Menstrual hygiene management in resource-poor countries. Obstet Gynecol Surv 72(6):356–376. https://doi.org/10.1097/ogx.0000000000000443

Kuhlmann AS, Peters Bergquist E, Danjoint D, Wall LL (2019) Unmet menstrual hygiene needs among low-income women. Obstet Gynecol 133(2):238–244. https://doi.org/10.1097/aog.0000000000003060

Kumar A, Srivastava K (2011) Cultural and social practices regarding menstruation among adolescent girls. Soc Work Public Health 26(6):594–604. https://doi.org/10.1080/19371918.2010.525144

Loughnan L, Mahon T, Goddard S, Bain R, Sommer M (2020) Monitoring menstrual health in the sustainable development goals. In: The Palgrave handbook of critical menstruation studies, pp 577–592. https://doi.org/10.1007/978-981-15-0614-7_44

Mahon T, Fernandes M (2010) Menstrual hygiene in South Asia: a neglected issue for WASH (water, sanitation and hygiene) programmes. Gend Dev 18(1):99–113. https://doi.org/10.1080/13552071003600083

Majeed J, Sharma P, Ajmera P, Dalal K (2022) Menstrual hygiene practices and associated factors among Indian adolescent girls: a meta-analysis. Reprod Health 19(1):148. https://doi.org/10.1186/s12978-022-01453-3

McCammon E, Bansal S, Hebert LE, Yan S, Menendez A, Gilliam M (2020) Exploring young women's menstruation-related challenges in Uttar Pradesh, India, using the socio-ecological framework. Sex Reprod Health Matters 28(1). https://doi.org/10.1080/26410397.2020.1749342

Meacham T (2009) Female purity (Niddah). Jewish women: a comprehensive historical encyclopedia. Jewish Women's Archive. https://jwa.org/encyclopedia/article/female-purity-niddah

Mukherjee A, Lama M, Khakurel U, Jha AN, Ajose F, Acharya S, Tymes-Wilbekin K, Sommer M, Jolly PE, Lhaki P, Shrestha S (2020) Perception and practices of menstruation restrictions among urban adolescent girls and women in Nepal: a cross-sectional survey. Reprod Health 17(1):81. https://doi.org/10.1186/s12978-020-00935-6

Olson MM, Alhelou N, Kavattur PS, Rountree L, Winkler IT (2022) The persistent power of stigma: a critical review of policy initiatives to break the menstrual silence and advance menstrual literacy. PLoS Glob Public Health 2(7):e0000070. https://doi.org/10.1371/journal.pgph.0000070

Oster E, Thornton R (2011) Menstruation, sanitary products, and school attendance: evidence from a randomized evaluation. Am Econ J Appl Econ 3(1):91–100. https://doi.org/10.1257/app.3.1.91

Parthasarathy S (2022) How sanitary pads came to save the world: knowing inclusive innovation through science and the marketplace. Soc Stud Sci 52(5):637–663. https://doi.org/10.1177/03063127221122457

Patkar A (2020) In: Bobel C, Winkler IT, Fahs B, Hasson KA, Kissling EA, Roberts T-A (eds) Policy and practice pathways to addressing menstrual stigma and discrimination. Palgrave Macmillan, London

Rossouw L, Ross H (2021) Understanding period poverty: socio-economic inequalities in menstrual hygiene management in eight low- and middle-income countries. Int J Environ Res Public Health 18(5):2571. https://doi.org/10.3390/ijerph18052571

Singh A (2006) Place of menstruation in the reproductive lives of women of rural North India. Indian J Commun Med 31(1):10. https://doi.org/10.4103/0970-0218.54923

Sommer M, Hirsch JS, Nathanson C, Parker RG (2015) Comfortably, safely, and without shame: defining menstrual hygiene management as a public health issue. Am J Public Health 105(7):1302–1311. https://doi.org/10.2105/ajph.2014.302525

Sonawane N, Kannake R (2020) A descriptive study to assess the knowledge, attitude and practices regarding menstrual health among the high school girls in Ashram Shaala of Tribal Area: in view to develop information booklet. Indian J Nurs Sci 5(1):106–112. https://doi.org/10.31690/ijns/44

Stangl AL, Earnshaw VA, Logie CH, van Brakel W, Simbayi C, Barré I, Dovidio JF (2019) The health stigma and discrimination framework: a global, crosscutting framework to inform research, intervention development, and policy on health-related stigmas. BMC Med 17(1):31. https://doi.org/10.1186/s12916-019-1271-3

Thapa S, Bhattarai S, Aro AR (2019) "Menstrual blood is bad and should be cleaned": a qualitative case study on traditional menstrual practices and contextual factors in the rural communities of far-western Nepal. SAGE Open Med 7:205031211985040. https://doi.org/10.1177/2050312119850400

UNICEF (2022) FACT SHEET: menstrual health and hygiene management still out of reach for many. www.unicef.org. https://www.unicef.org/press-releases/fact-sheet-menstrual-health-and-hygiene-management-still-out-reach-many

van Lonkhuijzen RM, Garcia FK, Wagemakers A (2022) The stigma surrounding menstruation: attitudes and practices regarding menstruation and sexual activity during menstruation. Women's Reprod Health 10(3):364–384. https://doi.org/10.1080/23293691.2022.2124041

Verma A, Patyal A, Meena JK, Mathur M (2021) Breaking the silence around menstruation: experiences from urban and rural India. Int J Commun Med Public Health 8(3):1538. https://doi.org/10.18203/2394-6040.ijcmph20210859

Wakefield MA, Loken B, Hornik RC (2020) Use of mass media campaigns to change health behaviour. Lancet 376(9748):1261–1271. https://doi.org/10.1016/s0140-6736(10)60809-4

White LR (2012) The function of ethnicity, income level, and menstrual taboos in postmenarcheal adolescents' understanding of menarche and menstruation. Sex Roles 68(1–2):65–76. https://doi.org/10.1007/s11199-012-0166-y

Xue R (2023) The research on the causes and countermeasures of shame in women's menstrual period. BCP Soc Sci Humanities 21:36–43. https://doi.org/10.54691/bcpssh.v21i.3419

Chapter 21
Gender-Parity-Specific Fertility Decline in India: A Spatiotemporal Study

Kakoli Das and Saswata Ghosh

Abstract India, a developing country, has been experiencing a fertility transition since the 1960s, with a significant acceleration in the past decade. Over the past 30 years, India's total fertility rate (TFR) has declined from 3.4 in 1992–1993 to 2.0 in 2019–2021. Hence, the present chapter focuses on understanding the intricate relationship between declining fertility desires and demographic factors, particularly gender and the number of previous offspring. It places particular emphasis on the acceptance of daughters within the cohort of nonmenopausal, nonsterilized mothers aged 15–45 years. Using data from NFHS-1 and NFHS-5 and employing descriptive analyses and multivariate models, our chapter reveals a 30 percentage-point increase (from 39.5% to 70.8%) in mothers' completing their childbearing up to parity 2. The reluctance to have another child increased by 10.7 percentage points (PPs) among mothers with one daughter, whereas families with two daughters saw such an increase by 35 percentage points between survey rounds. A multivariate analysis demonstrates that educated working mothers are more inclined to accept families with only girls. However, a contradictory decrease in the desire for additional children when mothers have exactly two daughters indicates a complex interplay aimed at avoiding having only girls successively. Additionally, awareness of rising childrearing costs and economic instability compel financially disadvantaged couples, particularly those not employed or engaged in primary sectors, to limit their family size to one or two children, regardless of gender composition. Thus, although fertility declines in India demonstrate a balanced gender-parity distribution, labeling it as gender equity in fertility outcomes demands further investigation.

Keywords Gender parity · Fertility · India

K. Das
Institute of Development Studies, Salt Lake, Kolkata, West Bengal, India

Vidyasagar University, West Medinipur, West Bengal, India

S. Ghosh (✉)
Institute of Development Studies, Salt Lake, Kolkata, West Bengal, India

21.1 Introduction

Son preference in India is a deep-seated societal phenomenon that has persisted for centuries, influencing various aspects of family dynamics and the very fabric of society (Guilmoto 2009, 2012; Das Gupta et al. 2003). This preference for male offspring is influenced primarily by the economic benefits of having at least one boy, patriarchal norms, religious beliefs, and overall societal expectations and by community pressure (Karve 1993; Dyson and Moore 1983). In many traditional societies, including India, sons are often seen as the primary caregivers during old age, the ones who carry on the family name, and the inheritors of ancestral property (Chellaiyan et al. 2018; Das and Ghosh 2021). Daughters, on the other hand, are sometimes considered a financial burden due to cultural practices such as dowry. The preference for sons has implications for various aspects of Indian society, including skewed sex ratios and gender-based discrimination (Weitzman 2015; Nanda et al. 2019) in intrahousehold resource allocation. Moreover, the practice of sex-selective abortion, despite being illegal, remains prevalent in some parts of the country (Retherford and Roy 2003; Nandi and Deolalikar 2013). Because of this, a noticeable gender imbalance has now emerged, with more men than women being born, surviving, and being valued. According to the Census of India 2011, the sex ratio is 940 girls and women per 1000 boys and men, indicating a skewed distribution (RGI 2011). However, a north–south dichotomy can be seen in the sex ratio over 3 decades (1981 to 2011), when the extent of son preference in the southeastern region was found to be lower than that in northwestern India, which is generally manifested through sex-selective abortions and poorer nutritional status among girls compared to boys (Das and Ghosh 2021; Ghosh et al. 2020).

Additionally, India's kinship system is also marked by a distinct son–daughter dichotomy that exhibits a preference for sons over daughters. In this structure, sons, along with daughters-in-law, assume the responsibility of supporting elderly parents, while daughters are actively discouraged from providing similar assistance (Desai and Temsah 2014; Nasir and Kalla 2006; Unnithan-Kumar 2010; Zaidi and Morgan 2016). Notably, daughters experience a separation between their natal and conjugal families, reinforcing traditional gender roles. Furthermore, practices characterized by male dominance, such as dowry and hypergamy, have transcended their original cultural boundaries and influenced communities beyond their geographic origins (Basu 1999; Diamond-Smith et al. 2008). In addition to differences in kinship systems, variations emerge in the valuation of daughters across different religious communities as well. Arguably, Muslim women exhibit lower levels of "daughter aversion," influenced by religious tenets and practices like birth control. In contrast, Hindu perspectives position daughters as ritually inferior to sons, a perception strengthened by obligations tied to the sacred nature of marriage and the prevalent practice of dowry (Borooah and Iyer 2004).

Moreover, against a backdrop of declining fertility rates in India (SRS 2023), the preference for sons has intensified despite the enduring acknowledgment of daughters for their roles in emotional companionship and caregiving (Arnold 2001; Diamond-Smith et al. 2008; Patel 2007). Patel (2020) refers to these families as "aspirational" because they strive to improve their economic and social status through a combination of low fertility and son preference. A compelling reason to reduce overall family size has also emerged from the gendered demographic dividend (Allendorf 2020).

However, evidence from recent research findings, across several Indian regions, indicates a potential diminishing trend in son preference, as manifested by normalizing (Tong 2022) or decreasing sex ratios at birth (number of boys per 100 girls) (Diamond-Smith and Bishai 2015; Guilmoto and Rahm 2021; Kaur et al. 2017). This trend aligns with a broader Asian phenomenon: the emergence of diverse, context-specific gender equity (Nagarajan and Sahoo 2019). In South Korea and Japan, a daughter preference has gained momentum (Asadullah et al. 2021; Chun and Das Gupta 2021), and Taiwan and certain areas of China exhibit increasing gender indifference (Fuse 2013; Lei 2013; Lin 2009). Notably, Bangladesh showcases a distinct societal desire for gender balance (Asadullah et al. 2021).

The observed decline in son preference can be attributed to the synergistic interplay of several factors. The increased diffusion of ideas promoting gender equality, fueled by socioeconomic development, policy interventions, and the women's movement, appears to be a key driver (Bongaarts and Watkins 1996; Casterline 2001; Chung and Das Gupta 2007; Tong 2022). Although socioeconomic forces, such as urbanization, education gains, and rising incomes, undoubtedly contribute to shifting demographics, these changes can mask underlying transformations in social norms (Chung and Das Gupta 2007; Eloundou-Enyegue et al. 2021; Kaur et al. 2017). Untangling the relative contributions of these factors remains a vital area of inquiry for understanding the complex dynamics of the change in gender preference. Hence, the focal point of this chapter lies in the examination of how fertility desires are shaped by gender and the number of previous offspring, with a specific focus on understanding the dynamics of daughter acceptance. Additionally, the research rigorously scrutinizes the determinants contributing to the observed rise in gender-balanced fertility rates within the sociocultural context of India.

21.2 Materials and Methods

21.2.1 Data and Variables

The present research is based on data extracted from the National Family Health Survey (NFHS), a large-scale, multiround nationwide survey designed to provide comprehensive information on Indian demographics, health, and family-planning practices. To understand how societal shifts have influenced reproductive choices, we compare findings from two NFHS rounds (NFHS-1 and NFHS-5), conducted across nearly 3 decades (1992–1993 and 2019–2021) (IIPS 1995; IIPS 2021). Our analysis focuses on a specific subset of currently married women aged 15–45 years who were nonmenopausal and nonsterilized at the time of the survey, ensuring consistency between the two datasets. For the first round (1992–1993), a subsample of 69,643 (weighted 678,538) women aged 15–45 was extracted, and for the 2019–2021 round, information on 62,516 (state-level data, weighted 599,773) women aged 15–45 was analyzed.

For ease of interpretation, comparative analyses for NFHS-1 and NFHS-5 have been separately carried out, individually focusing on each survey, thus allowing for the clearer identification of shifts in fertility preferences, both across different parities (family sizes) and within gender compositions (e.g., son preference/gender equality). This facilitates seeing how these preferences may have evolved.

To comprehend the influence of individual characteristics of mothers, household financial conditions, families' awareness of family size, and various socioeconomic factors on mothers' decisions about family size, various independent variables were selected. For the gender-parity composition, women were categorized on the basis of the number and sex composition of their living children at each parity, including parity 1 (0 sons, 1 son), parity 2 (0 sons, 1 son, 2 sons), and parity 3+ (0 sons, 1 son, 2 sons, 3 or more sons).

Additional factors included the respondents' age (continuous), their level of education (categorized as illiterate, primary, secondary, or above secondary), their working status (categorized as working or not working), their partner's employment status (categorized as not working, primary, secondary, or tertiary), their wealth index (categorized as poorest, poorer, middle, richer, and richest—calculated by using data from NFHS-5, except for the first round), their caste (categorized as SC, ST, or others), their religious affiliation (categorized as Hindu, Muslim, or others), and the prevalence of contraceptives. To incorporate contextual factors, apart from women's place of residence (rural/urban), a variable representing region was created and subsequently divided into three categories: north-central states, east-northeast states, and southwest states.

To capture the range of contraceptive practices, respondents were categorized into four groups on the basis of their method of choice: (1) not using any method; (2) relying on natural methods like withdrawal or rhythm; (3) using modern methods such as IUDs, pills, or condoms; and (4) having undergone sterilization. Sterilized women and sterilized men were dropped from the present analysis to meet its objectives.

To understand mothers' future family planning, a binary variable ("future child desire") was created on the basis of their reported intention to have another child. Initially, several sociodemographic factors like marital duration, partner's age, and partner's education were also included in the analysis. However, these were later excluded due to potential data redundancy ("multicollinearity") to ensure that the analysis focused on independent influences.

21.2.2 Analytical Model

This chapter employed both descriptive analysis and multivariate modeling techniques to explore how mothers' decisions about having another child are shaped by individual and socioeconomic factors, with a focus on prevailing gender-parity composition. Multivariate binary logit regression models were used to explain the factors responsible for gender-parity-specific fertility decline in India over 3 decades, especially for couples with one or two girls and who had no future desire for children. We estimated the adjusted probabilities (predictive marginal effects) of the predictor variables of interest. Later on, adjusted marginal effects (MEs for multivariate binary logit regression; net differentials) were converted into percentages with one decimal place for easy interpretation.

The logit model can be written as follows:

$$\log \frac{p}{1-p} = b_{0+} + b_1 x_1 + b_2 x_2 + b_3 x_3 + b_4 x_4 .. + b_8 x_8 + b_k x_k$$

where p denotes the predicted proportion of the response variable and the $x_1, x_2 ... x_n$ denotes the predictor variables in a model.

For a logit model, the marginal effect (ME) depends on the estimated probability, thus yielding the following:

$$g(p) = \log(p) - \log(1-p) \Rightarrow g'(p) = \frac{1}{p} + \frac{1}{1-p} = \frac{1}{p-(1-p)},$$

And here, the marginal effect is $m_j^{logit} = \beta_j \, p(1-p)$ where $p(1 - p)$ is zero at $p = 0$ and at $p = 1$

The analysis was carried out by using STATA 16.

21.3 Results

21.3.1 Change in Completed Fertility and Desired Family Size from NFHS-1 to NFHS-5

Table 21.1 displays the number of children born to mothers and the corresponding percentage of those who express a lack of desire for additional children in two NFHS rounds. A noticeable trend emerges, as evidenced by NFHS-1, where only 60% of completed fertility is associated with parity 3. In contrast, NFHS-5 reveals a significant increase, with nearly 85% of completed fertility observed up to parity 3. The data point to a rise of 30.7 percentage points in couples with only one child from NFHS-1 to NFHS-5. Conversely, couples with more than four children experienced a notable decline, that of 65 percentage points.

Table 21.1 Number of children born and childbearing preferences: changes from NFHS-1 to NFHS-5, India

Number of children born	NFHS-1	Nondesire for an additional child	NFHS-5	Nondesire for an additional child
One	17.2	18.2	35.8	32.9
Two	22.2	49.6	35.1	87.3
Three	21.0	59.1	15.3	93.2
Four or more children	39.5	75.9	13.9	94.7
Total		51.8		77.5

Source: Calculated from NFHS two rounds, NFHS-1 and NFHS-5

A clear correlation emerges between the number of currently living children and the percentage of women expressing a reluctance to have another child. The aversion to having an additional child among mothers with only one child surged by nearly 50 percentage points between rounds. In NFHS-5, approximately 93% of mothers express a disinclination for further children if they already have three, a substantial increase from the approximately 60% recorded during NFHS-1.

21.3.2 Gender-Parity Composition and Family-Size Choices

Table 21.2 reveals a notable shift that focuses on the trend of one-girl families. Families with only one daughter are on the rise. Between rounds, the proportion of mothers with just one girl and no desire for more children increased by nearly 10 percentage points. This preference for not having more children intensifies with increasing parity, irrespective of the children's gender. Notably, NFHS-5 data show a 33-percentage-point increase in two-daughter acceptance at parity 2, compared to 34 percentage points for one girl and one boy and 32 percentage points for two sons. However, the lowest desire for further children occurs at parity 2, when mothers have only two daughters, consistent across both survey rounds. At parity 3, more than 90% of mothers express a lack of desire for any more children, irrespective of the sex of the previous birth, a substantial increase from the initial NFHS survey.

21.3.3 Fertility Desires and Household Economic Conditions

Table 21.3 shows an interesting picture of changing fertility desires across economic classes in India. In NFHS-1, the urge for additional children decreased with both increasing family size (parity) and economic status. This suggested a strong

Table 21.2 Relationship between gender-parity composition and family-size decisions, NFHS-1 and NFHS-5, India

Gender-parity composition	Proportion of women reported		Unwillingness to have another child	
	Current gender-parity composition			
	NFHS-1	NFHS-5	NFHS-1	NFHS-5
Parity 1				
No son	8.7	10.1	16.0	26.7
One son	8.5	12.2	20.4	38.0
Parity 2				
No son	4.9	6.4	26.7	62.9
One son	11.4	22.6	56.8	91.3
Two sons	5.8	11.2	60.3	93.3
Parity 3				
No son	4.3	3.0	33.8	67.8
One son	16.8	13.7	63.3	94.3
Two sons	22.7	14.9	79.0	97.7
Three or more sons	16.8	5.9	82.5	96.5
Total			51.8	77.5

Source: Calculated from NFHS two rounds, NFHS-1 and NFHS-5

association between household finances and family-planning decisions. Poorer families, on average, tended to have more children than wealthier ones did.

Contrastingly, data from NFHS-5 reveal that fertility desires remain indifferent to economic standing. At parity 1, mothers, whether categorized as poor, middle class, or rich, exhibit nearly the same level of reluctance toward having any more children. Among the poorest families, a noticeable rise in the aversion to future children is observed, particularly those with only daughters. The percentage of such parents' choosing to stop childbearing after one or two daughters increased significantly (18.6 percentage points and 33.4 percentage points, respectively) in NFHS-5 compared to NFHS-1. The shift in the inclination to avoid future children registers the highest increase in the poorest and poorer households—even among parents with one boy and one girl and two successive boys at parity 2—compared to other economic classes. Interestingly, the wealthiest class exhibits the least change in their desire for further offspring.

21.3.4 *Influence of Women's Education on Changing Fertility Preferences Across Different Survey Rounds*

Figure 21.1 reveals a fascinating divergence in how education levels influence women's desires for additional children in India. Mothers with lower levels of education, particularly those who are illiterate or have primary education, are increasingly

Table 21.3 Change in association between gender-parity composition and reluctance to have additional children from NFHS-1 to NFHS-5, India

Gender-parity composition	NFHS-1					NFHS-5				
	Poorest	Poorer	Middle	Richer	Richest	Poorest	Poorer	Middle	Richer	Richest
Parity 1										
No son	8.8	11.6	14.1	17.3	28.9	20.7	26.5	26.9	28.2	28.8
One son	11.7	13.5	18.6	21.3	34.4	30.3	34.4	34.7	37.6	47.0
Parity 2										
No son	12.7	13.9	20.6	33.7	56.2	46.2	55.4	66.4	71.2	68.5
One son	32.0	37.8	52.9	65.3	84.6	82.2	90.1	92.2	92.8	95.1
Two sons	34.6	39.5	56.4	65.1	86.1	89.4	91.3	93.4	94.8	95.7
Parity 3										
No son	23.6	29.1	33.2	41.3	57.9	58.1	69.0	70.6	74.9	70.5
One son	51.8	51.5	67.0	72.9	88.9	91.4	93.9	94.9	96.3	96.7
Two sons	71.0	75.1	82.1	85.3	91.9	97.0	97.5	97.9	98.7	98
Three more sons	80.1	80.9	84.3	84.1	88.8	95.4	97.0	97.3	97.4	95.8
Total	22.1	22.8	23.7	15.0	18.4	19.3	20.7	20.6	20.2	19.3

Source: Calculated from NFHS two rounds, NFHS-1 and NFHS-5

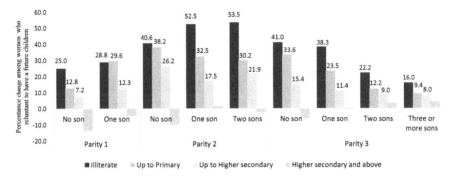

Fig. 21.1 Percentage-point difference in women's nondesire for a future child according to their educational attainment from NFHS-1 to NFHS-5, India. (*Source*: Constructed from NFHS two rounds, NFHS-1 and NFHS-5)

choosing to stop childbearing regardless of the gender of their previous birth. Among them, the reluctance to have more children, even when they have only female children, significantly increases across all parities and between rounds, particularly at parity 2 and parity 3, reaching around 41 percentage points. Furthermore, an evident increase is observed in the unwillingness to have an additional child among mothers with one boy and one girl or two boys at parity 2, with the highest increase observed among illiterate mothers, surpassing 50 percentage points.

Conversely, mothers with secondary education and above exhibit a contrasting trend, showing an increase in the desire for an additional child between survey rounds. Interestingly, among them, the reluctance to have another child when they have only one female child decreased by 13.6 percentage points from NFHS-1 to NFHS-5. Similarly, affluent mothers with two female children experienced a 10-percentage-point decrease in their nondesire for an additional child during the same period.

21.3.5 Influence of Spouse's Occupational Characteristics on Family-Planning Choices Between Survey Rounds

Like the influence of educational qualifications on mothers, mothers whose spouses are engaged in primary economic activities display reluctance to have another child, and this reluctance increases between survey rounds regardless of parity or the sex of previous children (Fig. 21.2). Despite 13.8-percentage-point and 41-percentage-point increases in the acceptance of female children at parities 1 and 2, respectively, this increase is less substantial than that for parities with at least one male child. Notably, among mothers with spouses in primary occupations, the combination of having one girl and one boy appears to be an ideal sex composition given that the difference between rounds of having another child is highest in this category.

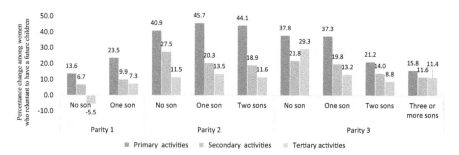

Fig. 21.2 Percentage-point difference in women's nondesire for a future child according to their spouse's economic activity from NFHS-1 to NFHS-5, India. (*Source*: Constructed from NFHS two rounds, NFHS-1 and NFHS-5)

Mothers with spouses employed in tertiary sectors appear less inclined to have only girls in any parity. This is evident at parity 1 with only a female child, where the reluctance to have another child decreased by 5.5 percentage points between survey rounds. At parity 2, the reluctance to have another child increased the least among mothers with two children in this category.

21.3.6 Religious Affiliation and the Waning Desire for Another Child

Figure 21.3 demonstrates that nondesire for a second child increased dramatically between the rounds regardless of whether the mothers were Muslims, with a consistent difference (8–9 percentage points) between two religious affiliations (Muslim and Hindu). For both religions, the percentage-point increase associated with not having a second child is comparable. However, Hindu women are more likely to stop having children if they have one son at parity 1 (18.6 percentage points) or no son at parities 2 and 3 (36.7 percentage points and 34.6 percentage points, respectively) (see Fig. 21.3).

21.3.7 Current Working Status of Mothers and the Shifts in Their Desire for Future Children Between Survey Rounds

Figure 21.4 demonstrates that regardless of the number of previous births or the sex of the previous child, working women tend to be more open to accepting daughters within their families. However, a noticeable trend of strong resistance emerges, evidenced by a higher increase in the percentage-point change in the reluctance toward having an additional child between two survey rounds, particularly when parents

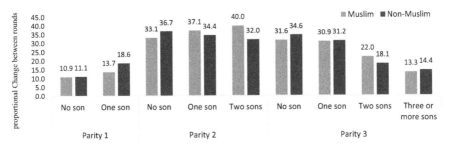

Fig. 21.3 Percentage-point difference in women's nondesire for a future child according to their religious affiliation from NFHS-1 to NFHS-5, India. (*Source*: Constructed from NFHS two rounds, NFHS-1 and NFHS-5)

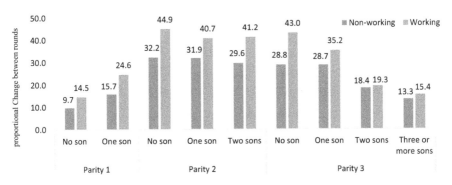

Fig. 21.4 Percentage-point difference in women's nondesire for a future child according to their working status from NFHS-1 to NFHS-5, India. (*Source*: Constructed from NFHS two rounds, NFHS-1 and NFHS-5)

have two successive girls, indicating an underlying concern among parents about avoiding having another child in such circumstances.

21.3.8 Media Exposure and Changing Fertility Choices Among Mothers

According to Fig. 21.5, mothers who encounter family-planning messages through mass media are less likely to desire additional children. Figure 21.5 highlights the significant role of mass media in influencing gender equality in fertility outcomes and restraining childbearing up to parity 2. The reluctance to have an additional child increases with the growing number of children, regardless of the sex of the previous children. While a preference for having a boy within their parity persists, mothers with only a female child or only female children are now exhibiting a reluctance to have another child, with an increase of 7 percentage points at parity 1, 27

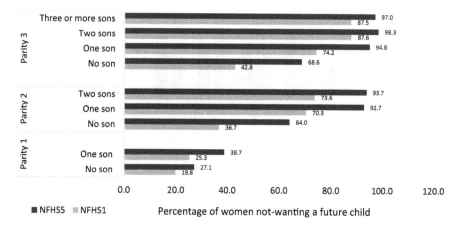

Fig. 21.5 Percentage-point difference in women's nondesire for a future child according to their exposure to mass media from NFHS-1 to NFHS-5, India. (*Source*: Constructed from NFHS two rounds, NFHS-1 and NFHS-5)

percentage points at parity 2, and 26 percentage points at parity 3 between survey rounds.

21.3.9 Region-Specific Decline in the Desire for an Additional Child

Examining the region-specific decline in the desire for an additional child in Table 21.4 reveals distinct patterns across different parts of India. In north-central India, the most significant increase in reluctance to have another child is observed among mothers with one male child and one female child, reaching 35% at parity 2, which is the highest among other parities. In the east-northeast (east–NE) areas, the highest increase between the two survey rounds is noted among mothers with two children, especially if they have two successive boys. In addition, in southeast India, the highest unwillingness to have an additional child is observed among mothers with two daughters, experiencing an increase of nearly 40 percentage points between survey rounds.

Notably, mothers who have only one daughter and choose to restrict their childbearing are more prevalent in east–NE India, whereas the increase in mothers who have two successive daughters and wish to restrict childbearing is found to be highest in southeast India, followed by the east–NE and north-central regions. A similar trend is evident at parity 3 when women have only female children.

After an examination of residential locations (Table 21.5), urban India shows and continues to show significant acceptance of daughters, as anticipated. A closer examination reveals that the increase in women's nondesire for additional children

Table 21.4 Region-specific decline in women's nondesire for an additional child from NFHS-1 to NFHS-5, India

Gender-parity composition	NFHS-1			NFHS-5		
	North-Central	East–NE	Southwest	North-Central	East–NE	Southwest
Parity 1						
No son	11.6	17.7	20.4	19.4	32.4	27.9
One son	17.9	19.9	24.1	35.9	40.8	37.6
Parity 2						
No son	19.0	25.3	40.2	39.4	60.8	79.6
One son	55.4	51.4	65.6	89.9	87.7	94.3
Two sons	62.8	53.1	64.5	92.6	91.2	94.8
Parity 3						
No son	28.2	33.6	45.4	56.1	67.8	79.7
One son	61.0	62.4	71.3	93.9	91.2	97.6
Two sons	79.5	75.8	84.8	98.1	96.5	98.3
Three or more sons	83.0	81.4	83.5	97.2	95.3	96.8

Source: Calculated from NFHS two rounds, NFHS-1 and NFHS-5

is higher in rural areas than in urban ones, regardless of parities. Furthermore, a discernible preference for sons, coupled with relatively higher acceptance of daughters, is evident, particularly in rural areas when compared to urban areas.

21.3.10 Multivariate Analysis

Table 21.6 shows the predictive margins of expected trends for mothers' reluctance to have another child in the future as well as their acceptance of having a female child or female children. The acceptance of families with only girls has significantly increased over the past three decades. This surge is attributed primarily to the individual characteristics of mothers, with a notable emphasis on their educational attainment. As mothers' education levels rise, a significant increase in the likelihood of accepting either one or two girls only in the family takes place. A deeper delve into the NFHS-5 data reveals that mothers with education at the higher secondary level and above are 88% more likely to embrace a family with only a girl, marking a substantial 40-percentage-point increase from the NFHS-1 findings. At parity 2, the difference for a family with two girls is a mere 9-percentage-point increase between the two survey rounds (from 66.1% to 75.9%), though it was already higher in the earlier round, and thus, a "level effect" was anticipated. However, the engagement of mothers in the labor force does not exhibit significance in predicting having only-girl families at parity 2 during NFHS-5.

Interestingly, the occupation of spouses and their inclination toward accepting families with one or two girls showed a significantly positive relationship during

Table 21.5 Rural–urban variation in women's nondesire for an additional child from NFHS-1 to NFHS-2, India

Gender-Parity composition	NFHS-1		NFHS-5	
	Rural	Urban	Rural	Urban
Parity 1				
No son	12.3	25.1	23.0	32.7
One son	16.0	30.1	34.9	43.3
Parity 2				
No son	19.2	45.2	57.3	72.9
One son	46.7	75.7	90.3	93.1
Two sons	49.5	77.8	92.9	94.0
Parity 3				
No son	28.8	49.4	66.1	72.4
One son	58.6	77.9	93.8	95.9
Two sons	76.9	85.9	97.8	97.4
Three or more sons	81.4	86.8	96.4	96.5

Source: Calculated from NFHS two rounds, NFHS-1 and NFHS-5

Table 21.6 Predictive margins of desiring of girls among students according to their background characteristics, India

Variable	One daughter and no desire for future children		Two daughters and no desire for future children	
	NFHS-1	NFHS-5	NFHS-1	NFHS-5
Respondent's age				
25 years	17.8***	61.8***	13.5***	38.8***
35 years	16.3***	18.3***	30.9***	72.6***
Respondent's education				
Illiterate	28.6	45.2	20.7	27.8
Up to primary	29.1**	34.7***	24.2***	41.5***
Up to higher secondary	35.7***	68.2***	44***	64.6***
Higher secondary and above	40.6***	88.1***	66.1***	75.9***
Respondent's working status				
Not working	38.2	62	32	54.9
Working	43.4***	65.2***	38.5***	54.4
Respondent's partner's occupation				
Not working	31.1	74.8	24.9	66.3
Primary activities	39.7***	63.8***	34.5***	61.1***
Secondary activities	37.1***	61.2***	32.6***	54.5***
Tertiary activities	40.6***	60.1***	45.5***	61.4*
Respondent's contraceptive use				
Not using any	48	85.7	34.7	56.4

(continued)

Table 21.6 (continued)

Variable	One daughter and no desire for future children		Two daughters and no desire for future children	
	NFHS-1	NFHS-5	NFHS-1	NFHS-5
Using natural methods	30.6***	44.2**	37.4**	46.9***
Modern reversible method	20.9***	47.8***	28.9***	57.2**
Respondent's exposure to social media				
No	42.8	53	34.8	58
Yes	37.7***	67.7	33.5***	53.2
Respondent's religion				
Hindu	46.2	67.4	44.8	55.9
Non-Hindu	18.1***	41.1***	25.4***	49***
Respondent's caste				
SC/ST (caste)	32.5	64.4	32.1	60.9
Others (no caste)	41.2***	62.2*	34*	52.6
Respondent's wealth quintile				
Poor	29.6	67.9	25.2	56.8
Middle	37.7***	68.9***	30.6***	59***
Rich	47.3***	62.3***	39.6***	52.4*
Respondent's place of residence				
Urban	44.2	77.9	36.2	60.7
Rural	36.5***	54.1***	31.8***	51.3***
Respondent's region				
North-central	27.4	35.4	22.3	37.2
East–NE	44.9***	87***	33.9***	67.5***
Southwest	53.8***	72.1***	53.8***	70.9***

Source: Calculated from NFHS two rounds, NFHS-1 and NFHS-5
Note: *** $p < 0.001$, ** $p < 0.01$, and * $p < 0.05$

NFHS-1. However, in NFHS-5, women with nonworking partners are more likely to accept families with only girls compared to their counterparts. Similarly, household assets are proportional to having only-girl families, and their significance diminishes during NFHS-5 at parity 2. Among mothers who do not use any contraception, the likelihood of acceptance is higher, with a 40-percentage-point increase for families with one girl and a 22-percentage-point increase for families with two girls between survey rounds. Although exposure to mass media is proportional to the acceptance of girls, it loses its significance in NFHS-5, irrespective of parity.

As expected, the likelihood of accepting families with only girls remains higher among Hindus in both survey rounds. Nevertheless, the gap between the two religious groups has narrowed during NFHS-5. For example, at parity 2, where a 20-percentage-point difference appears during NFHS-1, it has reduced to 6 percentage points in NFHS-5. At a contextual level, urban mothers and those from the east-northeast and southwest states are more likely to accept families with only a girl, regardless of the NFHS round or the number of girls.

21.4 Discussion

The objective of the chapter is to examine the evolving distribution of parity and the increasing prevalence of the "child-aversion" sentiment regarding additional children in India. The findings suggest a significant shift in childbearing preferences across India. Mothers increasingly opt for smaller families and restrict their childbearing up to parity 3, with a notable rise in their reluctance to have an additional child—particularly among mothers who have only girls, irrespective of parities. As India progresses, these encouraging trends suggest a move toward more-inclusive and more-egalitarian reproductive choices. However, a paradoxical decline in the desire for additional children when mothers have precisely two daughters indicates a complex interplay of factors influencing family-size decisions. It could be embedded in the fact that a female child is considered to be "undesired" not "unwanted" per se (Das and Ghosh 2021). Substantial large-scale evidence is lacking on whether girls are deprived of essential privileges, including immunization, nutrition, education, and overall well-being (Das and Roy 2021).

This study acknowledges the significant change in mindset observed when couples choose to have only one female child and skip further childbearing. However, in the context of parity 2, the majority of couples may opt to limit childbearing after the birth of two consecutive girls as a strategy employed to avoid an undesired sex composition (Ghosh and Begum 2015). Nevertheless, this practice does not inherently contribute to the realization of gender balance in fertility choices. Within the broader framework of fertility transition, imposing limitations at parity 2 becomes imperative (Behrman and Duvisac 2017; Kaur et al. 2017), even when the desired sex composition has not been achieved (Mutharayappa et al. 1997).

Bivariate and multivariate analyses reveal that in addition to individual factors, household, community, and contextual factors play crucial roles in this context. Beyond the gender-parity lens, India's poorest populations are experiencing a significant shift in family-size preferences, opting for fewer children than ever before. An exploration into fertility desires and economic conditions unveils a departure from historical trends as poorer families (Desai 2023), particularly those with only daughters, display an unexpected rise in aversion to future children. Multivariate analysis shows a similar trend. Surprisingly, the wealthiest class displays the least change in their desire for further offspring in bivariate analysis, adding a layer of complexity to the relationship between economic affluence and fertility preferences. Rising costs of living, particularly in education and healthcare, strain limited budgets, increasingly hindering couples from being able to raise large families. Therefore, they tend to stop at a parity that is economically beneficial to them. The sex composition of the previous child becomes secondary here. The scrutiny of a spouse's job as a determinant of family-planning choices supports a similar narrative. Mothers with spouses engaged in primary economic activities are reluctant to have another child, particularly with a specific preference for one girl and one boy. Tertiary sector employment appears to influence family-planning decisions differently, showing a less pronounced inclination against having only girls.

Social and cultural dynamics are transforming, with notable shifts propelled by increased female education and empowerment. The intricate nexus between women's education and shifting fertility desires delineates an intriguing divergence. That lower-educated mothers are increasingly opting to curtail childbearing contrasts sharply with their more-educated counterparts' expression of an augmented desire for an additional child. Nevertheless, in the contenxt of having a family with only girls, women's education emerges as a significant factor (see Table 21.6). This dichotomy suggests a paradigm shift in the influence of education on family-planning decisions. Benefiting from different central and state sponsored programs, female education has increased and has presumably resulted in women's empowerment at the societal level in India. Consequently, women are now prioritizing career aspirations alongside family commitments. The latest NFHS data reveal a rise in the average age of marriage for women, to 22.1 years (NFHS, 2019–2021), contributing significantly to the overall decline in fertility rates and in gender inequality in fertility choices. This trend is also evident among working mothers in this chapter's bivariate analysis. Although they may be open to having a daughter if they desire only one child and choose to stop thereafter, the acceptance becomes less favorable when they have two successive girls at parity 2. This indicates a shift in attitude or behavior among working mothers when faced with the prospect of having multiple daughters in succession. Despite a remarkable rise in women's education in India after 2000, their participation in the workforce has remained surprisingly stagnant, which has had a significant influence on balanced fertility choices among mothers. This paradox, where educational gains have not translated into economic empowerment, stems from a complex web of social, economic, and cultural factors (Chatterjee et al. 2018; Kaur et al. 2017).

This study also highlights the pivotal role of media exposure in shaping fertility choices, where mothers who encounter family-planning messages through mass media display a reduced likelihood to desire additional children. The increasing reluctance to have another child, irrespective of gender composition, signifies the evolving role of media in influencing gender equality in fertility outcomes. However, this variable loses its significance in recent data, prompting the exploration of other factors that influence mothers' preferences for having a family with only girls (Das et al. 2023; Desai 2023).

Region-specific variations in the desire for additional children add another layer of complexity, as north-central India witnesses a substantial increase in reluctance among mothers to have at least one boy in their parity. Other regions display unique patterns—emphasizing the acceptance of girls-only families—highlighting the need for a deeper understanding of regional dynamics. In eastern and southern India, a historical continuity in matrilineal and matrilocal traditions has persisted in certain communities, fostering a more inclusive and equitable view of gender roles (Eapen 2020; Gill 2013; Mitra 2014). On the other hand, northern India has a prevalent patrilineal and patrilocal social structure, where the family's lineage and inheritance traditionally pass through male descendants. This entrenched patriarchal framework may contribute to a relatively lower acceptance of daughters, given that they are often perceived as future members of another family (Vera-Sanso 1999; Sekher and Hatti 2007).

21.5 Conclusion

In conclusion, this study effectively navigates through multiple dimensions, contributing valuable insights to the evolving landscape of family-size choices, fertility desires, and family-planning decisions in India. The analysis establishes a changing distribution of parity and a rising prevalence of the "nondesire" sentiment toward additional children, especially among mothers with only-girl families. This discernible trend reveals a significant surge in one-girl families, accompanied by an increasing inclination toward limiting family size (fertility transition). However, aiming for an equal gender balance in fertility outcomes, on the basis of only achieving numerical equality, seems an appealing yet reductionist perspective. It may oversimplify the complex interplay of cultural, individual, and societal factors that intricately influence the perceived value of girls. Similarly, the growing prevalence of daughter-only families in India may indicate a psychological shift, but attributing it solely to an increased value placed on daughters could be premature. It might overlook the historical experiences of girls who are dealing with disparities in access to education, healthcare, and economic opportunities. Such an approach assumes a linear correlation between quantitative representation and actual qualitative well-being, neglecting the pervasive impact of discrimination. In India, daughters' marriages remain significant financial and emotional burdens for parents, reflecting their distinct gender roles within families. This dichotomy emerges as individual valuations of daughters clash with societal norms, constraining their perceived capacity to fulfill traditional familial duties. Furthermore, achieving genuine gender balance necessitates a fundamental restructuring of societal frameworks that perpetuate the devaluation of girls. This imperative requires challenging entrenched patriarchal norms, ensuring equitable access to resources and opportunities, and cultivating a cultural milieu characterized by genuine respect and appreciation for individuals, irrespective of gender. Only through such transformative efforts can we surpass superficial equivalence and establish a world where the intrinsic value of girls becomes an inherent and unwavering reality. Accurate assessments of whether daughters are "actually" valued for their intrinsic worth and potential, rather than solely for their existence, can be achieved only through further research and a readiness to challenge entrenched societal norms.

Declaration

Availability of Data and Materials The data and materials for this chapter are sourced from publicly available secondary sources accessible at https://dhsprogram.com/methodology/survey/survey-display-541.cfm. Interested individuals can register at the provided link to freely download the necessary data.

Ethics Approval and Consent to Participate This chapter is based on secondary data, which are available in the public domain. Therefore, ethical approval is not required to conduct this study.

Competing Interests The authors declare that they have no competing interests.

Funding This chapter did not receive any specific grant from funding agencies in the public, commercial, or not-for-profit sectors.

References

Allendorf K (2020) Another gendered demographic dividend: adjusting to a future without sons. Popul Dev Rev 46(3):471–499

Arnold F (2001) Son preference in South Asia. In: Sathar ZA, Phillips JF (eds) Fertility transition in South Asia. Oxford University Press, Oxford, pp 281–299

Asadullah MN, Mansoor N, Randazzo T, Wahhaj Z (2021) Is son preference disappearing from Bangladesh? World Dev 140(2021):105353

Basu AM (1999) Fertility decline and increasing gender imbalance in India, including a possible south Indian turnaround. Dev Change 30(2):237–263

Behrman J, Duvisac S (2017) The relationship between women's paid employment and women's stated son preference in India. Demogr Res 36(52):1601–1636

Bongaarts J, Watkins SC (1996) Social interactions and contemporary fertility transitions. Popul Dev Rev 22(4):639–682

Borooah V, Iyer S (2004) Religion and fertility in India: the role of son preference and daughter aversion [working paper in economics 0436]. University of Cambridge. RGI, 2021

Casterline J (ed) (2001) Diffusion processes and fertility transition: selected perspectives. National Academy Press, Washington, DC

Chatterjee S, Gupta SD, Upadhyay P (2018) Empowering women and stimulating development at bottom of pyramid through micro-entrepreneurship. Manag Decis 56(1):160–174

Chellaiyan VG, Adhikary M, Das TK, Taneja N, Daral S (2018) Factors influencing gender preference for child among married women attending ante-natal clinic in a tertiary care hospital in Delhi: a cross-sectional study. Int J Commun Med Public Health 5:1666–1670

Chun H, Das Gupta M (2021) 'Not a bowl of rice, but tender loving care': from aborting girls to preferring daughters in South Korea. Asian Popul Stud 18:1–21

Chung W, Das Gupta M (2007) The decline of son preference in South Korea: the roles of development and public policy. Popul Dev Rev 33(4):757–783

Das K, Ghosh S (2021) Rural–urban fertility convergence, differential stopping behavior, and contraceptive method mix in West Bengal, India: a spatiotemporal analysis. J Fam Hist 46(2):211–235

Das Gupta M, Zhenghua J, Bohua L, Zhenming X, Chung W, Hwa-Ok B (2003) Why is son preference so persistent in east and South Asia? A cross-country study of China, India and the Republic of Korea. J Dev Stud 40(2):153–187

Das K, Roy U (2021) Facts and reflections of changing child sex ratio in West Bengal during 2011-2011, India. Indian J Geogr Environ 17(18):63–73

Das K, Ghosh S, Shenk MK (2023) Responsibility, social aspirations, and contemporary low fertility: a case study of rural West Bengal, India. Asian Popul Stud:1–19

Desai S (2023) The global aspirational class and its demographic fortunes. Presidential address, population Association of America annual meeting, April 2023. Article forthcoming in demography

Desai S, Temsah G (2014) Muslim and Hindu women's public and private behaviors: gender, family, and communalized politics in India. Demography 51(6):2307–2332

Diamond-Smith N, Bishai D (2015) Evidence of self-correction of child sex ratios in India: a district-level analysis of child sex ratios from 1981 to 2011. Demography 52(2):641–666

Diamond-Smith N, Luke N, McGarvey S (2008) 'Too many girls, too much dowry': son preference and daughter aversion in rural Tamil Nadu, India. Cult Health Sex 10(7):697–708

Dyson T, Moore M (1983) On kinship structure, female autonomy, and demographic behavior in India. Popul Dev Rev 9(1):35–60

Eapen LM (2020) Son preference in India: is it a cultural bequest? In: International conference on gender research. Academic Conferences International, Reading, pp 76–IX

Eloundou-Enyegue PM, Giroux SC, Tenikue M (2021) Demographic analysis and the decomposition of social change. In: Klimczuk A (ed) Demographic analysis: selected concepts, tools, and applications, pp 182–195

Fuse K (2013) Daughter preference in Japan: a reflection of gender role attitudes? Demogr Res 28(36):1021–1052. https://doi.org/10.4054/DemRes.2013.28.36

Ghosh S, Begum S (2015) Influence of son preference on contraceptive method mix: some evidences from 'two Bengals'. Asian Popul Stud 11(3):296–311

Ghosh S et al (2020) Religion, contraceptive method mix and son preference among Bengali-speaking Community in Indian Subcontinent: a long view. In: Chattopadhyay A, Ghosh S (eds) Population dynamics in eastern India and Bangladesh. Springer, Singapore, pp 183–207

Gill MS (2013) Female foeticide in India: looking beyond son preference and dowry. Mank Q 53(3/4):281

Guilmoto CZ (2009) The sex ratio transition in Asia. Popul Dev Rev 35(3):519–549

Guilmoto CZ (2012) Sex ratio imbalances at birth: current trends, consequences and policy implications. UNFPA Asia Pacific Regional Office, Bangkok

Guilmoto CZ, Rahm L (2021) Why should prenatal sex selection ultimately decline? In: IUSSP International Population Conference, Hyderabad, December 8, India

International Institute for Population Sciences (IIPS) (1995) National Family Health Survey (NFHS-1), India, 1992–93: India. IIPS, Mumbai

International Institute for Population Sciences and East-West Center Program on Population (2021) International Institute for Population Sciences (IIPS) and ICF, National Family Health Survey (NFHS-5), India, 2019–21: India. IIPS, Mumbai

Karve I (1993) The kinship map of India. In: Uberoi P (ed) Family, kinship and marriage in India. Oxford University Press, Oxford, pp 50–73

Kaur R, Bhalla SS, Agarwal MK, Ramakrishnan P (2017) Sex ratio at birth—the role of gender, class and education: a technical report. UNFPA, New Delhi

Lei L (2013) Sons, daughters, and intergenerational support in China. Chin Sociol Rev 45(3):26–52

Lin TC (2009) The decline of son preference and rise of gender indifference in Taiwan since 1990. Demogr Res 20(16):377–402

Mitra A (2014) Son preference in India: implications for gender development. J Econ Issues 48(4):1021–1037

Mutharayappa R, Choe MK, Arnold F, Roy TK (1997) Is son preference slowing down India's transition to low fertility? NFHS Bulletin No. 4. International Institute for Population Sciences, Mumbai

Nagarajan R, Sahoo H (2019) Increasing acceptance of daughters in India: trends, regional differentials and determinants. J Popul Soc Stud 27(2):106–123

Nanda B, Ray N, Mukherjee R, Jairaj R (2019) Gender discrimination and violence against women: connecting the dots of declining child sex ratio (CSR) in India. Mainstream Wkly 16(22):30

Nandi A, Deolalikar AB (2013) Does a legal ban on sex-selective abortions improve child sex ratios? Evidence from a policy change in India. J Dev Econ 103:216–228

Nasir R, Kalla AK (2006) Kinship system, fertility and son preference among the Muslims: a review. Anthropologist 8(4):275–281

Patel T (2007) The mindset behind eliminating the female foetus. In: Patel T (ed) Sex-selective abortion in India: gender, society and new reproductive technologies. Sage, Thousand Oaks, CA, pp 135–174

Patel T (2020) New faces of the Indian family in the 21st century: some explorations. In: Patel T (ed) The contemporary Indian family. Routledge, London, pp 23–41

Retherford RD, Roy TK (2003) Factors affecting sex-selective abortion in India and 17 major states. International Institute for Population Sciences, Mumbai

RGI (2011) Office of the Registrar General & census commissioner, India. GOI, Census Data

Sample Registration System Statistical Report (2023) Office of the Registrar General, New Delhi. https://censusindia.gov.in/census.website/data/SRSSTAT. Accessed 19 Mar 2023

Sekher TV, Hatti N (2007) Vulnerable daughters in a modernising society: from son preference to daughter discrimination in rural South India. In: Watering the neighbour's garden: the growing demographic female deficit in Asia, pp 295–323

Tong Y (2022) India's sex ratio at birth begins to normalize. Pew Research Centre, Washington, DC

Unnithan-Kumar M (2010) Female selective abortion–beyond 'culture': family making and gender inequality in a globalising India. Cult Health Sex 12(2):153–166

Vera-Sanso P (1999) Dominant daughters-in-law and submissive mothers-in-law? Cooperation and conflict in South India. J R Anthropol Inst 5:577–593

Weitzman A (2015) Creating a crisis?: gender discrimination, sex ratios and their implications for the developing world. In: Development in crisis. Routledge, London, pp 100–114

Zaidi B, Morgan SP (2016) In the pursuit of sons: additional births or sex-selective abortion in Pakistan? Popul Dev Rev 42(4):693

Chapter 22
Intimate Partner Violence and Risk of Unintended Pregnancy: Findings from Rural India

Anshika Singh and Aditya Singh

Abstract Intimate partner violence (IPV) and unintended pregnancy (UP) are significant public health concerns with profound implications for women's well-being. Only limited evidence is available on the association between IPV and UP for rural areas of India. Therefore, this chapter aims to examine this specific association in the context of rural India. Data from the fifth round of the National Family Health Survey were examined to evaluate the relationship between IPV and UP among rural women aged 18–49. UP was the dependent variable, and the primary predictor variable was the IPV. A logistic regression analysis was employed to explore the association between IPV and UP while controlling for other factors influencing the likelihood of UP. The findings suggest that women who reported IPV were more prone to experience UP even after adjusting for relevant factors. The likelihood of UP was approximately 1.6 times higher among those subjected to either physical or sexual IPV and 2.6 times higher among those experiencing both sexual and physical IPV compared to women who never experienced IPV. The study reveals a significant association between UP and IPV in rural India, emphasizing the pressing need to enhance and adapt existing IPV interventions to mitigate the associated risk of UP. Efforts should be directed towards devising comprehensive strategies aimed at preventing and addressing IPV while also catering to the reproductive health needs of women in abusive relationships.

Keywords IPV · Physical violence · Sexual violence · Unintended pregnancy · Rural India

---

A. Singh · A. Singh (✉)
Department of Geography, Banaras Hindu University, Varanasi, Uttar Pradesh, India
e-mail: anshikasingh@bhu.ac.in; adityasingh@bhu.ac.in

22.1 Introduction

Intimate partner violence (IPV) encompasses actions by a partner or former partner that cause physical, sexual, or psychological harm. This includes physical aggression, coercion during sexual activity, psychological abuse, and controlling behaviours (United Nations 1993). According to recent WHO estimates, nearly one-third of women across the world suffer from physical abuse, sexual abuse, or both from their intimate partner (World Health Organization 2021). The rate of IPV varies significantly across countries. In developed countries, the rates range from 7% to 35%. However, the prevalence is even higher in developing countries, particularly among ever-married women. For instance, studies have reported rates of 45.3% in Bangladesh, 35.9% in Nigeria, 32% in India, 29.4% in China, and 26.3% in Nepal (Chang et al. 2022; Gautam and Jeong 2019; IIPS and MacroInternational 2022; National Institute of Population Studies (NIPS) and ICF 2019; Rayhan and Akter 2021).

IPV may cause various types (sexual, physical, and reproductive) of health problems for women (World Health Organization 2021). One of the major consequences of IPV is losing control over fertility and sexual decision-making, leading to unintended pregnancy, or UP (Pallitto et al. 2005). *Unintended pregnancy* can be defined as "a mistimed pregnancy"—that is, a woman did not want to become pregnant at the time—or as "an unwanted pregnancy with no plans to become pregnant" (Brown and Eisenberg 1995; Dutta et al. 2015).

Women experiencing IPV often face coercive control and manipulation from their abusive partners, which extends to reproductive choices and sexual autonomy. This control can manifest in various ways, such as forced or nonconsensual sexual activity, contraceptive sabotage, or restrictions on accessing reproductive healthcare. As a result, women affected by IPV may struggle to assert control over their fertility and make decisions aligned with their reproductive goals. The loss of autonomy in these intimate matters greatly increases the likelihood that women who live will have to grapple with the complex emotional, physical, and social implications of such circumstances (Miller et al. 2010). UP creates perplexing health problems, resulting in poor health outcomes for mothers and children (Iseyemi et al. 2017). Previous studies have found a significant association between induced abortion, maternal depression, psychological issues, and anxiety with UP (Dutta et al. 2015; Pallitto and O'Campo 2004).

Approximately 68% of the Indian population resides in rural areas, according to the Census of India 2011 (Ministry of Home Affairs, Government of India 2011). Rural women are more prone to IPV and UP than their urban counterparts are (Fig. 22.1) because of a lack of interventions and awareness about contraception, maternal health, and family planning, which are present in urban areas. However, rural areas still need such initiatives (Society for Women's Action and Training Initiatives (SWATI) 2020).

Previous studies have provided varying findings on the relationship between UP and IPV, with some indicating a significant link internationally and nationally

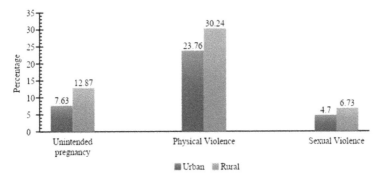

Fig. 22.1 Prevalence of unintended pregnancy, physical violence, and sexual violence in urban and rural areas of India, 2019–2021

(Acharya et al. 2019; Ajayi et al. 2021; Dixit et al. 2012; Garg et al. 2022; Ismayilova 2010; Pallitto and O'Campo 2004) and others reporting no significant association (Azevêdo et al. 2013). However, a dearth of research focusing on rural India to explore the connection between IPV and UP remains (Dehingia et al. 2020; Singh et al. 2013; Stephenson et al. 2008). Despite the significant proportion of the Indian population that resides in rural areas (68%) (Office of the Registrar General and Census Commissioner, India 2011), prior studies have not specifically targeted this demographic. Given the distinctive characteristics of rural populations, including their unique fertility patterns and social dynamics, this relationship must be separately investigated within rural contexts. Furthermore, the association between IPV and UP may exhibit complex and variable dynamics across different populations. In light of these considerations, the present study aims to assess, while considering a range of background characteristics, the association between UP and IPV among women aged 18–49 in rural India. By using data from the fifth wave of the National Family Health Survey (NFHS), this study conducted a comprehensive national-level analysis to address this critical gap in the literature.

22.2 Data and Methods

22.2.1 Source of Data

In the present chapter, the data used for analysis were obtained from NFHS-5 (2019–2021). It entails an extensive, multiphase survey carried out in a diverse sample of households across India. The NFHS focuses on reproduction, menstrual hygiene, family planning, maternal health, marriage and sexual activity, fertility preference, women's empowerment, domestic violence, and other health issues. NFHS employs a two-step, stratified sampling approach for data collection. Additional information on the sampling methods and procedures utilized by NFHS

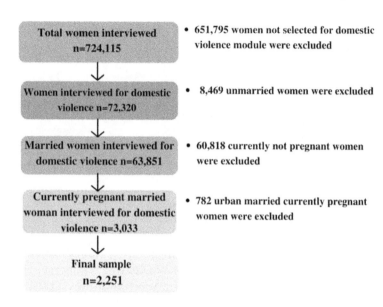

Fig. 22.2 Flowchart showing sample selection procedure

can be found in other specified sources. The dataset analysed in this chapter is accessible via the Demographic and Health Surveys (DHS) repository, accessible at https://dhsprogram.com/data/available-datasets.cfm, and can be acquired by submitting an online request.

In total, 747,176 women were interviewed in different states and union territories in India. Interviews were successfully conducted with 724,115 women, resulting in a response rate of 97%. The number of women who completed the domestic violence module was 72,320. In the end, 2251 women aged 18–49 years who were currently pregnant, resided in rural areas, and gave information on fertility preferences were selected for this chapter (Fig. 22.2). In adherence to the World Health Organization's ethical guidelines for gathering information on domestic violence, only one eligible woman from each household was selected for the module. This chapter used publicly accessible secondary data, which eliminates the need for ethical approval because identifiable survey participants are absent.

22.2.2 Dependent Variable

The primary concern of our chapter is fertility preference. Fertility preference is based on NFHS-5 questions. Respondents were asked, "Are you pregnant now?" If they replied yes, a further question was asked: "When you got pregnant, did you want to get pregnant at that time?" The possible responses were "then," "later," and "not at all." The response "then" was coded as "0" (intended pregnancy), and the other two categories, "later" and "not at all," were coded as "1" (unintended pregnancy).

22.2.3 Independent Variables

The main independent variables were the types of IPV reported by the women. The NFHS obtains these data by inquiring about certain physical and sexual IPV questions. These questions are available in the NFHS questionnaire for women, which can be accessed at https://dhsprogram.com. Women who reported sexual or physical IPV at any frequency ("sometimes," "often," or "not in the past 12 months") were considered to have experienced IPV. For the analysis, the types of IPV were grouped into three categories: "no IPV," "physical or sexual IPV," and "both physical and sexual IPV."

22.2.4 Control Variables

Through a rigorous review of the literature, control variables were considered because they had a significant association with fertility preference. The control variables included women's age, education, partner's education, household wealth quintile, religion, social group, number of children/parity, household population (number of members), exposure to mass media, region of residence, and ever having experienced physical IPV (no and yes) (Acharya et al. 2019; Dixit et al. 2012; Dutta et al. 2015; Garg et al. 2022; Ismayilova 2010; Miller et al. 2010; Pallitto and O'Campo 2004; Seifu et al. 2020; Stephenson et al. 2008).

22.2.5 Statistical Analysis

The bivariate analysis examined how UP (the dependent variable) varied across types of IPV (independent variables) and control variables. A chi-squared test was applied to assess the one-to-one association between the UP and independent variables.

In the initial stage of regression analysis, unadjusted odds ratios were calculated to examine the relationship between UP and the types of IPV. This allowed for an initial assessment of the relationship between these variables without considering any potential confounding factors. In the second stage, logistic regression models were constructed hierarchically, taking potential confounders into account. This method sought to mitigate the influence of additional factors that might affect the link between IPV and UP. By integrating these confounding variables into the analyses, we could evaluate the distinct impact of IPV on UP while controlling for other variables.

The first model in this chapter incorporated distal determinants that indirectly impact women's reproductive behaviour. These determinants included variables such as the education of respondents and their partners, wealth index, religion, social group, the number of household members, mass-media exposure, region of residence, and the main independent variables (the types of IPV). Statically significant distal variables (those with p-values <0.05) were incorporated into the final model alongside proximal determinants and types of IPV. On the other hand, the proximal determinants directly influence fertility preferences and include variables such as age and parity. These factors were considered in the final model to account for their potential influence on UP. In assessing the importance of variables within the ultimate model, variables exhibiting p-values <0.05 were deemed to possess a notable correlation with UP. The statistical examination for this chapter's study was carried out utilizing Stata 13 software (StataCorp.2013 2013).

22.3 Results

22.3.1 Respondent's Background Characteristics

Around half of the sampled women were between 25 and 34 years old (Table 22.1). Over 50% of the sampled women and their partners had achieved a secondary level of education. Nearly 31% of the sampled women belonged to the poorest households. Slightly less than three-fourths of women were Hindu. Almost 40% of the sampled women belonged to the Other Backward Class (OBC) category. Nearly 32% of women were nulliparous, and one-third had only one child. Approximately 55% of women resided in a household with four to six members. Only 5% of respondents had high mass-media exposure. Nearly one-fourth of women belonged to the central region of India. A little over 20% of women reported experiencing physical IPV.

Table 22.1 Sample characteristics

Variable	n (2251)	%
Age (in years)		
18–24	1048	46.6
25–34	1069	47.5
>35	134	6.0
Woman's education		
No education	482	21.4
Primary	293	13.0
Secondary	1217	54.1
Higher	259	11.5
Partner's education		
No education	323	14.4

(continued)

Table 22.1 (continued)

Variable	n (2251)	%
Primary	284	12.6
Secondary	1294	57.5
Higher	350	15.6
Wealth index		
Poorest	716	31.8
Poorer	632	28.1
Middle	428	19.0
Richer	320	14.2
Richest	155	6.9
Religion		
Hindu	1663	73.9
Muslim	279	12.4
Christian	221	9.8
Others	88	3.9
Social group		
SC	469	20.8
ST	573	25.5
OBC	878	39.0
Others	331	14.7
Parity		
None	726	32.3
One child	758	33.7
Two children	421	18.7
Three children	180	8.0
Four or more children	166	7.4
Number of household members		
1–3 members	575	25.5
4–6 members	1256	55.8
7+ members	420	18.7
Mass-media exposure		
No exposure	744	33.1
Low exposure	932	41.4
Medium exposure	447	19.9
High exposure	128	5.7
Region		
North	408	18.1
Central	592	26.3
East	506	22.5
Northeast	352	15.6
West	163	7.2
South	230	10.2
Ever experienced physical IPV		
No	1752	77.8
Yes	499	22.2
Total	2251	100

22.3.2 Physical IPV Among Currently Pregnant Women

Table 22.2 illustrates the occurrence of physical IPV among pregnant women in rural India, categorized according to their demographic characteristics. Older women, those aged 35 years and above, exhibited a slightly higher prevalence of experiencing physical violence. Furthermore, women lacking education, as well as those whose partners were similarly uneducated, were more prone to experiencing physical IPV. Additionally, physical violence was more prevalent among women from the poorest wealth quintile, Hindu women, and those from Scheduled Caste (SC) communities. The likelihood of physical violence was notably elevated among women with four or more children and those residing in households with more than four members. Furthermore, women who were not exposed to mass media were more susceptible to physical violence by their intimate partners. Notably, the proportion of women experiencing physical IPV differs across the regions of India, with the highest rates observed in the central region and the lowest in the northern region.

Table 22.2 Prevalence of physical violence, sexual violence, and unintended pregnancy according to background characteristics among rural women in India, 2019–2021

Variable	Physical violence		Sexual violence		Unintended pregnancy	
	Yes	p-value	Yes	p-value	Yes	p-value
Age (in years)		0.126		0.073		0.001
18–24	18.0		3.0		10.6	
25–34	23.4		5.8		13.3	
>35	26.8		5.4		44.5	
Woman's education		<0.001		<0.001		<0.001
No education	31.8		9.2		24.5	
Primary	28.1		1.8		18.2	
Secondary	17.9		3.5		8.9	
Higher	5.8		0.7		7.8	
Partner's education		<0.001		0.002		0.001
No education	31.7		9.1		23.1	
Primary	26.8		2.1		21.1	
Secondary	19.3		3.8		11.2	
Higher	8.9		2.2		4.9	
Wealth index		<0.001		<0.001		<0.001
Poorest	30.6		7.7		21.0	
Poorer	22.1		3.3		14.7	
Middle	13.8		2.9		7.1	
Richer	9.3		1.6		6.6	
Richest	11.4		1.2		2.9	
Religion		0.341		0.290		0.044
Hindu	21.6		4.6		12.2	

(continued)

Table 22.2 (continued)

Variable	Physical violence Yes	p-value	Sexual violence Yes	p-value	Unintended pregnancy Yes	p-value
Muslim	16.3		3.0		20.2	
Christian	13.2		0.6		7.9	
Others	14.4		2.4		1.4	
Social group		0.427		0.271		0.594
SC	23.6		6.2		14.1	
ST	20.1		4.2		11.0	
OBC	20.5		3.8		12.1	
Others	16.3		2.6		16.5	
Parity		<0.001		<0.001		<0.001
None	11.9		2.2		5.4	
One child	21.0		4.2		11.2	
Two children	27.6		2.4		18.2	
Three children	32.9		11.3		27.1	
Four or more	38.9		11.6		40.8	
Number of household members		0.882		0.181		0.022
1–3 members	19.1		3.9		8.5	
4–6 members	20.8		3.3		11.7	
7+ members	20.7		5.8		18.3	
Mass-media exposure		<0.001		0.059		0.004
No exposure	29.7		6.2		19.8	
Low exposure	17.3		3.8		12.7	
Medium exposure	15.9		2.2		5.3	
High exposure	10.1		3.3		10.0	
Region		0.004		0.065		<0.001
North	10.2		3.3		7.8	
Central	28.1		6.7		12.3	
East	23.7		5.2		21.1	
Northeast	20.7		3.2		14.1	
West	13.2		0.9		5.7	
South	16.3		2.8		3.1	

22.3.3 Sexual IPV Among Currently Pregnant Women

Table 22.2 also indicates that the proportion of women who experienced sexual IPV was relatively higher among women aged 25–34 and those with uneducated partners than among other women. Similarly, women lacking education and those whose partners were uneducated were more susceptible to sexual violence. Additionally, sexual violence was more prevalent among women living in the poorest households, Hindu women, and those belonging to Scheduled Caste (SC) communities. Women with four or more children had a notably higher prevalence of experiencing sexual violence. Moreover, women residing in households with seven or more members and those not exposed to mass media were more prone to sexual violence. The proportion of women who experienced sexual IPV was higher in the central region than in other regions. Moreover, women who had encountered physical IPV were notably more prone of experiencing sexual violence too.

22.3.4 Unintended Pregnancy Among Currently Pregnant Women

Table 22.2 also showcases the occurrence of UP. UP was higher among women who were aged over 35, lacking education, and from the poorest households. Additionally, women with four or more children, households comprising seven or more members, and those with no access to mass media were significantly more prone to UP. Moreover, women whose partners were uneducated and Muslim women showed a higher prevalence of UP. Furthermore, UP was higher among women who had encountered physical IPV. The prevalence of UP was relatively higher in the eastern region.

22.3.5 Association Between Intimate Partner Violence (IPV) and Unintended Pregnancy (UP)

In Table 22.3, the initial model presents the unadjusted odds ratio of UP for various types of IPV. It reveals that the probability of UP among women subjected to both physical and sexual IPV was over three times greater than that among women who had not encountered IPV.

The second model investigated the underlying factors associated with unintended pregnancies, encompassing aspects such as forms of IPV, the educational attainment of partners, social background, and household size. The findings demonstrated that women who had encountered both sexual violence and physical violence were nearly three times more likely to experience UP than those who hadn't faced IPV. Furthermore, women whose partners had secondary education had a 10% reduced probability of UP than those whose partners had no formal education. Additionally, ST women exhibited a 50% lower likelihood and OBC women a 22% lower likelihood of UP than did SC women. Lastly, women from households containing seven or more members had two times higher odds of UP than those in households with one to three members. The final model incorporated the predictors of UP which are statistically significant. These predictors were identified in the second model, along with the proximal independent variables. The adjusted odds ratios for various factors, including types of IPV, age, parity, partner's education, and social group, remained statistically significant. In line with the earlier model's

Table 22.3 Odds ratios showing factors affecting unintended pregnancy, India, 2019–2021

Variable	OR	p-Value	95% CI	OR	p-Value	95% CI	OR	p-Value	95% CI
IPV									
No IPV	®			®			®		
Physical or sexual	2.10	<0.001	(01.56–02.83)	1.85	<0.001	(01.35–02.52)	1.64	0.002	(01.20–02.24)
Both physical and sexual	3.26	<0.001	(01.96–05.42)	2.92	<0.001	(01.72–04.97)	2.55	0.001	(01.50–04.35)
Age (in years)									
18–24	–			–			®		
25–34	–			–			0.49	<0.001	(00.35–00.69)
>35	–			–			0.56	0.047	(00.31–00.99)
Parity									
None	–			–			®		
One child	–			–			2.60	<0.001	(01.68–04.03)
Two children	–			–			4.82	<0.001	(02.97–07.83)
Three children	–			–			8.51	<0.001	(04.77–15.19)
Four or more children	–			–			10.31	<0.001	(05.53–19.23)
Woman's education									
No education	–			®			–		
Primary	–			1.05	0.839	(00.68–01.62)	–		
Secondary	–			1.04	0.836	(00.71–01.54)	–		
Higher	–			0.94	0.856	(00.48–01.84)	–		
Partner's education									
No education	–			®			®		
Primary	–			1.63	0.037	(01.03–02.59)	1.76	0.015	(01.12–02.77)
Secondary	–			0.90	0.639	(00.59–01.39)	0.96	0.855	(00.65–01.42)
Higher	–			1.00	0.998	(00.54–01.84)	1.15	0.605	(00.68–01.96)

(continued)

Table 22.3 (continued)

Variable	OR	p-Value	95% CI	OR	p-Value	95% CI	OR	p-Value	95% CI
Wealth index									
Poorest	–			®			–		
Poorer	–			0.82	0.260	(00.57–01.16)	–		
Middle	–			0.71	0.149	(00.45–01.13)	–		
Richer	–			0.74	0.284	(00.43–01.28)	–		
Richest	–			0.58	0.173	(00.26–01.27)	–		
Religion									
Hindu	–			®			–		
Muslim	–			1.14	0.554	(00.74–01.76)	–		
Christian	–			1.19	0.635	(00.58–02.41)	–		
Others	–			0.52	0.223	(00.18–01.49)	–		
Social group									
SC	–			®			®		
ST	–			0.50	0.004	(00.32–00.81)	0.57	0.007	(00.38–00.86)
OBC	–			0.78	0.169	(00.55–01.11)	0.79	0.186	(00.56–01.12)
Others	–			0.94	0.792	(00.58–01.52)	1.02	0.939	(00.65–01.59)
Number of household members									
1–3 members	–			®			®		
4–6 members	–			1.62	0.009	(01.13–02.32)	1.05	0.803	(00.71–01.55)
7+ members	–			2.29	0.000	(01.51–03.49)	1.35	0.186	(00.86–02.12)
Mass-media exposure									
No exposure	–			®			–		
Low exposure	–			0.80	0.193	(00.58–01.12)	–		
Medium exposure	–			0.97	0.884	(00.63–01.49)	–		
High exposure	–			0.54	0.151	(00.24–01.25)	–		

Region				
North	–	®		–
Central	–	1.13	0.600	(00.72–01.79)
East	–	1.35	0.205	(00.85–02.16)
Northeast	–	1.28	0.458	(00.67–02.44)
West	–	0.67	0.294	(00.32–01.42)
South	–	0.56	0.105	(00.28–01.13)

® reference, *OR* odds ratio, *CI* confidence interval

results, women who had experienced both sexual violence and physical violence were approximately two and a half times more likely to experience UP than those women who had not encountered IPV before. Regarding age, women aged 25–34 and those over 35 had 50% lower odds of experiencing UP than women aged 18–24. Additionally, the likelihood of UP notably rose with increasing parity. Women with three children were eight times more likely to have UP and those with four or more children ten times more likely to have UP than those women who were without children. Likewise, as per the earlier model, women whose partners had completed secondary education had a 4% lower likelihood of experiencing UP than those women whose partners had no formal education. Moreover, ST women and OBC women exhibited approximately 40% and 20% reduced likelihoods, respectively, of facing UP than SC women. Even after accounting for both distal and proximal determinants of UP, the effect of IPV on UP continues to be significant and robust. The statistical analysis demonstrates that IPV has a strong and independent effect on the likelihood of women's experiencing UP, even when other factors are included.

22.4 Discussion

The main aim of this chapter is to measure how IPV influences UP rates in rural India. This chapter's findings revealed a higher incidence of UP among individuals who had experienced both physical IPV and sexual IPV. Moreover, certain demographic categories exhibited a significantly higher chance of UP. These groups encompassed women aged 15–24, women with four or more children, women whose spouses lacked formal education or had completed only primary schooling, and women classified as Scheduled Caste (SC). Previous studies' findings support our finding of IPV's association with UP (Acharya et al. 2019; Garg et al. 2022; Ismayilova 2010; Pallitto and O'Campo 2004). An environment characterized by patriarchal dominance and fear is often inhabited by women who experience both sexual and physical IPV. These circumstances can significantly diminish their capacity to control their reproductive rights. The power dynamics within such relationships can restrict women's ability to make autonomous decisions on contraception, family planning, and pregnancy. The presence of violence and fear may limit their access to the information, resources, and support systems necessary for exercising reproductive autonomy. Consequently, these women may face heightened challenges in asserting their reproductive rights and experiencing desired and planned pregnancies. Addressing the underlying factors contributing to patriarchal dominance and providing comprehensive support services can help empower these women and promote their reproductive agency (Pallitto and O'Campo 2004).

Our observations indicate that IPV significantly affects UP. To effectively reduce UP, campaigns that raise awareness about the detrimental effects of IPV on its victims' mental, physical, and psychological well-being must be organized. These campaigns can help highlight the importance of addressing IPV as a pressing issue requiring policymakers' and society's attention.

Interventions should focus on changing the social norms perpetuating male dominance and contributing to IPV. This requires concerted efforts to promote gender equality, challenge harmful stereotypes, and foster healthy relationships based on mutual respect and consent. Policymakers should prioritize formulating and implementing laws and policies aimed at empowering women and increasing their decision-making power, particularly concerning their reproductive rights and health.

One crucial aspect is to address the social norms and power dynamics perpetuating male dominance and contributing to IPV. Efforts should be made to challenge harmful stereotypes and promote gender equality. By altering these societal expectations, we can foster a more encouraging and fairer atmosphere for women, enabling them to take charge of their reproductive decisions.

Policymakers play crucial roles in dealing with IPV and its impact on women's reproductive health. The formulation and implementation of laws and policies should prioritize protecting and empowering women who have experienced IPV. This includes increasing their decision-making power and access to necessary resources and support services. The effective enforcement of existing legislation, such as The Protection of Women from Domestic Violence Act, is crucial in providing legal protection and assistance to victims of IPV (Chowdhury et al. 2022; Stephenson et al. 2008). The Protection of Women against Domestic Violence Act of 2005, enacted by the Indian Parliament, is crafted to shield women from domestic abuse. It prohibits a range of abuses, encompassing physical, sexual, emotional, and economic maltreatment of women, all of which are extensively delineated in the legislation. The act aims to ensure the well-being of women within familial environments, shielding them from harm inflicted by male family members. Section 498A of the Indian Penal Code, falling under criminal law, specifically addresses instances where partners or their relatives mistreat women, covering various forms of abuse, such as physical and psychological harm. Additionally, the Government of India had introduced One Stop Centres to support women affected by violence in diverse settings, including private and public spheres, communities, workplaces, and places where they are around their families. These centres provide assistance and avenues for resolution to women facing physical, sexual, emotional, psychological, and economic abuse, irrespective of factors such as age, social status, caste, education, marital status, ethnicity, or cultural background. One Stop Centres provide a range of integrated services in a single location, including police support, medical care, legal assistance, counselling, psychosocial support, and temporary accommodation for women affected by violence or facing distressing situations.

In addition to legal measures, comprehensive support systems should be in place to address the unique needs of women who have experienced IPV (Singh et al. 2018). Counselling services should be available to both girls/women and boys/men, focusing on family planning, contraceptives, and the potential consequences of UP (Garg et al. 2022). These counselling sessions can help individuals make informed decisions on their reproductive health and develop strategies to protect themselves from UP in IPV (Seifu et al. 2020).

Women who have experienced IPV may face additional barriers in exercising their reproductive rights and accessing appropriate healthcare. Tailored interventions and strategies should be developed to address these challenges, taking into account this population's specific circumstances and needs. By providing targeted support and resources, we can empower these women and mitigate IPV's adverse reproductive health outcomes.

This chapter's strength lies in its focus on rural women, a population often underrepresented in research despite facing unique challenges related to UP. By examining this group, this chapter provides valuable insights into the experiences of rural women with limited resources for and awareness of reproductive health. Using a standardized methodology adds to the reliability and comparability of the findings. Additionally, including variables through a careful literature review ensures that relevant factors influencing UP are considered. Nevertheless, this chapter has certain limitations. First, we could not include certain variables, such as alcoholism, contraceptive use, the number of sexual partners, and the gender of the most recent live-birth child in the analysis of this chapter, due to a huge number of missing observations. These variables could provide further insights into the factors associated with UP. Subsequent research can attempt to integrate these factors to achieve a more thorough assessment of the subject matter. Furthermore, although this chapter identifies associations between variables, causation cannot be determined from this type of chapter design alone. The findings in this chapter should be interpreted cautiously, recognizing that other unmeasured factors or confounding variables may contribute to the observed associations.

22.5 Conclusion

In conclusion, the findings of this study underscored a notable association between IPV and UP among women in rural India. Even after adjusting for relevant factors, women who reported IPV demonstrated a heightened susceptibility to UP. Specifically, the likelihood of experiencing UP was significantly elevated among those subjected to either physical IPV or sexual IPV or both forms of IPV when compared to women who had not encountered IPV. These results emphasize the urgent necessity of augmenting and tailoring existing IPV interventions to effectively address the associated risk of UP. Efforts must be directed towards the development of comprehensive strategies aimed at both preventing and mitigating IPV while concurrently attending to the reproductive health needs of women ensnared in abusive relationships. By prioritizing these initiatives, we can strive towards fostering safer and healthier environments for women in rural India, where they are empowered to make informed decisions on their reproductive health, free from the pervasive threat of intimate partner violence.

Declaration

Availability of Data and Materials The data and materials for this chapter are sourced from publicly available secondary sources accessible at https://dhsprogram.com/methodology/survey/

survey-display-541.cfm. Interested individuals can register at the provided link to freely download the necessary data.

Ethics Approval and Consent to Participate This chapter is based on secondary data, which are available in the public domain. Therefore, ethical approval is not required to conduct this study.

Competing Interests The authors declare that they have no competing interests.

Funding This chapter did not receive any specific grant from funding agencies in the public, commercial, or not-for-profit sectors.

References

Acharya K, Paudel YR, Silwal P (2019) Sexual violence as a predictor of unintended pregnancy among married young women: evidence from the 2016 Nepal demographic and health survey. BMC Pregnancy Childbirth 19(1):1–10

Ajayi AI, Odunga SA, Oduor C, Ouedraogo R, Ushie BA, Wado YD (2021) "I was tricked": understanding reasons for unintended pregnancy among sexually active adolescent girls. Reprod Health 18(1):1–11

Azevêdo ACC, de Araújo TVB, Valongueiro S, Ludermir AB (2013) Intimate partner violence and unintended pregnancy: prevalence and associated factors. Cad Saude Publica 29(12):2394–2404

Brown SS, Eisenberg L (eds) (1995) The best intentions: unintended pregnancy and the well-being of children and families, vol 274. National Academies Press, Washington, DC, p 1332

Chang X, Yang Y, Li R (2022) The characteristics of husbands and violence against women in Wuhan, China: a cross-sectional study. BMC Womens Health 22(1):1–7

Chowdhury S, Singh A, Kasemi N, Chakrabarty M (2022) Economic inequality in intimate partner violence among forward and backward class women in India: a decomposition analysis. Vict Offenders 19(6):1–27. https://doi.org/10.1080/15564886.2022.2080312

Dehingia N, Dixit A, Atmavilas Y, Chandurkar D, Singh K, Silverman J, Raj A (2020) Unintended pregnancy and maternal health complications: cross-sectional analysis of data from rural Uttar Pradesh, India. BMC Pregnancy Childbirth 20(1):1–11. https://doi.org/10.1186/s12884-020-2848-8

Dixit P, Ram F, Dwivedi LK (2012) Determinants of unwanted pregnancies in India using matched case-control designs. BMC Pregnancy Childbirth 12(1):1. https://doi.org/10.1186/1471-2393-12-84

Dutta M, Shekhar C, Prashad L (2015) Level, trend and correlates of mistimed and unwanted pregnancies among currently pregnant ever-married women in India. PLoS One 10(12):1–11. https://doi.org/10.1371/journal.pone.0144400

Garg P, Verma M, Sharma P, Coll CVN, Das M (2022) Sexual violence as a predictor of unintended pregnancy among married women of India: evidence from the fourth round of the National Family Health Survey (2015–16). BMC Pregnancy Childbirth 22(1):1–9. https://doi.org/10.1186/s12884-022-04673-4

Gautam S, Jeong HS (2019) Intimate partner violence in relation to husband characteristics and women empowerment: evidence from Nepal. Int J Environ Res Public Health 16(5). https://doi.org/10.3390/ijerph16050709

IIPS and MacroInternational (2022) National Family Health Survey (NFHS-5), 2019–21 India Report 1–713. http://rchiips.org/nfhs/NFHS-5Reports/NFHS-5_INDIA_REPORT.pdf

Iseyemi A, Zhao Q, McNicholas C, Peipert JF (2017) Socioeconomic status as a risk factor for unintended pregnancy in the contraceptive CHOICE project. Obstet Gynecol 130(1):609–615

Ismayilova L (2010) Intimate partner violence and unintended pregnancy in Azerbaijan, Moldova, and Ukraine. In: DHS working papers no. 79, December 28

Miller E, Decker MR, McCauley HL, Tancredi DJ, Levenson RR, Waldman J, Schoenwald P, Silverman JG (2010) Pregnancy coercion, intimate partner violence and unintended pregnancy. Contraception 81(4):316–322. https://doi.org/10.1016/j.contraception.2009.12.004

Ministry of Home Affairs, Government of India (2011) Census of India 2011. Office of the Registrar General and Census Commissioner, India. https://censusindia.gov.in/census.website/

National Institute of Population Studies (NIPS), & ICF (2019) Pakistan demographic and health survey demographic and health survey. https://www.dhsprogram.com/pubs/pdf/FR354/FR354.pdf

Office of the Registrar General and Census Commissioner, India (2011) Census of India 2011

Pallitto CC, O'Campo P (2004) The relationship between intimate partner violence and unintended pregnancy: analysis of a national sample from Colombia. Int Fam Plan Perspect 30(4):165–173. https://doi.org/10.1363/3016504

Pallitto CC, Campbell JC, O'campo P (2005) Is intimate partner violence associated with unintended pregnancy? A review of the literature. Trauma Violence Abuse 6(3):217–235. https://doi.org/10.1177/1524838005277441

Rayhan I, Akter K (2021) Prevalence and associated factors of intimate partner violence (IPV) against women in Bangladesh amid COVID-19 pandemic. Heliyon 7(3):e06619. https://doi.org/10.1016/j.heliyon.2021.e06619

Seifu CN, Fahey PP, Hailemariam TG, Atlantis E (2020) Association of husbands' education status with unintended pregnancy in their wives in Southern Ethiopia: a cross-sectional study. PLoS One 15:1–11. https://doi.org/10.1371/journal.pone.0235675

Singh A, Singh A, Mahapatra B (2013) The consequences of unintended pregnancy for maternal and child health in rural India: evidence from prospective data. Matern Child Health J 17(3):493–500. https://doi.org/10.1007/s10995-012-1023-x

Singh S et al (2018) Abortion & unintended pregnancy in six Indian states: findings and implications for policies and programs, New York. https://doi.org/10.1363/2018.30009

Society for Women's Action and Training Initiatives (SWATI) (2020) Making rural healthcare system responsive to domestic violence: notes from Patan in Gujrat. Econ Pol Wkly 55(17)

StataCorp.2013 (2013) Stata statistical software: release 13. StataCorp LLC, College Station, TX

Stephenson R, Koenig MA, Acharya R, Roy TK (2008) Domestic violence, contraceptive use, and unwanted pregnancy in rural India. Stud Fam Plann 39(3):177–186. https://doi.org/10.1111/j.1728-4465.2008.165.x

United Nations (1993) Declaration on the elimination of violence against women. https://www.ohchr.org/en/instruments-mechanisms/instruments/declaration-elimination-violence-against-women. Accessed 21 Jan 2024

World Health Organization (2021) Violence against women prevalence estimates, 2018. In: World report on violence and health. WHO, Geneva

Chapter 23
Male Involvement in Maternal Healthcare (MHC) Services: A Religious Differential Approach

Bikash Barman and Koyel Majumder

Abstract The whole world is trying to achieve the third United Nations' Millennium Development Goal (improve maternal health) by combating maternal mortality and infant mortality, which are severe global problems in underdeveloped and developing countries and may cause the improper utilization of maternal healthcare services. The proper utilization of maternal healthcare (MHC) services helps to reduce delivery complications and the risk of maternal and infant death. Male involvement (the involvement of the male spouse of a woman) is one of the essential factors in the utilization of maternal healthcare services. The present study attempts to show the degree of male involvement and the controlling factors for male participation among the Muslim women of the Maldah district in West Bengal. This study was carried out by using the primary data collected from 816 Muslim spouses from families where the women had at least one live birth within the past 5 years of beginning the survey. Bivariate (chi-square analysis) and multivariate analysis (binary logistic regression analysis) were used to show the results. The results show that the involvement of spouses in the utilization of MHC services is negligible; nearly 33% and about 20% of spouses go to health facilities with their pregnant partners for antenatal care (ANC) and postnatal care (PNC), respectively. About 20% of spouses know the importance of MHC services for mothers and newborns. The involvement of men is conditioned by their education, age at marriage, occupation, place of residence, standard of living and mass-media exposure. The chi-square analysis shows a significant association between various sociodemographic factors and male involvement in the utilization of MHC services, and the results of the binary logistic regression analysis show significant differences in the likelihood of participation among spouses depending on their sociodemographic characteristics.

Keywords Male involvement · Antenatal care · Delivery care · Postnatal care · Binary logistic regression

---

B. Barman (✉)
Department of Geography, Malda Women's College, Malda, West Bengal, India

K. Majumder
Department of Geography, University of Gour Banga, Malda, West Bengal, India

© The Author(s), under exclusive license to Springer Nature Singapore Pte Ltd. 2024
P. Chouhan et al. (eds.), *Sexual and Reproductive Health of Women*,
https://doi.org/10.1007/978-981-97-8418-9_23

23.1 Introduction

The proper utilization of maternal healthcare (MHC) services may reduce the risk of maternal and infant mortality, which now acts as a serious public health concern in underdeveloped and developing countries (Andanje 2016). India is also facing such problems, where many women do not receive the required maternal healthcare services during their pregnancy, at delivery and after delivery, which leads to maternal health vulnerability (Andanje 2016; August et al. 2016). The World Health Organization places more emphasis on spousal involvement in the utilization of maternal healthcare (MHC) services, mainly among rural and low-educated women who are disadvantaged in terms of their utilization of maternal healthcare services (Bishwajit et al. 2017; Mohammed et al. 2019). Male involvement is another important aspect of the utilization of MHC services, which means "a process of change in the social and behavioural domains required of men plays a critical role in reproductive healthcare, aimed at ensuring the wellbeing of women and their children" by the United Nations' report at the International Conference on Population and Development (ICPD) (Dudgeon and Inhorn 2004; Mbadugha et al. 2019). To achieve the United Nations' Sustainable Development Goals (SDGs) and Millenium Development Goals, gender-based inequalities need to be mitigated and male partner participation (male involvement) in the utilization of maternal healthcare services improved (Mersha 2018; Navaneetham and Dharmalingam 2002). During pregnancy and within 42 days after delivery, death is related to maternal mortality and is similar to the duration of the pregnancy. Maternal mortality is from any cause related to pregnancy or its management, but it excludes those with accidental or incidental causes. The poor maternal situation that occurs in any region is caused by social, cultural, and religious factors, among others (Okeke et al. 2016). According to the World Health Report in 2005, maternal deaths happen between 11% to 17% of the time at delivery and between 50% to 71% after delivery; in the postpartum period, 45% of maternal deaths happen within 24 h of delivery and more than 66.66% within the first week of delivery; Andanje 2016). Two international conferences were held, the first one in Cairo in 1994, which was an international conference on population, and the second one in Beijing in 1995, which was an international conference on women that called global attention to the importance of male involvement in maternal health (Mohammed et al. 2019). Before the International Conference on Population and Development (ICPD) in Cairo (1994), men were thought to be nonactors whose role in reproductive health programmes was irrelevant. But recently, attention to the role of a male partner in a mother's reproductive health increased after the recognition that a woman's healthcare choices can be highly influenced by men's attitudes, knowledge and behaviour (Gibore et al. 2019). Men's perception plays a crucial role in maternal healthcare in reducing infant and maternal mortality. Also, maternal healthcare decisions include where pregnant women go (e.g. a health centre) and are influenced by men's decisions (Muheirwe and Nuhu 2019). Direct male involvement in maternal healthcare is an important factor in the utilization of the services of skilled birth attendants at the time of delivery (Mangeni et al. 2012). Maternal health is viewed as a gender-based issue, and gender may influence male involvement in maternal healthcare. Presumably, both men and women have important individual roles in progressing families and society (Kululanga et al. 2012). Still, men are usually hesitant to shift gender responsibilities (Singh et al. 2014). Continuously monitoring male involvement will not worsen gender inequality or negatively affect women's reproductive rights (Mersha 2018). Cultural beliefs and practices obstruct men's participation in communities, and that obstruction continues to promote gendered belief systems. Men's attitudes also determine their participation. Biased attitudes and a lack of knowledge erect a barrier to male involvement in antenatal care (ANC) (Ongeso and Okoth 2018). In highly patriarchal societies, men are the heads of the family, and they play a crucial role in decision-making on which health facilities their pregnant wives go to, where they will be delivered, etc. (Yidana et al. 2018; Mondal and Murhekar 2018). However, men's knowledge about antenatal care and men's positive gender attitudes increase maternal healthcare utilization and women's decision-making on their healthcare. In contrast, their presence at the time of antenatal care visits increases the chance of institutional delivery instead of home delivery (Chattopadhyay 2012; Kululanga et al. 2012). One of the key factors, male spouse involvement in antenatal care, is used to discover pregnancy-related complications early and quickly obtain a referral. However, in India, the main focus is on pregnant women and healthcare workers instead of male involvement in maternal healthcare, due to scarce data on male involvement in maternal healthcare and men's awareness of various danger signs of pregnancy (Chakrabarti and Sarkar 2017). In India, the one who determines a women's ANC visits and her place of delivery is usually the same: her male partner. Some factors that affect male involvement in antenatal care visits are the pregnant women's partner's education, age, place of residence, caste, religion, number of living children, etc. (Sinha 2016). Male partners, depending on their sociodemographic characteristics, influence their pregnant partner's decision on which health centre she goes to for ANC services. Some men believe that it is detrimental to follow their wives to an ANC clinic; not only that, but some men also believe that she exposes her privacy to her spouse at home if he goes to an antenatal care clinic (Kiptoo and Kipmerewo 2017; Chakrabarti and Sarkar 2017). Many factors affect male involvement in maternal health services, such as socioeconomic, cultural, health and place-of-residence factors. However, in the case of rural and urban areas, different factors affect male involvement in maternal health services differently (Chattopadhyay 2012). The level or degree of male involvement in maternal healthcare services is associated with men's level of education, type of residence, and mass-media exposure (e.g. TV and radio). The aim of the national health policy programme should be to focus on improving male involvement in reproductive care by improving men's knowledge and awareness (Ghose et al. 2017). The home-based life-saving skilled programme, where intervention employing community health workers to educate the community, is both feasible and effective in improving male involvement in maternal healthcare (August et al. 2016; Okeke et al. 2016). The present study focuses on the degree of male involvement and associated factors in the utilization of maternal healthcare services among the Muslim community in the Maldah district of West Bengal.

23.2 Data Source and Methods

23.2.1 Data

This study was completed with the help of primary data, which were collected from 816 respondents in the Maldah district. The focus group discussion included the male partners of reproductive-age women who had at least one live birth within the past 5 years. In some cases, due to the absence of male partners during the survey, their spouses were taken as respondents.

23.2.2 Methods

The present study adopted the stratified multistage random sampling technique. In the first stage, the developed blocks and underdeveloped blocks were computed on the basis of the composite Z score of the selected social, cultural, economic and health indicators (31 indicators) of the 15 blocks of the Maldah district. In the first stage, four blocks (two developed blocks and two underdeveloped blocks) were used on the basis of their rank in the composite Z score. The second stage was also classified into two categories, i.e. urban areas and rural areas. In this context, a census town was considered an urban area when no municipality or notified town area or cantonment was nearby. In the third stage, some households from census towns were used in the study; on the other hand, rural areas from the selected villages of each block were taken into consideration as a sample (Fig. 23.1).

The descriptive analysis, bivariate analysis (chi-square) and multivariate analysis (binary logistic regression) were incorporated in the present study to adequately describe and present the results.

23.2.3 Variable

Male involvement in antenatal care (ANC), in delivery care and in postnatal care (PNC) were regarded as separate outcome variables, whereas different sociodemographic factors were used as explanatory variables, which play significant roles in male involvement in the utilization of MHC services among the Muslim women in the Maldah district. The explanatory variables were as follows: age (1 = 20–29 years, 2 = 30–39, 3 = 40–49 or 4 = 50 and above), age at marriage (1 = <18 years, 2 = 18 or above 18), birth order (1, 2, 3, 4 or higher), men's

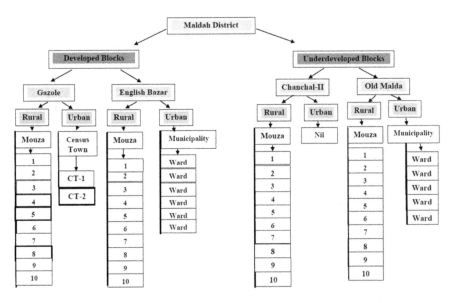

Fig. 23.1 Sample design

education (1 = illiterate, 2 = primary, 3 = secondary and 4 = higher), men's occupation (1 = not in workforce, 2 = agricultural activities, 3 = sales, 4 = services, 5 = clerical/technical and 6 = don't know), place of residence (1 = urban and 2 = rural), family structure (1 = nuclear and 2 = joint), standard of living (1 = low, 2 = medium and 3 = high), mass-media exposure (1 = no exposure, 2 = partial exposure and 3 = full exposure) and distance to nearest hospital from home (1 = < 3 km, 2 = 3–5 km and 3 = > 5 km).

To construct the standard of living index (SLI), six indicators were used, i.e. whether a household had a pucca house in an urban area or a pucca or semipucca house in a rural area (1 = yes, 2 = no); whether a household in a rural area had some land or whether a household in an urban area had a watch, sofa, fan, refrigerator, pressing iron, water pump and washing machine (1 = yes, 2 = no); whether a household had electricity (1 = yes, 2 = no); whether a household had a drinking water facility in the house (1 = yes, 2 = no); whether a household had at least one adult literate member (1 = yes, 2 = no); and whether a household had a radio, transistor, cell phone, television, bicycle and car (1 = yes, 2 = no). After the field survey, the SLI was calculated from all the values of these indicators with the help of a composite Z score, and finally, the SLI was categorized into three categories, i.e. low, medium or high.

To construct the mass-media exposure variable, four indicators were used, i.e. listening to a radio (1 = yes, 0 = no), reading a newspaper (1 = yes, 0 = no), watching television (1 = yes, 0 = no) and engaging with social media like Facebook, WhatsApp, etc. (1 = yes, 0 = no). With the help of a composite score after completing the field survey, the mass-media exposure (no exposure, partial exposure or full exposure) variable was constructed.

23.2.4 About the Study Area

The study area is Maldah (also spelt as Malda or Maldaha), which lies between 24°40′20″N and 25°32′08″N and whose longitude range is from 87°45′50″E to 88°28′10″E, lying 350 km north of Kolkata, the state capital. The total area of the district is 3733 km^2. It shares a boundary with Bihar and Uttar Dinajpur in the north, Murshidabad in the south, Bangladesh in the east and Jharkhand and Bihar in the west. It shares a 165.5 km international boundary with Bangladesh (Socioeconomic and Caste Census 2011). The total population of the district is 39.89 lakh, as per the 2011 census, which contains 4.37% of the state's total population. Maldah occupies the eleventh and sixth positions in terms of total population and child population (0- to 6-year-old population) in West Bengal, respectively. As per the 2011 census, 13.6% of the population lives in an urban area, and the decadal growth rate of the population is 21.2% in the state. The population density of this district is comparatively higher (1069 persons/km^2) than the state average (947 persons/km^2), which has made the district densely populated. The sex ratio is 944 women/1000 men, which seems to be lower than the state average (950 women/1000 men), which clearly demonstrates gender inequality due to son preference and low female literacy. The literacy rate of this district is 61.7%, where male literacy is 66.0% and female literacy is 57%. A considerable gap is found between male literacy and female literacy, mainly among the Muslim population; male literacy is 51%, whereas female literacy is only 38%. The district comprises 15 community development blocks and two municipalities, i.e. English Bazar Municipality and Old Maldah Municipality. On the basis of the mean composite Z score of 15 community development blocks, two blocks were selected as developed blocks, whose scores are high, i.e. English Bazar and Gazole, and two blocks were selected as underdeveloped blocks, whose scores are lower than those of the other blocks, i.e. Chanchal-II and Old Maldah (Map 23.1).

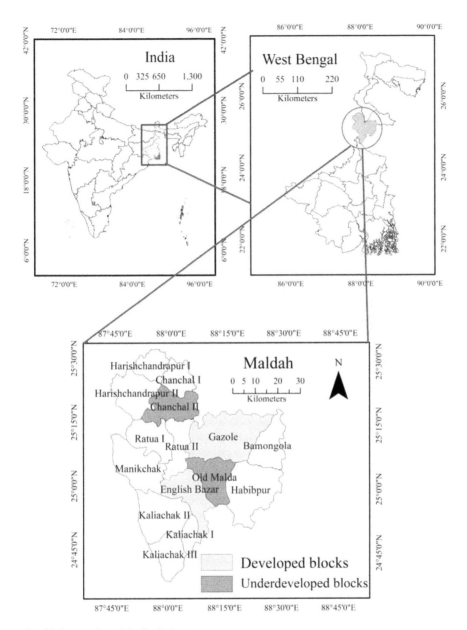

Map 23.1 Location of the Study Area

23.3 Results

23.3.1 Sociodemographic Characteristics of Men in Maldah

Table 23.1 depicts the percentage distribution of various sociodemographic characteristics: men's age, age at marriage, birth order, education, occupation, place of residence, family structure, standard of living, mass-media exposure and distance to a hospital from home and visiting a health facility for an ANC and a PNC with their pregnant wife, among Muslim men aged 20–50+ years who had at least one live birth in the past 5 years at the time of the field survey (2020–2021).

In Table 23.1, in the age group 30–39 years, 43.2% of respondents belonged to that age group, and 86.8% were married at 18 or after 18 years. Most of the respondents (56.8%) had secondary education, and illiterate respondents constituted 9.6%. Most (44.3%) of the respondents' occupations were in agriculture, followed by sales (31%). On full exposure to mass media (listening to radio, reading newspapers, watching television), men's percentage was 16.6%. Only 14.4% of men's standard of living was high. Most (42.2%) of men lived >5 km away from a hospital, and only 19.2% were situated <3 km away from a hospital. Only 32.4% and 19.6% of men visit a health facility with their pregnant wives for ANC visits and PNC visits, respectively.

23.3.2 Knowledge About MHC Services

Table 23.2 displays the percentage distribution of men among the Muslim population who know the importance of different maternal healthcare services. The results show that a minimal number of male partners know about the necessity of the various aspects of using maternal healthcare services. About 20% of men know that MHC services are vital for both a mother and her newborn; nearly 80% of men do not know that at least four ANC visits are mandatory for pregnant women because such visits help to detect different complications related to pregnancy and infant health. Overall, 20% of men know the importance of tetanus toxoid (TT) injections and iron–folic acid (IFA) tablets during pregnancy, which help to increase the immunity of pregnant and nursing women, reduce the risk of anaemia and help to fight against various diseases.

23.3.3 Knowledge About Danger Signs During Pregnancy

Figure 23.2 shows the percentage distribution of men who know danger signs during pregnancy, such as leg swelling (64.8%), prolonged labour (52.2%) and abdominal pain (49.5%), among others. The highest and lowest knowledge about danger signs during pregnancy were on the topics of leg swelling (64.8%) and high blood pressure (34.6%), respectively.

Table 23.1 Sociodemographic characteristics of men in Maldah

Respondent's characteristics	Category	Percentage ($n = 816$)
Age	20–29 years	37.4
	30–39 years	43.2
	40–49 years	14.8
	50+ years	4.6
Age at marriage	<18 years	13.3
	18 or above 18 years	86.8
Birth order	1	30.4
	2	38.6
	3	14.6
	4 and higher	16.4
Education	Illiterate	9.6
	Primary	14.9
	Secondary	56.8
	Higher	18.7
Occupation	Not in workforce	4.8
	Agricultural	44.3
	Sales	31.0
	Services	14.3
	Clerical/technical	4.8
	Don't know	0.9
Place of residence	Urban	34.0
	Rural	66.0
Family structure	Nuclear	46.8
	Joint	53.2
Standard of living	Low	56.2
	Medium	29.3
	High	14.4
Mass-media exposure	Low	31.6
	Medium	51.9
	High	16.6
Distance to a hospital from home	<3 km	19.2
	3–5 km	38.6
	>5 km	42.2
Visits a health facility for an ANC visit with pregnant wife	Yes	32.4
	No	67.6
Visits a health facility for a PNC visit with pregnant wife	Yes	19.6
	No	80.4

Source: Field survey, 2020–2021

Table 23.2 Knowledge about the importance of MHC services

Knowledge about MHC services	Percentage Yes	No
MHC services are important for both a mother and her newborn	17.4	82.6
MHC services reduce the risk of maternal mortality	14.6	85.4
MHC services reduce the risk of delivery complications	16.3	83.7
At least four antenatal care visits are mandatory for pregnant women	20.2	79.8
At least two tetanus toxoid injections are mandatory for pregnant women	19.8	80.2
At least 100 IFA tablets are mandatory during pregnancy	22.7	77.3
Janani Suraksha Yojana	21.5	78.5
Free ambulance services for delivery	26.3	73.7
Institutional delivery is safer than at-home delivery	29.8	70.2
The role of a spouse during pregnancy	20.9	79.1
Delivery complications, maternal mortality and infant mortality	18.6	81.4

Source: Field survey, 2020–2021

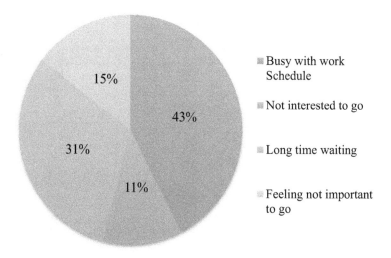

Fig. 23.2 Percentage of men who know danger signs during pregnancy

23.3.4 Reasons for Not Visiting a Health Facility for ANC Visits

Figure 23.3 shows the percentage distribution of men who do not attend health facilities for ANC visits for different reasons. For those who do not attend health facilities for ANC visits with their pregnant wives, 42.5% of men say that they are busy with work; 31.5% of men say that they have to wait a long time at the health facility and therefore do not visit the health facility; 11.4% and 14.6% of men say that they are not interested and believe that going to a health facility is not essential for them, respectively.

Fig. 23.3 Percentage of men who did not visit a health facility for ANC visits for different reasons

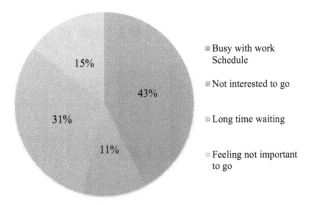

Table 23.3 Type of care given to a wife by her husband at the time of pregnancy

Type of care	Percentage ($n = 816$)
Water was carried out from well/tube well	13.6
Gave the medicine at the time	16.7
Went to a health facility with his wife	33.2
Reminded her of the date and time of next visit	22.5
Arranged mode of transportation	56.8
Decided on where to go for an ANC visit	21.4
Provided funds for ANC visit	75.5
Stayed with his wife during labour	14.3
Performed household chores when she was unable	9.2
Provided funds for her upkeep	74.9
Provided healthy food	54.5
Sang a song for mental wellbeing	5.5

Source: Field survey, 2020–2021

23.3.5 Pregnancy Care Given to a Wife by Her Husband

Table 23.3 represents the percentage distribution of men who took different types of care of wives at the time of pregnancy. It is found that 33.2% of men go to a health facility with their wives. It is also found that provide funds for ANC visits, 74.9% of men provided funds for their wife's upkeep is 74.9% men. Helped with household chores when wives were outside and sang a song for mind refreshment of wives were 9.2% and 5.5% men respectively.

23.3.6 Preparation for Delivery During Pregnancy

Birth preparedness is one of the most critical indicators of the proper utilization of delivery care, of the safe delivery of a newborn and of reducing risk during pregnancy. Figure 23.4 shows that 68.6% of men undertook preparations during

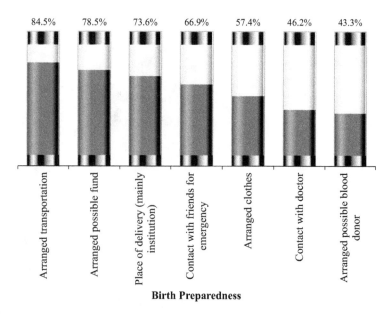

Fig. 23.4 Percentage of men who prepared for delivery during pregnancy

pregnancy and delivery (mainly institution); 73.5% and 79.5% of men arranged transportation and possible funds, respectively, during pregnancy; only 38.3% of men arranged for blood donors; and 41.2% of men kept in contact with the doctor during pregnancy.

23.3.7 Determinants of Male Involvement in the Utilization of MHC Services

23.3.7.1 Determinants of Male Involvement in the Utilization of ANC Services

Antenatal care is the treatment-seeking behaviour of women during pregnancy, which is the most vital for the minimization of maternal mortality and infant mortality. Male involvement in antenatal care services increases the mental satisfaction and the physical strength of pregnant women. Table 23.4 depicts the results of bivariate and multivariate analyses on various individual characteristics and male involvement in antenatal care among the Muslim women of Maldah. The chi-square and p-value show the degree of association between the other explanatory variables and outcome variables, respectively. The likelihood of male involvement in antenatal care is found to be higher among men who are 40–49 years old [$\chi^2 = 106.54$, AOR = 2.206, 95% CI = 1.783–2.846 and $p < 0.01$] than among other age groups of men, and it is found to be higher among men who married at 18 or above 18 years

Table 23.4 Male involvement in the utilization of antenatal care services

Men's characteristics	Category	Antenatal care Yes	No	AOR	95% CI
Age	20–29 years	17.5	82.5	1.00	–
	30–39 years	31.4	68.6	1.321**	(0.428–2.042)
	40–49 years	51.8	48.2	2.206***	(1.783–2.846)
	50+ years	33.3	66.7	1.104*	(0.316–2.076)
Chi-square and p-value		106.54; 0.004			
Age at marriage	<18 years	34.6	65.4	1.00	–
	18 or 18+ years	56.8	43.2	3.682**	(1.073–5.617)
Chi-square and p-value		176.49; 0.000			
Birth order	1	46.6	53.4	1.00	–
	2	42.7	57.3	0.864**	(0.374–1.628)
	3	30.3	69.7	0.661***	(0.140–1.546)
	4 and higher	23.8	76.2	0.367**	(0.124–1.207)
Chi-square and p-value		72.31; 0.031			
Education	Illiterate	21.2	78.8	1.00	–
	Primary	41.8	58.2	2.421*	(1.123–2.973)
	Secondary	56.7	43.3	3.057**	(1.890–3.769)
	Higher	68.2	31.8	5.694***	(3.249–6.642)
Chi-square and p-value		149.58; 0.000			
Occupation	Not in workforce	24.7	75.3	1.00	–
	Agricultural	25.4	74.6	0.556*	(0.247–1.637)
	Sales	59.9	40.1	1.492*	(1.057–2.573)
	Services	65.4	34.6	4.730**	(2.258–5.482)
	Clerical/technical	74.8	25.2	3.649**	(2.103–4.237)
	Don't know	21.4	78.6	0.739*	(0.417–3.213)
Chi-square and p-value		78.50; 0.246			
Place of residence	Urban	64.2	35.8	1.00	–
	Rural	36.8	63.2	0.726***	(0.349–1.678)
Chi-square and p-value		115.40; 0.000			
Family structure	Nuclear	32.2	67.8	1.00	–
	Joint	29.5	70.5	0.834*	(0.345–1.496)
Chi-square and p-value		80.08; 0.017			
Standard of living	Low	23.4	76.6	1.00	–
	Medium	31.7	68.3	2.360**	(1.107–2.945)
	High	45.0	55	3.572**	(1.768–4.576)
Chi-square and p-value		108.82; 0.001			
Mass-media exposure	No exposure	27.8	72.2	1.00	–
	Partial exposure	34.9	65.1	2.875**	(1.643–4.725)
	Full exposure	49.8	50.2	3.270**	(2.057–4.848)
Chi-square and p-value		94.27; 0.003			

Source: Prepared by the researcher by using field survey data, 2020–2021
Note: AOR = adjusted odds ratio; *** $p < 0.01$, ** $p < 0.05$ and * $p < 0.1$; and ® = reference category

$[\chi^2 = 176.49$, AOR = 3.682, 95% CI = 1.073–5.617 and $p < 0.05]$ than among child-marriage men. Education and occupation play significant roles in the involvement of men in their wives' antenatal care services. In the study area, the higher-educated men $[\chi^2 = 149.58$, AOR = 5.694, 95% CI = 3.249–6.642 and $p < 0.01]$ and the men who are engaged in service sector activities $[\chi^2 = 78.50$, AOR = 4.730, 95% CI = 2.258–5.482 and $p < 0.05]$ are more likely to engage in antenatal care services. Male involvement in antenatal care services varies depending on men's place of residence and family structure; the urban men who belonged to nuclear families are more involved with the treatment-seeking behaviour of their wives during pregnancy than the rural men $[\chi^2 = 115.40$, AOR = 0.726, 95% CI = 0.349–1.678 and $p < 0.01]$ and joint family $[\chi^2 = 80.08$, AOR = 0.834, 95% CI = 0.345–1.496 and $p < 0.1]$ men are. Men's standard of living plays an essential role in determining the degree of their involvement in antenatal care services. Men who have a high standard of living $[\chi^2 = 108.82$, AOR = 3.572, 95% CI = 1.768–4.576 and $p < 0.1]$ are more involved in treatment-seeking behaviour during pregnancy than men who have a low standard of living in Maldah. Mass-media exposure helps to determine the importance of antenatal care services in safe delivery and for mothers and newborns. The likelihood of involvement in antenatal care services is three times higher among men who are fully exposed to mass media $[\chi^2 = 108.82$, AOR = 3.270, 95% CI = 2.057–4.848 and $p < 0.05]$ than among men who are not exposed to mass media (Fig. 23.5).

23.3.7.2 Determinants of Male Involvement in the Utilization of Delivery Care Services

Birth preparedness during pregnancy plays a vital role in safe delivery, which reduces the risk of delivery complications and the risk of infant mortality. Male involvement in delivery care indicates their full involvement in various allied activities, such as appointment arrangements with doctors, the arrangement of ambulances, the arrangement of money, the arrangement of possible blood donors, the arrangement of medicine and the arrangement of clothes, among others. Table 23.5 shows the significant variation in the likelihood of male involvement in delivery care services according to various sociodemographic factors (age, age at marriage, birth order, education, occupation, place of residence, standard of living, family structure and mass-media exposure) among the Muslim women of Maldah. Men who married at 18 or above 18 years $[\chi^2 = 194.54$, AOR = 3.832, 95% CI = 1.678–4.672 and $p < 0.05]$ are more likely to be involved in delivery care services than are men who married at under 18 years and men who had a high birth order $[\chi^2 = 87.49$, AOR = 0.369, 95% CI = 0.172–2.349 and $p < 0.1]$. Men's education and occupation significantly determine their involvement in delivery care services, which shows that higher-educated men $[\chi^2 = 162.10$, AOR = 4.973, 95% CI = 3.142–5.678 and $p < 0.01]$ and men employed in the service sector $[\chi^2 = 89.54$, AOR = 3.465, 95% CI = 1.642–4.952 and $p < 0.1]$ are more likely to get involved in various delivery care services. Rural men $[\chi^2 = 143.43$, AOR = 0.820, 95% CI = 0.524–2.108 and

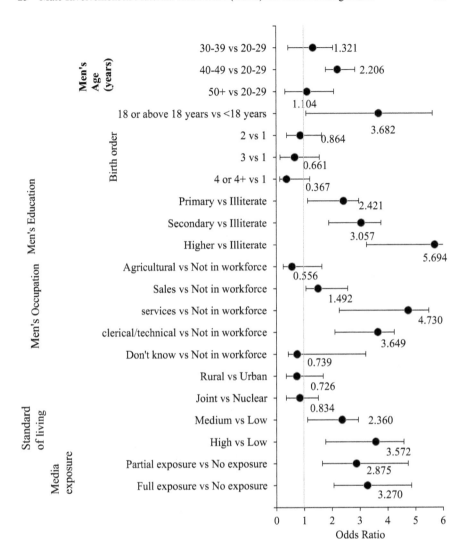

Fig. 23.5 Forest plot showing the determinants of male involvement in the utilization of antenatal care services

$p < 0.05$] from joint families [$\chi^2 = 76.59$, AOR = 0.634, 95% CI = 0.368–2.375 and $p < 0.1$] are less involved in delivery care services than urban men from nuclear families are. Men's standard of living and their level of mass-media exposure positively influence their involvement in delivery care services in the Maldah district. Men who have a high standard of living [$\chi^2 = 76.59$, AOR = 0.634, 95% CI = 0.368–2.375 and $p < 0.1$] and those who are fully exposed to mass media [$\chi^2 = 76.59$, AOR = 0.634, 95% CI = 0.368–2.375 and $p < 0.1$] are more likely to get involved in birth preparedness (see Fig. 23.6).

Table 23.5 Male involvement in the utilization of delivery care services

Men's characteristics	Category	Delivery care Yes	No	AOR	95% CI
Age	20–29 years	51.4	48.6	1.00	–
	30–39 years	42.7	57.3	1.721**	(1.137–2.497)
	40–49 years	54.7	45.3	2.103*	(1.214–3.316)
	50+ years	34.8	65.2	1.726	(1.108–2.532)
Chi-square and p-value		*164.47; 0.000*			
Age at marriage	<18 years	36.8	63.2	1.00	–
	18 or 18+ years	66.5	33.5	3.832**	(1.678–4.672)
Chi-square and p-value		*194.54; 0.004*			
Birth order	1	68.8	31.3	1.00	–
	2	62.4	37.6	0.920***	(0.375–2.143)
	3	56.5	43.5	0.792**	(0.367–2.274)
	4 and higher	43.3	56.7	0.369*	(0.172–2.349)
Chi-square and p-value		*87.49; 0.215*			
Education	Illiterate	32.2	67.8	1.00	–
	Primary	49.6	50.4	1.869*	(1.243–3.107)
	Secondary	66.3	33.7	2.683***	(1.672–4.105)
	Higher	75.8	24.2	4.973***	(3.142–5.678)
Chi-square and p-value		*162.10; 0.000*			
Occupation	Not in workforce	33.5	66.5	1.00	–
	Agricultural	30.7	69.3	0.709**	(0.372–2.104)
	Sales	66.8	33.2	1.628	
	Services	73.5	26.5	3.465*	(1.642–4.952)
	Clerical/technical	75.5	24.5	2.691	
	Don't know	32.5	67.5	0.624*	(0.311–2.243)
Chi-square and p-value		*89.54; 0.319*			
Place of residence	Urban	88.4	11.6	1.00	–
	Rural	62.5	37.5	0.820**	(0.524–2.108)
Chi-square and p-value		*143.43; 0.002*			
Family structure	Nuclear	72.5	27.5	1.00	–
	Joint	62.7	37.3	0.634***	(0.368–2.375)
Chi-square and p-value		*76.59; 0.310*			
Standard of living	Low	43.3	56.7	1.00	–
	Medium	51.8	48.2	2.539*	(1.536–3.693)
	High	66.6	33.4	4.729***	(2.634–5.690)
Chi-square and p-value		*134.54; 0.003*			
Mass-media exposure	No exposure	40.2	59.8	1.00	–
	Partial exposure	56.7	43.3	2.384**	(1.423–2.964)
	Full exposure	65.4	34.6	3.976**	(1.979–5.642)
Chi-square and p-value		*148.49; 0.000*			

Source: Prepared by the researcher by using field survey data, 2020–2021
Note: AOR = adjusted odds ratio; *** $p < 0.01$, ** $p < 0.05$ and * $p < 0.1$; and ® = reference category

23.3.7.3 Determinants of Male Involvement in the Utilization of Postnatal Care Services

Postnatal care is important after delivery to reduce newborn health vulnerabilities, and it also reduces the infant mortality rate. The utilization of postnatal care depends on the degree of male involvement, which is a strong predictor of the proper utilization of PNC services for both a mother and her newborn. The degree of spousal participation varies depending on the controlling factor (Table 23.6), such as age, age at marriage, birth order, education and occupation, among the Muslim women of Maldah. The involvement of men aged 40–49 years [χ^2 = 94.68, AOR = 1.876, 95% CI = 1.264–3.503 and $p < 0.1$] in postnatal care services is higher than that of any other age group. Men's participation in postnatal care is higher among those men who married at 18 years or after 18 years of age [χ^2 = 79.67, AOR = 2.729, 95% CI = 1.579–3.973 and $p < 0.05$] than among those who married at under 18 years. With increased birth order, the involvement of men in postnatal care services

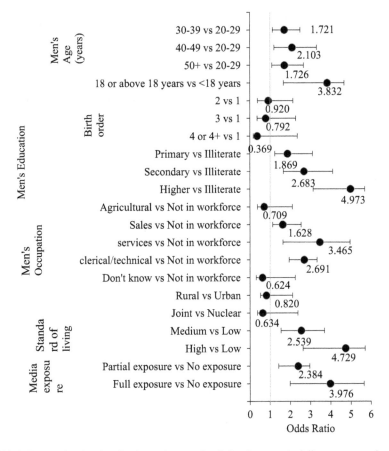

Fig. 23.6 Forest plot showing the determinants of male involvement in delivery care services

Table 23.6 Male involvement in postnatal care

Men's characteristics	Category	Postnatal care Yes	No	AOR	95% CI
Age	20–29 years	24.7	75.3		
	30–39 years	20.2	79.8	1.563**	(1.216–2.634)
	40–49 years	24.6	75.4	1.876*	(1.264–3.503)
	50+ years	16.6	83.4	1.273	
Chi-square and p-value		94.68; 0.005			
Age at marriage	<18 years	26.4	73.6		
	18 or 18+ years	46.6	53.4	2.729**	(1.579–3.973)
Chi-square and p-value		79.67; 0.036			
Birth order	1	39.9	60.1		
	2	36.6	63.4	0.850***	(0.320–2.059)
	3	24.8	75.2	0.632**	(0.363–2.108)
	4 and higher	19.8	80.3	0.301*	(0.164–2.265)
Chi-square and p-value		75.04; 0.0315			
Education	Illiterate	14.2	85.8		
	Primary	24.8	75.2	1.731*	(1.258–3.127)
	Secondary	33.6	66.4	2.176***	(1.579–3.972)
	Higher	48.8	51.2	3.282***	(2.075–5.467)
Chi-square and p-value		87.43; 0.215			
Occupation	Not in workforce	20.2	79.8		
	Agricultural	23.5	76.5	0.603**	(0.279–2.107)
	Sales	49.9	50.1	1.14	
	Services	50.8	49.2	2.355*	(1.578–4.207)
	Clerical/technical	44.8	55.2	2.108	
	Don't know	14.3	85.7	0.523*	(0.327–1.976)
Chi-square and p-value		69.81; 0.426			
Place of residence	Urban	52.3	47.7		
	Rural	28.2	71.8	0.439**	(0.321–1.428)
Chi-square and p-value		81.20; 0.341			
Family structure	Nuclear	49.8	50.2		
	Joint	27.5	72.5	0.570***	(0.279–2.307)
Chi-square and p-value		64.49; 0.319			
Standard of living	Low	19.8	80.2		
	Medium	23.5	76.5	1.783*	(1.425–3.647)
	High	41.4	58.6	3.472***	(2.257–5.642)
Chi-square and p-value		86.40; 0.327			
Mass-media exposure	No exposure	26.5	73.5		
	Partial exposure	32.1	67.9	1.946**	(1.247–2.638)
	Full exposure	44.2	55.8	2.970**	(1.637–5.520)
Chi-square and p-value		90.21; 0.345			

Source: Prepared by the researcher by using field survey data, 2020–2021

Note: AOR = adjusted odds ratio; #Model-3 = postnatal care *** $p < 0.01$, ** $p < 0.05$ and * $p < 0.1$ ® = reference category

decreases, and birth order is inversely related to education. The involvement of men who are highly educated [χ^2 = 87.43, AOR = 3.282, 95% CI = 2.075–5.467 and $p < 0.01$] and those who are employed in the service sector [χ^2 = 69.81, AOR = 2.355, 95% CI = 1.578–4.207 and $p < 0.1$] in postnatal care services is higher than that of men who are illiterate or completed primary education and who are engaged in any other sector, respectively. Rural men's involvement [χ^2 = 81.20, AOR = 0.439, 95% CI = 0.321–1.428 and $p < 0.05$] men from joint families' involvement [χ^2 = 81.20, AOR = 0.439, 95% CI = 0.321–1.428 and $p < 0.05$] in postnatal care services is lower than that of those men who live in a nuclear family and in an urban area. Those men who have a high standard of living [χ^2 = 86.40, AOR = 3.472, 95% CI = 2.257–5.642 and $p < 0.01$] and high exposure to mass media [χ^2 = 90.21, AOR = 2.970, 95% CI = 1.637–5.520 and $p < 0.1$] have higher involvement in postnatal care services than do those men who have a low standard of living and low exposure to mass media (see Fig. 23.7).

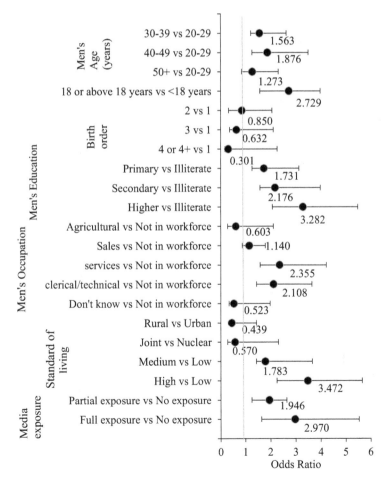

Fig. 23.7 Forest plot showing the determinants of male involvement in postnatal care

23.4 Discussion

Male involvement in the utilization of MHC services in India is a topic of critical importance, mainly in rural India, because it plays a substantial role in improving maternal and child health outcomes (Ongeso and Okoth 2018). In India, traditionally, maternal healthcare has been perceived as being predominantly in the female domain, where men are constantly being sidelined in the healthcare process (Singh et al. 2014). Recent research has found that active partner participation in maternal healthcare services during three phases can lead to numerous benefits for both a mother and her newborn (Yidana et al. 2018). The utilization of MHC services is a crucial indicator in newborn health and safe delivery; the proper utilization of maternal healthcare services depends on adequate male involvement, which has been reflected in many previous studies, and male involvement is an important issue that has been shown since 1994 at a conference in Cairo, the International Conference on Population and Development (ICPD) (UNFPA 1995; WHO 2002; Hossain et al. 2007). The essential key aspect of male involvement in the utilization of MHC services is providing support to pregnant women. This support, from the beginning—i.e. antenatal visits, the selection of a place for delivery and postnatal care—to performing household chores and childcare, reduces maternal stress and helps to improve the overall wellbeing of a mother and her newborn (Greene and Biddlecom 2000; Wendy Holmes 2013; Mullany et al. 2007). The present study shows the degree of male involvement in the utilization of essential maternal healthcare services among the Muslim community. The results show that among the Muslim community, the involvement of men in the utilization of MHC services is low; only 32.4% of the men are present with their wives for ANC. Men's knowledge about danger signs during pregnancy is also low, and education influences the knowledge about danger signs and plays an essential role in the level of male involvement in MHC services. A significant portion of the respondents (26%) do not go to health facilities with their wives for an antenatal checkup, because they think that doing so is not essential. Educational attainment is the crucial driving force behind participation in the utilization of MHC services. The present study reveals that the level of involvement of highly educated men and men who work in the service sector is comparatively high not only in ANC services but also in delivery care and PNC services. However, the percentage of such men remains deficient. In contrast, nearly 80% of men had no proper knowledge about the importance of essential health-seeking behaviour during pregnancy, at delivery and after delivery for both a mother and her newborn. In the study area, husbands were not so engaged in the various health-seeking behaviour of their wives due to the men's not having proper knowledge, their occupation and their cultural norms, all of which are reflected in their expressed views:

> I always want to engage with the different works related to my wife during pregnancy at home, but I have no way to being engaged with her because, on the one hand, I have no clear knowledge about the dos and don'ts during pregnancy and on another hand, I work as a daily labourer and have to work all day outside the home. (Participant in the FGD).

I think my participation in the utilization of maternal healthcare services is not so necessary, whereas my mother and sister's participation is necessary. Because I feel that if I go to the health centres with my wife, she might be scared and uncomfortable about all the complications in front of me. My mother and sister always take care of her. They go to the hospital or health centre whenever needed. I give money to my wife, and if there's anything serious, then I take her to hospital. (Participant in the FGD).

The spouses who went to healthcare services were more likely to engage in all the aspects of the utilization of MHC services during pregnancy, at delivery and during the post-delivery period. Poorer husbands were not so involved with their wives during the antenatal phase compared to rich husbands. Similar findings were also shown by Chattopadhyay (2012), Singh et al. (2014) and Mohammed et al. (2019) in their respective articles. Furthermore, men with knowledge of complications during pregnancy, at delivery and during the postpartum period were more likely to engage in three phases of maternal healthcare services. The study found that the main reason for the low level of male involvement in maternal healthcare was the pressure of earning a living, which is directly related to affording ANC services. MHC services have been delivered by private health centres also, and the use of private clinics is high among those who have a high standard of living and even among those who can choose an institutional delivery and are fully involved in delivery care. However, poor people and people who have a low standard of living visit a public healthcare unit for MHC services; among them, institutional delivery and the level of male involvement are low. A similar finding was obtained in India according to a study on NFHS-2 data by Jungari and Paswan (2020). Mass-media exposure helps people to learn about the importance of the various treatment-seeking behaviours and helps them to make better decisions on delivery preparedness and on choosing where to visit for antenatal care checkups and delivery. In the study area, the number of husbands who have been highly exposed to mass media on male involvement in reproductive healthcare services is comparatively higher than the values of all other metrics; even among them, choosing institutional delivery is also high because many government schemes (Janani Suraksha Yojana, free ambulance, etc) have attracted people to such institutions for safe delivery.

23.5 Conclusion

In conclusion, the participation of men in the utilization of MHC services is meagre among the Muslim community of the Maldah district of West Bengal. Men's involvement is not satisfactory in these communities, due to their lack of proper knowledge, gender discrepancies, their engagement in daily labour, their disbelief in the necessity of their involvement and both social and cultural norms. Men who had adequate education and knowledge about danger signs during pregnancy were more likely to be involved in different activities related to their wives during pregnancy, and they performed household chores. Hence, increased education and increased awareness of the importance of male involvement with their wives during the three phases of maternal healthcare services is essential for decreasing maternal and infant mortality.

Various community-based programmes have to be organized to raise awareness of the importance of male involvement and provide support and resources to encourage them to actively participate in the utilization of maternal healthcare services. Moreover, policymakers have to play a role in creating a suitable environment for male involvement by implementing policies that support gender equality, increase access to healthcare services and promote adequate awareness and education so that their governments can achieve the Sustainable Development Goals related to healthcare services and gender equality.

Declaration

Data Availability The data analysed in this chapter are available from the corresponding author upon reasonable request. The corresponding author takes responsibility for the integrity and accuracy of the data analysis.

Ethical Approval and Consent to Participate Verbal consent was obtained from all adult study participants, and we also obtained verbal consent from parents and key informants for minor (below 18 years) participants.

Competing Interest The contributors declare that they have no competing interests.

Funding This research did not receive any specific grant from funding agencies in the public, commercial or not-for-profit sectors.

References

Andanje RK (2016) Male partner involvement in promoting skilled attendance at childbirth in matayos sub-county, Busia county, Kenya

August F, Pembe AB, Mpembeni R, Axemo P, Darj E (2016) Community health workers can improve male involvement in maternal health: evidence from rural Tanzania. Glob Health Action 9(1):30064

Bishwajit G, Tang S, Yaya S, Ide S, Fu H, Wang M et al (2017) Factors associated with male involvement in reproductive care in Bangladesh. BMC Public Health 17(1):1–8

Chakrabarti S, Sarkar D (2017) Awareness and involvement of male spouse in various aspects of antenatal care: observation in a rural area of West Bengal. Int J Commun Med Public Health 4(4):1179–1182

Chattopadhyay A (2012) Men in maternal care: evidence from India. J Biosoc Sci 44(2):129

Dudgeon MR, Inhorn MC (2004) Men's influences on women's reproductive health: medical anthropological perspectives. Soc Sci Med 59(7):1379–1395

Gibore NS, Bali TA, Kibusi SM (2019) Factors influencing men's involvement in antenatal care services: a crosssectional study in a low resource setting, Central Tanzania. Reprod health 16(1):52

Greene ME, Biddlecom AE (2000) Absent and problematic men: demographic accounts of male reproductive roles, 2000. Popul Dev Rev 26(1):81–115

Hossain MB, Phillips JF, Khorshed ABM, Mozumdar A (2007) The effect of husbands' fertility preferences on couples' reproductivebehaviour in rural Bangladesh. J Biosoc Sci 39:745–757

Jungari S, Paswan B (2020) Supported motherhood? An examination of the cultural context of male participation in maternal health care among tribal communities in India. J Biosoc Sci 52(3):452–471

Kiptoo SJ, Kipmerewo M (2017) Male partner involvement in antenatal care services in Mumias east and west sub-counties, Kakamega County, Kenya. IOSR J Nurs Health Sci 6(4):37–46

Kululanga LI, Sundby J, Malata A, Chirwa E (2012) Male involvement in maternity health care in Malawi. Afr J Reprod Health 16(1):145–157

Mangeni JN, Nwangi A, Mbugua S, Mukthar VK (2012) Male involvement in maternal healthcare as a determinant of utilisation of skilled birth attendants in Kenya. East Afr Med J 89(11):372–383

Mbadugha CJ, Anetekhai CJ, Obiekwu AL, Okonkwo I, Ingwu JA (2019) Adult male involvement in maternity care in Enugu state, Nigeria: a cross-sectional study. Eur J Midwifery 3:16

Mersha AG (2018) Male involvement in the maternal health care system: implication towards decreasing the high burden of maternal mortality. BMC Pregnancy Childbirth 18(1):1–8

Mohammed BH, Johnston JM, Vackova D, Hassen SM, Yi H (2019) Therole of male partner in utilization of maternal health care services in Ethiopia: a community-based couple study. BMC Pregnancy Childbirth 19(1):1–9

Mondal N, Murhekar MV (2018) Factors associated with low performance of Accredited Social Health Activist (ASHA) regarding maternal care in Howrah district, West Bengal, 2015–16: an unmatched case control study. Clin Epidemiol Global Health 6(1):21–28. https://doi.org/10.1016/j.cegh.2017.05.003

Muheirwe F, Nuhu S (2019) Men's participation in maternal and child health care in Western Uganda: perspectives from the community. BMC Public Health 19(1):1–10

Mullany BC, Becker S, Hindin MJ (2007) The impact of including husbands in antenatal health education serviceson maternal health practices in urban Nepal: results from a randomized controlled trial. Health Educ Res 22(2):166–176

Navaneetham K, Dharmalingam A (2002) Utilization of maternal health care services in southern India. Soc Sci Med 55(10):1849–1869

Okeke EC, Oluwuo SO, Azil EI (2016) Women's perception of males' involvement in maternal healthcare in Rivers state, Nigeria. Int J Health Psychol Res 1:9–21

Ongeso A, Okoth B (2018) Factors influencing male involvement in antenatal care among clients attending antenatal clinic: a case of Kenyatta National Hospital, Kenya. Int J Adv Res 6(5):72–82

Singh D, Lample M, Earnest J (2014) The involvement of men in maternal health care: cross-sectional, pilot case studies from Maligita and Kibibi, Uganda. Reprod Health 11(1):1–8

Sinha KC (2016) Male involvement and utilization of maternal health services in India. Int J Sci Res Publ 4(11):1–13

UNFPA (1995) Male's participation in women's reproductive and sexual health. United Nations Fund for Family Planning Acivities, decumentotechnico no 28, New York

Wendy Holmes JD (2013) Stanley Lunchers. Engaging men in reproductive, maternal and newborn health compass. http://www.who.int/pmnch/knowledge/publications/summaries/ks26/en/

World Health Organisation (2002) Programing for male involvement inreproductive health: report of the meeting of WHO regional advisers in reproductive health. WHO, Geneva

Yidana A, Ziblim SD, Yamusah B (2018) Male partner involvement in birth preparedness and utilization of antenatal care services: a study in the west Mamprusi municipality of northern Ghana. World J Public Health 3(3):69

Chapter 24
A Survey on Awareness of Ongoing Family-Planning Programs and Policies Among Teacher Educators in Odisha, India

Tanushri Mohanta, Chaitali Sarangi, Moumita Pradhan, and Agradeep Mohanta

Abstract In India, family-planning policies and programs are developed and administered by the Ministry of Health and Family Welfare. In addition to the government's new initiative, factors such as better healthcare, more opportunities for women to get education, and more women in the labor force have contributed to declining birth rates in several Indian cities. This chapter intends to investigate the level of knowledge and awareness of family-planning programs among teacher educators in Odisha, India. The survey also demonstrates that no difference appears in the degree of knowledge among urban, rural, and semiurban teacher educators regardless of their location. Simultaneously, it suggests that although teacher educators are aware, 60% of them admit that they have not used different methods of family-planning programs at their own level. As a result, the survey suggests that considerably more orientation is needed for teacher educators because although they have information, their application of it is lacking. All teacher educators from urban, semiurban, and rural areas are eager to promote such a program at their institutions because it would benefit society.

This survey is designed to examine teacher educators' awareness of ongoing family-planning initiatives and policies in Odisha, India. This work fills a major gap in the literature by concentrating on this important demographic group's awareness and understanding of family-planning activities. This chapter provides useful insights for policymakers, educators, and stakeholders interested in improving reproductive health education in the education system. The scope of related work could be expanded in future research by comparing awareness levels among teacher educators across different regions of Odisha or among educators from other states in India. Longitudinal studies, qualitative investigations, and impact assessments

T. Mohanta · C. Sarangi · M. Pradhan
Radhanath Institute of Advanced Studies in Education, Cuttack, Odisha, India

A. Mohanta (✉)
Department of Botany, Maharaja Sayajirao University of Baroda, Vadodara, Gujarat, India

© The Author(s), under exclusive license to Springer Nature Singapore Pte Ltd. 2024
P. Chouhan et al. (eds.), *Sexual and Reproductive Health of Women*, https://doi.org/10.1007/978-981-97-8418-9_24

are further research pathways that could enhance evidence-based strategies for increasing family-planning awareness among Odisha teacher educators.

Keywords Teacher educators · Teacher education institutions · Family-planning programs and policies

24.1 Introduction

India was the first developing country to launch a state-sponsored family-planning program with the objective of decreasing fertility and moderating the population growth rate. Since the program's inception, fertility levels have declined throughout the country, at varying paces depending on the region; overall, the total fertility rate decreased from 6.4–6.6 lifetime births per woman in the early 1970s to 3.4 lifetime births per woman in the mid-1990s. Since the 1960s, however, the Indian population has continued to grow by approximately 2% annually and has more than doubled in size, from 439 million in 1961 to an estimated 930 million in 1996. The population is expected to grow beyond 1.5 billion before it stabilizes (Visaria et al. 1999).

Increases in modern methods of contraception determine the relative effectiveness of family-planning policies in the developing nations. By extension, traditional contraceptive techniques are associated with conventional attitudes and a lack of willingness to limit reproduction. Contraceptive use differences in India, however, show that the most "modern" women (those who have a college degree and live in cities) are the ones who are most likely to use traditional methods of birth control, and they are also the ones who use them most effectively (Basu 2005).

The usage of modern contraception has grown by 15.4% nationwide in India. On a subnational level, the outcomes are varied. Between 1990 and 2015, 13 states—Andhra Pradesh, Arunachal Pradesh, Haryana, Assam, Jharkhand, Maharashtra, Meghalaya, Tripura, Nagaland, Odisha, Rajasthan, Uttar Pradesh, and West Bengal—showed a significant improvement in the prevalence of modern contraceptives. Rajasthan saw the biggest increase, of 33.9% (New et al. 2017).

During the 2015–2016, 1.48 lakh sterilizations were performed in total (1.42 lakh sterilizations for women and 6035 sterilizations for men). Male sterilization was trending upward in 2015–2016. In spite of the criticism, Chhattisgarh had the higher number of male sterilizations (1097). Bihar recorded the best result in terms of total female sterilizations, at 25,906, ahead of Madhya Pradesh (21,322) and Odisha (17,751). Of the 3.51 lakh intrauterine contraceptive devices, or IUCDs (interval and postpartum IUCD), that were inserted, 12% were postpartum IUCDs and 88% interval IUCDs. While Madhya Pradesh had the highest number of postpartum IUCD insertions (14,313), Uttar Pradesh had the highest number of interval IUCD insertions (43,370), followed by Odisha (41,138) and West Bengal (38,293) (https://nhm.gov.in/images/pdf/programs/family-planing/annual-report/annual-report-fp-division-2015-16.pdf; Misra et al. 2021).

In the context of female marriages occurring at relatively young ages, teenage pregnancy and motherhood are significant topics. In addition to being significant from the standpoint of conception, this also has implications for a mother's and her child's health. The educational, social, and economic statuses of young women are significantly impacted by teenage pregnancy. The prevalence of low-birth-weight newborns, an increase in infant mortality, and high rates of maternal death and morbidity are all frequently linked to teen pregnancies. Odisha's rate of teenage pregnancy is 43.4% (46.1% in urban areas and 43.1% in rural areas; AHS 12–13). Delaying girls' marriage until they are 18 years old and preventing their first pregnancy for at least 2 years after marriage are crucial steps in reducing teen pregnancies. India's family-planning (FP) target for 2020 was to add 4.8 crore additional users of family-planning techniques (40% of the worldwide goal of 12 crore). As part of the national commitment, Odisha needed to add 19 lakh new users by 2020 (which was 3.9% of India's commitment) by improving the quality of family-planning service delivery while decreasing local variations in reproductive, maternal, newborn, child plus adolescent health (RMNCH+A) services through integrated, focused, and participatory public health interventions. As a part of its FP 2020 promise, the state needed to add twice as many new users as it did previously—i.e., 19 lakh additional users over a period of 8 years (2012–2020) (Family-Planning Roadmap Odisha, 2016–2017).

Odisha won the first award for population stabilization-related best practices among the eight empowered action group (EAG) states at the National Summit on Best Practices, organized by the government of India in 2013 (Annual Activity Report: 2022–2023; https://health.odisha.gov.in/). Beyond offering technical assistance or expanding access to contraception options, women's health is more important. Agency, choice, and access to high-quality reproductive treatments for women are extremely important. Not only does everyone have the human right to access to high-quality family planning, but such family planning is also critical to the growth of the country as a whole and to the welfare of individuals and society at large.

Several key policy and programmatic choices have been made by the government of India throughout the years to provide a suitable policy climate for family planning. In India, family-planning policy and implementation are handled by the Ministry of Health and Family Welfare. Fertility rates have decreased in many Indian cities because of a recently launched government program as well as better healthcare facilities, more education for women, and greater female engagement in the economy. Even though India's fertility rate is declining, some regions of the country continue to have substantially higher fertility rates. Several studies have shown that even with the decrease in fertility, India's reproductive health status is still low (Visaria et al. 1999).

Studies have found that among Hindu women with two or more children and those from low- to extremely low-income households, at least 80% used a terminal method of contraception; in contrast, only roughly 5% of Hindu women with one or more children and from very high-income households used a terminal method of contraception. Comparatively, only about 8% of Hindu women who belonged to households with low and extremely low standards of living and who had at least two surviving children used a modern method of contraception, whereas over 70% of women from households with very high standards of living, one surviving child, and more than 12 years of schooling did. However, compared to just 9% of non-Muslim women who had at least two surviving children and belonged to households with an at least an ordinary quality of living, over 40% of women without surviving children used a conventional method of contraception (Chaurasia 2014). Some studies have discovered that after a year of giving birth, just 25% of women had used an advanced form of contraception. Most of the women in the group underwent sterilization, primarily at the time of delivery (Bansal et al. 2022). Moreover, 55% of participants knew about oral contraceptives, 22% knew about emergency contraceptives, 17% knew about intrauterine devices (IUDs), and 77% were aware of male condoms. Although a considerable number of people knew about contraception, few really used it. Men's condoms (6.3%) and tablets (5.2%) were the most often used forms of contraception, with just 16% reporting ever having used any kind of birth control. People's usage of various contraceptives was impacted by their knowledge of, attitudes toward, and beliefs about contraception. Male condoms would lessen sexual pleasure, according to over half of young married men (56%), and two-thirds claimed that they would cause a man's penis to fall off and vanish within a woman's body. But over one-third of the these young married men felt positively about contraception. They said that taking contraception or insisting on using it was likely to lead to promiscuity and that contraception was not exclusively a woman's concern (Singh and Jaswal 2022).

The objective of the present work is to focus on three important aspects of the awareness of teacher educators as they pertain to ongoing family-planning programs and policies. First, this chapter assesses the level of awareness among teacher educators in Odisha about existing family-planning programs and policies. Second, it attempts to determine the comparative level of awareness about the various family-planning programs and policies among urban, semiurban, and rural teacher educators in Odisha, India. Third, it aims to determine teacher educators' perception of the promotion of awareness of family-planning programs and policies among student teachers and at teacher education institutions in Odisha. Family planning is a key concern for moving from a developing country to a developed country like India. If our country's population is under control, then our country's economy, global status, and wealth distribution will improve. Researchers have discovered that most of the research was undertaken for the general population, with no studies conducted for teacher educators in India, notably in Odisha. A teacher-training institute plays an important role in society in that any country's progress is fostered in its classroom, and teachers influence the outcomes of children by molding children's behavior. Teacher educators play a critical role in developing the knowledge, attitudes, and actions of future educators and generations. Their knowledge and understanding of family-planning programs and policies are critical for incorporating relevant content into educational curricula and effectively communicating information to students and communities. Enhancing teacher educators' understanding of family-planning programs and their awareness of them can have a big impact on public health by creating an atmosphere where students and communities feel supported in making decisions about their reproductive health. This can therefore help lower the rates of maternal and infant mortality, advance gender parity, and improve Odisha's general health results. Despite the importance of family-planning programs in enhancing public health outcomes and socioeconomic development, teacher educators in Odisha may lack a complete understanding of family-planning activities. This chapter seeks to bridge the knowledge gap by rigorously analyzing awareness levels among this specific demographic. Social justice and educational equity are promoted by ensuring that educators are knowledgeable about family-planning policies and initiatives. This chapter also assists in providing educators with the knowledge and tools that they need to meet the various needs of students and communities, especially in the marginalized or underserved parts of Odisha.

24.2 Methodology

The researchers of this chapter used a descriptive survey research design to conduct its research. The mixed-method research design was also used.

24.2.1 Population

Teacher educators from different teacher-training institutes in Odisha, India, are considered as the population of the research in this chapter.

24.2.2 Sample

In total, 150 teacher educators from all teacher-training institutions in Odisha, India—50 from rural, 50 from urban, and 50 from semiurban areas—were surveyed to collect the data in this chapter.

24.2.3 Tools

Data were collected through semistructured interviews with teacher educators via telephonic contact. Open-ended and closed questionnaires were given to teacher educators in the form of Google forms so that they would have easy access and to save time. Focus group discussion (FGD) with some teacher educators was also conducted to collect in-depth information. A pilot study that included two or three teacher educators from each college from rural, urban, semiurban areas was conducted. Some questions were added to the focus group discussion on the basis of the analysis of data from the questionnaire.

24.3 Results of Analyses

The first objective of this research is to determine the level of awareness among teacher educators in Odisha about existing family-planning programs and policies. Quantitative data from all the teacher educators from different teacher-training institutes in Odisha were collected and analyzed. The following Figs. 24.1, 24.2, 24.3, 24.4, 24.5 and 24.6 display the various results of the performed analyses.

These data indicate that almost all teacher educators have knowledge and awareness of family-planning programs.

The second objective of this chapter is to find out the comparative levels of awareness of the various family-planning programs and policies in India among urban, semiurban, and rural teacher educators in Odisha. These data were analyzed and interpreted, and the results of these tasks appear in Table 24.1.

Table 24.1 indicates that 92% of urban teacher educators gave correct answers to the questions posed to them to test their knowledge and awareness levels. More specifically, 94% of semiurban teacher educators gave correct answers. Similarly, 90% of rural teacher educators gave correct answers. These two rates indicate that almost all teacher educators, irrespective of their locality, are aware of available family-planning programs.

Table 24.2 indicates that 38% of urban teacher educators have used various contraceptive methods and 62% don't. Similarly, 40% of semiurban teacher educators have used them and 60% haven't. Simultaneously 34% of rural teacher educators have used them and 66% haven't. These three results indicate that all teacher educators from urban, semiurban, and rural areas have maximum knowledge and

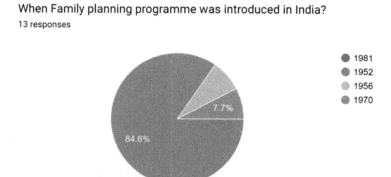

Fig. 24.1 Respondents who gave the correct answer (in red)

Which was the first country in the world to have launched a National Programme for family planning?

13 responses

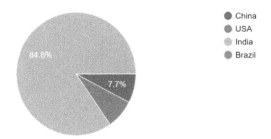

Fig. 24.2 Respondents who gave the correct answer (in orange)

Have you ever use any contraception method to prevent pregnancy?

13 responses

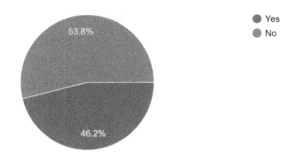

Fig. 24.3 Percentages of those who have used and have not used family-planning programs

awareness about family-planning programs, but still, very few have used them in their daily lives, irrespective of their locality.

The third objective of the research work is to find out teacher educators' perceptions of the promotion of awareness of family-planning programs and policies among student teachers and at teacher-training institutions in Odisha. The data were analyzed and interpreted, and the results of these tasks appear in Table 24.3.

Table 24.3 indicates that all teacher educators from urban, semiurban, and rural areas are willing to promote such family-planning programs at their institutions.

Out of these which one is not a contraceptive method?
13 responses

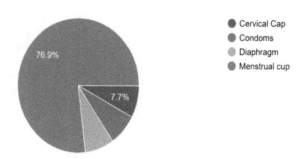

Fig. 24.4 Those who gave the correct answer (in green)

Identify the side effects related to excessive uses of contraceptive pills?
13 responses

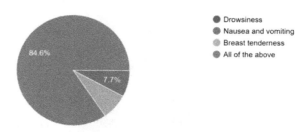

Fig. 24.5 Those who gave the correct answer (in green)

24.3.1 Major Findings

The major finding from the data analysis and interpretation is that teacher educators have maximal knowledge and awareness of family-planning programs. This chapter also reveals no difference among the urban, rural, and semiurban teacher educator's awareness levels—i.e., their awareness was irrespective of their locality. Simultaneously, it also indicates that although teacher educators are aware, 60% of them are not using the various methods of family-planning programs. Thus, the analysis indicates that much more orientation is required for teacher educators because although they have knowledge, their application is missing. Regarding the promotion of various family-planning programs among teacher educators at various teacher-training institutes in Odisha, the analysis indicates that all teacher educators from urban, semiurban, and rural areas are willing to promote such family-planning programs at their institutions. Awareness campaigns in teacher-training programs will help Indian society in three major ways: Awareness can help teacher educators themselves; it can be transmitted to student teachers; and both can transmit awareness to adolescent students. By affecting these three strata of Indian society,

Does your teacher training institute provide any types of awareness programs on family planning for student teachers?
13 responses

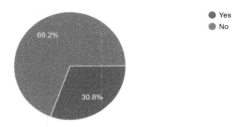

Fig. 24.6 Percentages of those who agreed and or disagreed that their teacher-training institute provided any type of program for family-planning awareness

Table 24.1 Effect of the knowledge and awareness levels of urban, semiurban, and rural teacher educators on family-planning programs

Category	Participants (n)	Correct answer provided by the participants (number and percentage)	Wrong answer provided by the participants (number and percentage)
Urban	50	46 (92%)	4 (8%)
Semiurban	50	47 (94%)	3 (6%)
Rural	50	45 (90%)	5 (10%)

awareness campaigns can have widespread impacts on Indian society by encouraging the use and implementation of family planning.

24.4 Discussion

In light of the first objective of the research, the data indicate that almost all teacher educators have knowledge and awareness of family-planning programs. The data pertaining to the second objective appear in various tables and figures. Table 24.1 and Fig. 24.7 show that 92% of urban teacher educators and 94% of semiurban teacher educators correctly answered the questions designed to assess their level of knowledge and awareness of family-planning programs. In a similar vein, 90% of rural teacher educators provided the correct answers. These results suggest that almost all teacher educators, regardless of where they work, are aware of family-planning initiatives. According to Table 24.2 and Fig. 24.8, 38% of urban teacher educators have used various forms of birth control, while 62% have not. Comparably, 60% of semiurban teacher educators have not used them, whereas 40% have. In addition, 34% of rural teacher educators have used them, whereas 66% have not. Regardless of their location, very few teacher educators from urban, semiurban, and rural areas have used family-planning programs in their everyday lives even though

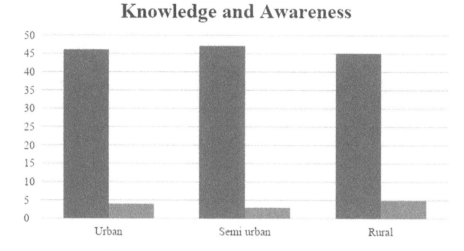

Fig. 24.7 Various knowledge and awareness levels of teacher educators in urban, semiurban, and rural areas

Table 24.2 Users of various contraceptive methods under family-planning programs from urban, semiurban, and rural areas

Category	Participants (n)	Users of contraceptive methods (number and percentage)	Nonusers of contraceptive methods (number and percentage)
Urban	50	19 (38%)	31 (62%)
Semiurban	50	20 (40%)	30 (60%)
Rural	50	17 (34%)	33 (66%)

Table 24.3 Willingness of teacher educators to promote family-planning programs at their respective institutions

Category	Participants (n)	Participants want to promote these programs (number and percentage)	Participants don't want to promote these programs (number and percentage)
Urban	50	49 (98%)	1 (2%)
Semiurban	50	50 (100%)	0
Rural	50	50 (100%)	0

they have maximal levels of information on and awareness of them overall. Data pertaining to the third objective, which appear in Table 24.3 and Fig. 24.9, show that all teacher educators in urban, semiurban, and rural areas are willing to support a family-planning program at their institutions.

Open-ended questionnaires help researchers to ascertain the perception of teacher educators on the promotion of awareness of family-planning programs and policies among student teachers and at teacher-training institutions in Odisha. The

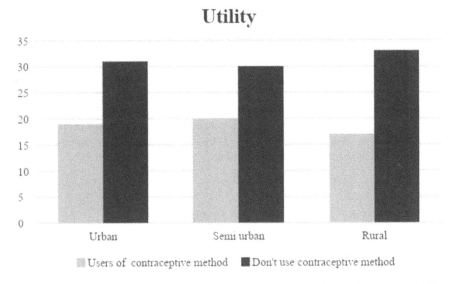

Fig. 24.8 Urban, semiurban, and rural users of various contraceptive methods under family-planning programs

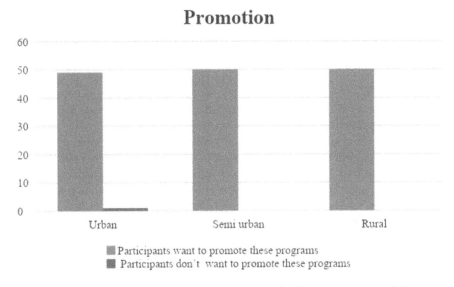

Fig. 24.9 Willingness of teacher educators to promote family-planning programs at their respective institutions

responses to various questions on promoting awareness campaigns at teacher-training institutions show that teacher educators at all levels are interested in promoting family-planning programs at their respective institutions. They mentioned various reasons, such as the economic growth and development of the country, adult awareness, increasing awareness in society through teachers, and transmitting awareness to adolescent students, among others.

Data triangulation from focus group discussion and open-ended questionnaires shows that 90% of respondents from urban, rural, and semiurban areas are interested in having these programs at their institutions and for their student teachers. They mentioned seminars, group discussions, debates, essay competitions, and expert lectures as the media to promote such programs. Many of them mentioned that these kinds of programs are rare and that such awareness has not been given to adult teachers or to adolescent students. They also emphasized promoting awareness programs at teacher-training institutions.

24.4.1 *Chapter Limitations and Strengths and Recommendations for Future Research*

The research work is limited to the teacher educators at teacher-training institutes in Odisha, India. This chapter focuses specifically on teacher educators, which may not provide a comprehensive assessment of awareness levels within the broader population. Other stakeholders, such as teachers, healthcare providers, and community leaders, may also play significant roles in influencing people's awareness of and the implementation of family-planning programs. The findings may have less generalizability to other regions or contexts outside of Odisha, India. Factors influencing people's awareness of family-planning programs and policies can significantly vary depending on cultural, socioeconomic, and geographic factors. The survey relies on self-reported data from teacher educators, which may be subject to bias. Participants may provide socially desirable responses or overstate their awareness of family-planning programs and policies.

The topic addresses a critical aspect of public health and education in Odisha, India, where understanding family-planning programs among teacher educators is crucial for effective implementation. This chapter fills a gap in the existing literature by providing empirical data on the awareness levels of family-planning programs specifically among teacher educators, a group that plays a vital role in disseminating information to future generations. The survey methodology ensures that the data collection included a representative sample of teacher educators in Odisha, employing appropriate sampling techniques and survey instruments to gather reliable and valid data. Focusing on Odisha ensures that this chapter captures the nuances and intricacies of family-planning awareness within the specific sociocultural, economic, and educational context of the region, making the findings more applicable and actionable for policymakers and practitioners. The researchers revealed that the majority of the research was conducted for the general public, with no studies conducted for teacher educators in India, particularly in Odisha. A teacher-training institute plays a significant role in society because any country's fate is decided in its classroom, and instructors impact the growth of students by molding their conduct. Thus, only teacher educators who are aware of various family-planning initiatives, as well as those who have accurate information on and an accurate understanding of them, can inform future generations and pass on their expertise to teens. In this way, a developing awareness of family-planning programs can occur from the ground up.

The scope of related work could be expanded in future research by comparing awareness levels among teacher educators across different regions of Odisha or among educators from other states in India. Comparative analysis can assist in the discovery of geographical differences, best practices, and areas for targeted action. Follow-up surveys could be conducted at regular intervals to monitor changes in teacher educators' awareness levels over time. This longitudinal method could shed light on the efficacy of programs, changes in policy implementation, and emerging trends in family-planning awareness. Developing and executing capacity-building programs or training workshops for teacher educators could improve their knowledge and skills in providing family-planning education. The efficacy of these programs in raising awareness and encouraging positive behavioral outcomes among instructors and students should be evaluated. By investigating these potential future directions, future work can contribute to ongoing initiatives that aim to promote family-planning awareness and education among Odisha teacher educators, ultimately resulting in improving public health outcomes and educational equity in the region.

24.5 Conclusion

In this work, an approach was taken to study the awareness level of teacher educators of family-planning programs in Odisha, India. An attempt was also made to study their willingness to promote such programs at their institutions. Almost all teacher educators had sufficient knowledge and awareness, but at the same time, they did not apply them in their daily lives, so the utility of these programs is missing at even this level. Most of them mentioned that they were willing to promote such programs because their will help Indian society at large. First, awareness will help teacher educators; next, awareness will be transmitted to student teachers; and finally, awareness will be transmitted to adolescent students, which is vital in our modern era. Because such a study had not been carried out before, the researchers determined not only that this study was needed to benefit not only teacher educators but also that, through teacher educators, increased awareness will have long-lasting impacts on the implementation of family-planning programs in Indian society. This chapter contributes valuable insights for policymakers, educators, and stakeholders involved in enhancing reproductive health education in the education system.

Declaration

Data Availability The data analyzed in this chapter are available from the corresponding author upon reasonable request. The corresponding author takes responsibility for the integrity and accuracy of the data analysis.

Ethical Approval and Consent to Participate Informed consent was obtained from each respondent before participation in the survey, and the privacy and confidentiality of responses given by the study participants were maintained.

Competing Interest The contributors declare that they have no competing interests.

Funding This research did not receive any specific grant from funding agencies in the public, commercial, or not-for-profit sectors.

References

Bansal A, Shirisha P, Mahapatra B, Dwivedi LK (2022) Role of maternal and child health services on the uptake of contraceptive use in India: a reproductive calendar approach. PLoS One 17(6):e0269170

Basu AM (2005) Ultramodern contraception: social class and family planning in India. Asian Popul Stud 1(3):303–323

Chaurasia AR (2014) Contraceptive use in India: a data mining approach. Int J Popul Res 2014:1–11

Misra S, Goli S, Rana MJ, Gautam A, Datta N, Nanda P, Verma R (2021) Family welfare expenditure, contraceptive use, sources and method-mix in India. Sustainability 13(17):9562

New JR, Cahill N, Stover J, Gupta YP, Alkema L (2017) Levels and trends in contraceptive prevalence, unmet need, and demand for family planning for 29 states and union territories in India: a modelling study using the family planning estimation tool. Lancet Glob Health 5(3):e350–e358

Singh J, Jaswal S (2022) Marriage practices, decision-making process and contraception use among young married men in rural Odisha, India. Cult Health Sex 24(7):1000–1015

Visaria L, Jejeebhoy S, Merrick T (1999) From family planning to reproductive health: challenges facing India. Int Fam Plan Perspect 25:S44–S49

Index

A
Adolescent girls, 5–14, 18, 23, 162, 163, 165–167, 169, 171–174, 284, 366
Antenatal care services, 200, 270–287, 299, 307, 424–427
Anthropometry, 4–14

C
Community-based programmes, 434
Contraceptive discontinuation, 104–112, 116, 118
Contraceptive use, 43, 97, 111, 112, 122–137, 142–152, 155, 156, 165, 386, 410, 438

E
Effective preventative strategies, 5, 186

F
Family planning programs, 438–449

G
Gender dynamics, 363, 365–366
Gender-parity, 180, 376–380, 385, 386, 388, 441
General health questionnaire, 3, 12

H
Healthcare behaviors, 26–27, 30, 294, 330
Healthcare infrastructure, 71, 201, 202, 261, 337
Homeless livelihood vulnerability, 18–31

I
Institutional deliveries, 193–197, 199, 201, 202, 246, 251, 252, 255–258, 263, 264, 283, 293, 299, 303, 336, 342–346, 350, 351, 353, 415, 433
Intimate partner violence (IPV), 396–410

M
Maternal and child healthcare (MCH), 336–353
Maternal health vulnerability, 414
Maternal mortality, 78, 167, 192, 194, 199, 201, 202, 244, 261, 264, 271, 286, 292, 318, 336, 414, 422, 424
Menstrual cycles, 36–38, 60, 163, 181, 185, 362, 363
Menstrual hygiene products, 362, 363, 366–368
Menstruation stigma, 361–364, 366–369
Mental well-being, 5, 11–12, 25, 364, 365

P
Parent-adolescent communication, 161–174
Perceived social support, 22, 211, 216, 223–229, 234
Postnatal care utilization, 308, 353

Q
Quality of life, 23, 29, 38–39

R
Ritual impurity, 363–365

S
Sexual diseases, 180–186
Sexual intercourse, 164, 165, 167–169, 171–173, 360
Skilled healthcare providers, 201, 202, 284
Social exclusion, 361–365
Socioeconomic inequality, 31, 60–71, 368

Spatial analysis, 19, 317–331
Spatial dependence, 321
Spatial heterogeneity, 319, 349, 352

T
Teacher educators, 438–449
Traditional contraceptives, 145–148, 151, 154, 156, 438

W
Wealth status, 43, 62, 106, 112, 117, 130, 135, 151, 155
Women homelessness, 24

www.ingramcontent.com/pod-product-compliance
Lightning Source LLC
Chambersburg PA
CBHW050505100225
21662CB00001B/25